Contemporary Medical Office Procedures

Second Edition

Doris D. Humphrey, Ph.D.
President
Career Solutions Training Group

NOTICE TO THE READER

Cover Credit: Kristina Almquist

Publishing Team:
Publisher: David C. Gordon
Senior Acquisitions Editor: Marion Waldman
Developmental Editor: Helen V. Yackel
Editorial Assistant: Sarah Holle

Project Editor: Melissa Conan
Production Coordinator: Mary Ellen Black
Art and Design Coordinator: Vincent Berger

COPYRIGHT © 1996
By Delmar Publishers
A division of International Thomson Publishing Inc.

The ITP logo is a trademark under license

Printed in the United States of America

For more information, contact:

Delmar Publishers
3 Columbia Circle, Box 15015
Albany, New York 12212-5015

International Thomson Publishing Europe
Berkshire House 168-173
High Holborn
London, WC1V7AA
England

Thomas Nelson Australia
102 Dodds Street
South Melbourne 3205
Victoria, Australia

Nelson Canada
1120 Birchmount Road
Scarborough, Ontario
Canada M1K 5G4

International Thomson Editores
Campos Eliseos 385, Piso 7
Col Polanco
11560 Mexico D F Mexico

International Thomson Publishing GmbH
Königswinterer Strasse 418
53227 Bonn
Germany

International Thomson Publishing Asia
221 Henderson Road
#05-10 Henderson Building
Singapore 0315

International Thomson Publishing - Japan
Hirakawacho Kyowa Building, 3F
2-2-1 Hirakawacho
Chiyoda-ku, Tokyo 102
Japan

Delmar Publishers' Online Services
to access Delmar on the World Wide Web, point your browser to:
http://www.delmar.com/delmar.html
to access through Gopher: gopher://gopher.delmar.com
(Delmar Online is part of "thomson.com", an Internet site
with information on more than 30 publishers of the
International Thomson Publishing organization.)
For information on our products and services:
email: **info @ delmar.com or call 800-347-7707**

3 4 5 6 7 8 9 10 XXX 01 00 99 98 97

Library of Congress Cataloging-in-Publication Data

Humphrey, Doris.
    Contemporary medical office procedures / Doris D. Humphrey. — 2nd ed.
        p. cm.
    Includes bibliographical references and index.
    ISBN 0-8273-7420-8
    1. Medical assistants. 2. Medical offices—Automation.
I. Title.
    [DNLM: 1. Medical Secretaries. 2. Office Management. 3. Office Automation. W 80 H926c 1996]
    R728.8.H845 1996
    651'.961—dc20
    DNLM/DLC
        for Library of Congress   95-6199
                                                              CIP

Contents

$62.95

Part I   Today's Medical Environment   1

Part II   Patient Relations   83

Part III   Computers and Information Processing in the Medical Office   147

Preface

One of the most intriguing, perplexing, and time-consuming issues facing the United States today is reform of the health care system. Medical assistants enjoy an exciting opportunity during this period of transition because new, broader professional roles may develop as a result. In *Contemporary Medical Office Procedures,* Second Edition, you will learn about health care reform issues that may impact your career as a medical assistant.

What's unique about this book?

Contemporary Medical Office Procedures, Second Edition, is a guide for what is to come and a resource for what is happening now in the medical assisting profession.

- **This text was written with health care system reform in mind.** After finishing the book, you should be able to discuss the most current issues in a thoughtful, insightful manner.
- **Bioethical and legal issues brought about by advancing technology are covered in depth.** References are made to interesting cases; discussion is provided regarding potential medical breakthroughs and clear, simple explanations are given for some of the most complex medical ethics issues.
- **Skills that lead to career success are highlighted in several different chapters.** Communication ability, technology skills, and employability are interwoven throughout the text to emphasize the importance that employers place on these three requirements for success.
- **"Healthspeak" sections in each chapter define many of the words you will encounter while reading.** This helps you understand the material without having to refer to a medical dictionary.
- **Administrative tasks are discussed from both a manual and computerized perspective.** You will be prepared to perform whether you go into a traditional practice or a highly technological practice.
- **The most recent national research from leading training and government organizations addresses what employers demand of workers.** You won't have to guess about how to prepare for entry-level and continuing employment in the 2000s.
- **Students form a partnership at the beginning of the text with a mentoring practice.** By observing, listening, analyzing, interviewing, and researching a successful practice, you tie classroom activities to "real life." You actually create a personal portfolio by the end of the course.

• **Concepts from *The Medical Manager* are blended into the narrative and the exercises of *Contemporary Medical Office Procedures,* Second Edition.** If you used *The Medical Manager* in a previous course, you will be able to review and practice what you learned by applying your knowledge to new situations in this course. **Warning:** You should not use *The Medical Manager* for *Contemporary Medical Office Procedures* applications until your instructor advises that you have completed all *The Medical Manager* requirements. Otherwise, you could destroy valuable data. Material referring to *The Medical Manager* will be denoted with the *Medical Manager* icon shown at the beginning of this paragraph.

the type of work you are required to complete. In *Contemporary Medical Office Procedures,* Second Edition, you will be asked to form teams, solve problems, make decisions, interview, analyze, present panel discussions, and engage in other work typical of what is found in the real world. This allows you to practice real skills before you go to work.

• **Portfolio assessment calls for integrating what you learn throughout the book.** At the end of the course, you will have a portfolio of "proof" that you "can do" what is required of medical assistants. Portfolio assessments are found at the end of Parts I, II, III, IV, and V. These real-life applications build on what you learn as you read and complete the exercises in the text. Instructions for completing portfolio assessments are provided in the next section called *How to Create Your Portfolio.*

Why is this book considered so contemporary?

Although you hear a great deal about reform in health care, you may not have heard as much about reform in education. Education methods are changing dramatically in order to prepare students to work in the more demanding, performance-based economy of the future. Employers want newly hired employees to be able "to do" their work immediately, not just "to know how to do" the work. Therefore, education based on performance of tasks has assumed a powerful role in preparing students for employment.

• **Performance-based competencies related to the 1990 DACUM (Developing A CUrriculuM) for medical assisting are listed at the beginning of each chapter.** By studying these competencies developed by the American Association of Medical Assistants (AAMA), you will see what you are expected to be able "to do" as a medical assistant.

• **Performance-based assessments *measure* what you can do.** If you compare the exercises in this text with those from other books, you will see a definite difference in

How is this book organized?

Contemporary Medical Office Procedures, Second Edition, is organized around topics that relate to health care and medical assisting employment concerns. The book is divided into five parts. Each part focuses on a major area that influences a medical assistant's responsibilities.

• **Today's Medical Environment** provides material that is essential for anyone entering the health care field today. Starting with an introduction to medical specialties and subspecialties, this unit continues with an overview of the duties of all medical staff. Then it provides a thorough look at the ethics and laws under which physicians and health care employees should practice.

• Excellent **Patient Relations** are essential to the success of any medical practice. This unit provides examples, suggestions, and procedures for interacting with patients in person and over the telephone for routine matters, emergencies, scheduling, and general information.

- **Computers and Information Processing in the Medical Office** takes you through office management, the role of the computer, and arranging for the physician's professional activities.
- **Computers and Financial Management in the Medical Office** covers pegboard accounting, computerized practice management, health insurance, and billing and collection.
- The last section, **Becoming a Career Medical Assistant,** covers the skills identified in important national studies as essential to all workers. Combined with the skills named in the AAMA DACUM and the Registered Medical Assistants (RMA) competencies listed in the Teacher's edition, this unit describes exactly what is needed to be successful in the 2000s job market.

Who should use this text?

Contemporary Medical Office Procedures, Second Edition should be used by anyone planning a career in medical assisting, medical office management, medical financing and insurance, and computer-related medical work. The book can be viewed both as introductory, for people who need a broad overview of medical office procedures, and specialized, for those who must learn specific information regarding office functions. *Contemporary Medical Office Procedures,* Second Edition can be a powerful reference tool and should occupy a place of prominence on every medical assistant's desk.

What isn't included?

Health care reform is in a state of great transition, with both the federal government and state governments changing and refining plans continuously. While *Contemporary Medical Office Procedures,* Second Edition provides excellent general information regarding reform measures, you should read and listen to the news media to learn what is occurring in your area of the country.

Acknowledgments

Thanks and appreciation are extended to the following people and facilities:

Capital Region Orthopaedic Associates, Albany, New York, and their employees who allowed the use of their facilities for many of the new photographs in this new edition.

Uniform Village, Inc., Albany, New York, for providing the uniforms used for the photographs.

To the Instructor or Trainer

Contemporary Medical Office Procedures, Second Edition was created to address the issues that are most important to medical assistants in the future. The three biggest issues are (1) health care reform, (2) changing skills required for success, and (3) computerization of medical offices. As no textbook can remain current enough to include all the health care reform measures being considered, you should use this book as a guide to issues that should be discussed in your classroom. Understanding the changing success skills identified in the Secretary's Commission on Achieving Necessary Skills (SCANS) report, DACUM, RMA Guidelines, and American Society of Training and Development (ASTD) reports is essential for the soon-to-graduate medical assistant. You should make sure that Parts II and V receive attention equal to that of technology and clinical procedures. Although computerization of medical offices has accelerated, every town has medical offices that are not computerized yet. This book covers both manual and computerized methods for handling many medical office procedures functions. In order for your students to be well prepared no matter what medical environment they enter, you will want to instruct in both methods.

The most recent curriculum reform measures are built into *Contemporary Medical Office Procedures,* Second Edition, including performance-based competencies, performance-based assessment, and portfolio development. The underlying philosophy of performance-based education is that students should be able "to do" or "demonstrate" at the end of a course what they will have to do when they go to work. Performance-based learning integrates real-life experiences and classroom activities, so that students develop problem-solving and decision-making skills built about realistic situations.

A unique concept that allows students to develop a mentoring relationship with a local practice is introduced in this book. The mentoring practice serves as the real-life laboratory for shadowing, observation, research, analysis, team building, problem solving, and decision making. As the only authentic measurements in a performance-based learning environment are those that incorporate real-life experiences, many of the activities are built around the students' mentoring experience. In a problem-solving, decision-making, team-oriented environment, many different solutions to activities will be "right," as problems can be solved in many different ways. The process of arriving at the answers is just as important as which "right" answer is used. This is a new way of learning, both for students and teachers, and some people are uncomfortable with it, as with anything new. You should nurture and support these innovative techniques because, as research shows, students become more knowledgeable when they integrate textbook material with real-life learning.

How to Create Your Portfolio

To fulfill the requirements of your medical assisting course, you will engage in a challenging educational experience called portfolio assessment. When your portfolio is complete, it will provide evidence of your administrative skills and abilities as a medical assistant. The portfolio may be utilized in job interviews as documentation of your work readiness since it will contain a broad representation of your work in this course.

Guidelines for Compiling a Portfolio

At the end of Parts I–V of *Contemporary Medical Office Procedures,* Second Edition, several portfolio activities will be presented. You are to complete all activities and store them in a portfolio or folder. Special supplies will be indicated. Supplies can be obtained from your instructor or an office supply store.

Portfolio Description

Portfolios are used for two very important reasons. The first is that instructors assess portfolios to determine whether students are able to tie together the various components of learning that occur during training. Therefore, portfolio assignments are placed at the end of each part of this book. All the chapters in each part are important to the successful completion of the exercises.

Employers represent the second important reason for compiling a portfolio. The contents of a portfolio indicate the level of problem-solving ability, understanding, and knowledge that a prospective employee brings to a position. The employer can determine from the portfolio, resume, and interview combined whether an applicant's skills generally match the requirements of the position.

Art students for years have carried their portfolios to interviews to show the caliber of their work. However, only in the recent past have portfolios begun to appear in interviews for other types of employment.

In this text, you are asked to develop the following items for your portfolio:

PART I

- Letter requesting a mentoring practice
- Response from the mentoring practice
- Organization chart for the mentoring practice
- Analysis of the activities and attitudes of the medical staff
- Audiotape or summary of interview with the managing partner

PART II

- Manual scheduling of appointments
- Printed list of one day's appointments
- Analysis of scheduling methods of mentoring practice
- Interview with senior medical assistant
- Interview with three patients
- Analysis of interpersonal skills of staff based on patient interviews
- Team consensus of interpersonal skills needed by medical assistants

PART III

- Software analysis and application in the medical office
- Panel presentation of results of software analysis

- Team plan for implementation of software application
- Informational brochure on current medical topic
- Training plan for staff

PART IV

- Computerized and/or manual scheduling, posting, daily report, and insurance form production

PART V

- Interview for fictitious medical assistant position
- Summary of the mentor's critique and personal critique of interviewing performance

Today's Medical Environment

The U.S. health care system is quite often front-page news. The cost of health care in the United States has grown at a rate far greater than the cost of other goods and services. New diseases, such as acquired immuno-deficiency syndrome (AIDS), and a return of diseases once thought to have been eradicated, such as tuberculosis, have contributed to the increase. Another factor leading to the rise in expenditures is the extended life span of U.S. citizens, because an older population consumes more medical services.

Medical costs have skyrocketed so much in the last ten years that many families, especially those in which workers have lost employer-paid benefits, receive below-standard care or no care at all. Entire segments of the U.S. population have life expectancies, infant mortality rates, and diseases comparable to some third-world countries. In addition, many patients wait too long to seek treatment for routine illnesses and must be rushed to a hospital emergency room or trauma center. This is a very expensive practice, and may be too little, too late.

The delivery and financing of quality health care are issues currently being debated among physicians, economists, commentators, politicians, and patients. The discussions are often emotionally charged, as they directly involve questions such as: "Will Medicare continue to cover my mother's expensive prescription medicine?", "Why are some medications available abroad which we cannot purchase here?", "Why should my health care become more expensive in order to subsidize the costs for drug addicts who do not take responsibility for their own health?", "Why are all of us affected because of the costs of malpractice insurance?" President Bill Clinton's stature in this country will depend to a large degree on how successful he is at implementing health care reforms. His agenda embraces the position that affordable health care should be available to every citizen, with no restrictions for pre-existing medical conditions.

Since the 1930s, the United States has followed a worldwide trend of greater government financing of health services. Many countries, such as the United Kingdom, Canada, and Germany, provide comprehensive government health services for all citizens at limited or no cost to the individual. In the United States, our traditions of individual payment responsibility and abundant choice have meant less government involvement than in many other countries.

In the years between World War II and the introduction of Medicare and Medicaid in 1965, the federal government paid about 20 percent of each health care service. By 1975, this figure had grown to 40 percent; today, over 60 percent of every health care dollar is paid by public funds. This is a 300 percent increase in only thirty years.

Our high cost of health care is attributable to several factors, including (1) an aging population that requires treatment for additional years, (2) a culture that places its elderly in public nursing homes instead of caring for them privately, (3) a dramatic increase in earlier diagnosis and treatment, (4) technology that keeps people alive longer, (5) fear of malpractice suits which may lead physicians to use unnecessary or duplicative tests, (6) the expectation among citizens that everyone should have the highest level of medical care possible, even in the case of terminal illness, and (7) duplication among hospitals of expensive equipment and facilities, such as magnetic resonance imaging (MRI) scanners, helicopters, trauma centers, and intensive care units.

As a medical assistant, your opportunities for employment are outstanding. Projections indicate that more than five out of ten jobs in the future will be related in some way to health care. These positions may be clinical or administrative. They will be as varied as paramedic, delivery driver for blood products, nurse, receptionist, laboratory technician, medical technologist, medical office assistant, physical therapist, physician, human resource director for a medical facility, home health care worker, and hundreds of others. The opportunities are limitless; in fact, many of the jobs you may perform are not yet in existence. Much of the medical equipment you will use has not yet been invented.

Although you may be most familiar with private physician practices and general hospitals, other delivery systems will play a prominent role in the future. Of particular importance in the Clinton reform movement are health maintenance organizations (HMOs) and independent provider associations (IPAs).

Ambulatory centers, regional and national research organizations, extended care centers, therapy and rehabilitation centers, testing and research laboratories, and specialized clinics for the treatment of specific diseases are examples of other facilities and organizations that support health care. In each of these settings, the need

exists for well-trained clinical and administrative support staff.

The medical environment is filled with ethical dilemmas, and as you pursue your career you may have strong opinions about these issues. For example, recent ethical debates involve the use of fetal brain tissue for some treatments. Advances in genetic engineering allow physicians to bypass disease cycles in some patients.

The issue of euthanasia makes headlines, sometimes prompted by the appearance of Dr. Jack Kevorkian, the so-called "angel of death" or "suicide doctor," at the bedside of patients desiring to commit suicide because of terminal illnesses. The state of Michigan rushed a law against assisted suicide through its legislature as a response to Dr. Kevorkian's actions, and the issue will probably remain in legal limbo for some time to come. Supporting Dr. Kevorkian in this debate is a group known as "The Hemlock Society." (Socrates, you may recall, was condemned to die by drinking hemlock, a poison derived from the hemlock tree.) The Hemlock Society is comprised of many ordinary citizens who think that terminally ill patients should be able to die with dignity and without pain.

This is a momentous time to be enrolled in a health services course of study. During the next several years, you will be involved personally in many of the radical changes occurring in the health care delivery and financing systems. As you read the chapters in this part, follow the news for the latest developments involving genetic research, technological advances, the effects of personal habits on health, and the political and economic implications of our health care systems. The debate will make you a better health care employee and enhance your ability to make informed decisions about your future.

Chapter 1

The Medical Environment

TYLER, TEXAS

Every morning over breakfast, I read the paper to find out what's next in health care services that will affect my work. You see, I started this job just about the time the debate began on health care reform. Since then, we've been on a roller coaster ride. A lot of people are grumbling, even though everyone agrees that reform is needed.

My bosses, Dr. Albert, Dr. Jones, and Dr. Harlan, have a thriving group practice specializing in neurology. Now, with the movement toward managed competition, they are investigating other ways to structure the practice. We want to continue to offer high-quality medical care while making it more affordable to patients and allowing a reasonable income for the doctors.

That takes some creativity, but I think my doctors knew that health care services were due for an overhaul. The office staff and physicians were under a mountain of paper, mostly concerning insurance payments. In addition, some patients who needed treatment were not covered by insurance and couldn't afford to pay, which was a real dilemma. Now, the doctors attend health care reform meetings about once a week. They are currently looking into a health maintenance organization, but I know they will investigate other forms of professional structure before they make any decision about our office.

Andrea Cook
Medical Assistant

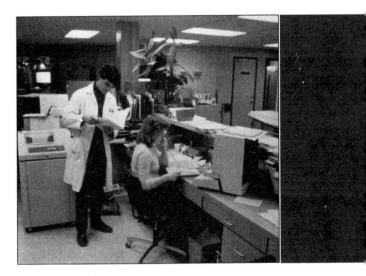

PERFORMANCE BASED COMPETENCIES

After completing this chapter, you should be able to:

1. Analyze the projected reforms in health care and support and debate two of the most important issues. (DACUM 1.9)
2. Detail the advantages of a managed care system and supplement your points with examples. (DACUM 2.6)
3. Compare and contrast the responsibilities a specialist and a subspecialist may have in treating the same patient. (DACUM 2.7)
4. Correlate each of the body systems to the appropriate specialties. (DACUM 2.10, 4.6)

Concern about financing the cost of quality health care for all Americans is resulting in rapid changes. Knowledge and information about health care are increasing almost as fast as costs, and, in some cases, contribute to rising expenditures. New treatments and medications are continually becoming available. State-of-the-art technology is used to diagnose every conceivable type of illness, from strokes to acquired immunodeficiency syndrome (AIDS).

Concerns about the rise in health care costs and increased regulations have led many solo practitioners to merge with other physicians into large group practices. Some hospitals and physicians are establishing large networks capable of meeting every possible patient need from the cradle to the grave. Other hospitals are electing to develop one segment of their business in a certain specialty or procedure. For example, one hospital in a large city may become the principal treatment center for heart disease. By concentrating on the care of one body system, it can reduce costs while providing quality service.

Medical Offices

Medical offices may be privately owned and operated by one or more physicians or by a for-profit private company employing its own physicians. They may also be established by local, state, or federal governments. Usually, government-controlled medical offices are larger than private practices and employ many physicians. Often, they serve "uncompensated care" patients who are unable to pay. They are located in metropolitan areas or in a wing of a city-owned or state-owned hospital.

The number of medical assistants employed in solo practices is decreasing yearly, as physicians merge practices. A 1991 survey by the American Association of Medical Assistants (AAMA) shows that although most medical assistants are still employed in solo physician practices there has been a growth in the number of positions in large, multiple-specialty prac-

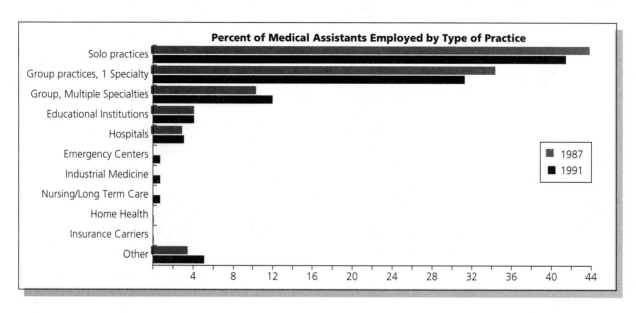

FIGURE 1-1

tices. Figure 1-1 contrasts the employment trends over a recent five-year span.

MEDICAL PRACTICES

A medical doctor is a physician with years of training in the diagnosis, treatment, and prevention of disease. After four years of college or university education, four years of medical school, and at least three years of specialty training under supervision, called residency, a physician is ready to begin his or her career. Physicians who prefer to practice alone open solo- or single-physician practices. Physicians who prefer to practice with associates join a group.

Solo-Physician Practice

When a physician maintains a solo practice, arrangements must be made with another physician to treat patients when the primary care physician is unavailable. The practice is limited in the number of patients it can effectively serve. Solo-physician practices usually charge based on a fee-for-service. In this form of payment, the patient or insurance company pays the full bill for each visit.

Many patients prefer the warm, close relationship they enjoy with the physician and staff of a single-physician practice. Patients like to know they will see the same physician each time they visit, and they develop a loyalty to the practice (Figure 1-2). Some experts consider a close relationship with the physician an important factor in patient health.

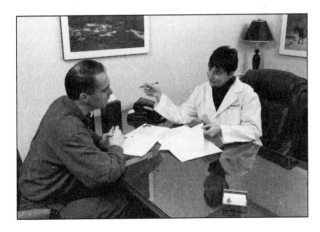

FIGURE 1-2 Patients may become more comfortable when they consult with the same physician several times.

Group Practice

Several physicians may associate as partners to share the expenses of operating a practice. The high costs of medical technology, paperwork, premiums for malpractice insurance, and expenditures for office space are more affordable when shared. For this reason, physicians who combine offices and staffs recognize an immediate savings.

In the last few years, the importance of accurate medical records and other documentation has increased because more malpractice lawsuits are being filed against physicians. As a result, medical transcriptionists are now hired to transcribe case histories, laboratory test results, doctors' notes, and other medical reports. When a group of physicians shares the services of one or more transcriptionists, the practice saves money by not duplicating personnel.

A group practice offers advantages to the physician beyond the economics of operating the office. By forming a group, physicians assure their patients that a doctor will always be available, even when the primary care physician is not. Group physicians are able to offer their patients more advanced levels of diagnosis and treatment. One of the most important gains is the immediate availability of laboratory testing for patients. For example, blood or urine may be tested and analyzed while the patient waits, avoiding a return trip or a trip to another facility. When saving time is important, the services of a group practice provide a strong incentive for the patient.

Physicians in a group practice usually have more flexible schedules because they alternate times when they are "on call." One of the greatest disadvantages of a medical career is the lack of time flexibility; a physician in a single practice is always on call, frequently receiving calls in the middle of the night. In a group practice where the physicians practice the same specialty, the time required to be on call is reduced.

A group practice also offers the new physician the advantage of associating with experienced doctors and building a practice more quickly. When established physicians in a group have all the patients they can treat effectively, they commonly assign new patients to the most recent member of the group.

The new physician in a group practice also saves part of the expense of opening a new office by joining an established group. These days, many doctors enter practice owing large amounts of money from student loans.

Ambulatory Centers

Ambulatory centers, also known as "urgent care centers," are usually private, for-profit centers that offer routine medical services for extended hours, some for twenty-four hours a day. They are in direct competition with private physician practices. This idea has sometimes been called "franchised" medicine because centers with the same name owned by one company have sprung up in cities all around the country. Ambulatory centers are often staffed by salaried physicians who do not participate in the profits of the company. Some experts predict an increase in the number of ambulatory centers; furthermore, they see competition for less expensive services drawing patients away from traditional practices.

Clinics

Clinics usually are set up to serve a specific medical need or a specific geographic area. Large group practices are often considered clinics. When a clinic serves a specialty, such as cardiology or pediatrics, all physicians who work in the clinic practice the same specialty or offer related services. By combining the knowledge and skill of several physicians, the clinic can provide advanced levels of patient care. Wellness centers, sports-injury clinics, rehabilitation facilities, and women's clinics are examples of specialty practices.

Clinics that serve geographic areas may offer their patients a broad range of specialties. Often located in the center of large cities or in isolated locations, these clinics provide medical assistance to patients of all ages for most illnesses and diseases. When a medical problem is beyond the scope of the physicians staffing the clinic, the patient is referred to another medical facility.

Clinics may be private, as with large group practices, or they may be operated by a government entity. Public health clinics historically have provided low-cost inoculations for school-

age children. Clinics for patients unable to pay are operated by some city governments.

Medical Centers

Medical centers offer many of the same services as clinics because they treat a variety of illnesses; however, they are usually much larger. Except for their names, it is sometimes difficult to distinguish between a large medical center and a hospital. Medical centers may be private or public, but because of their size and operating costs, most large medical centers are supported by public funds.

Managed Competition Organizations

Controlling health care costs and making services more affordable is the goal of managed competition. Under this type of plan, insurance buyers band together in large "alliances" to bargain with competing networks of physicians, hospitals, and other health care providers for the best care at the best price. Theoretically, managed competition bargaining will encourage lower costs and greater efficiency by establishing a schedule of fees and reducing unnecessary tests. Critics of managed competition complain that insurance company auditors, instead of doctors, may make the decisions about when patients should or would be allowed more care.

Three types of managed competition attract the most attention. They are health maintenance organizations, preferred provider organizations, and independent physician associations. Figure 1-3 contrasts these three types of managed competition organizations.

MEDICAL INSTITUTIONS

Medical institutions differ in the services they offer. Whereas some medical institutions exist solely to diagnose and treat disease, others do research or offer rehabilitation.

Research Centers

Research centers seek to broaden medical knowledge and to find answers to major health questions. Equipped with the latest medical technology, research centers are staffed by physicians, scientists, laboratory technicians, teachers, and others in related occupations. Research cen-

Health Maintenance Organizations

Health maintenance organizations (HMOs) are formed with an eye to controlling costs. HMOs sell health care at a fixed, prenegotiated price, usually to insurance carriers, large companies, or other groups who band together to purchase health care for everyone in the group. HMOs offer all types of care, often under one roof. The emphasis is on preventive care or wellness, since the HMO receives the same monthly payment whether the subscriber or member has been sick or well during the month.

Most of the physicians providing care in the HMOs are hired employees who receive a standard salary, no matter how many patients are seen, treatments performed, or tests ordered. If the cost of providing health services for all patients in a group during a month is greater than the fee paid for services, the HMO loses money. Conversely, if the HMO contains costs, it is profitable. HMOs compete with one another for large contracts.

Preferred Provider Organizations

A preferred provider organization (PPO) could be called a health care price club, where individuals receive discounts because they are members of an organization that buys in volume. PPOs discount their health care services to large employers, union members, or major insurance companies when they refer all their members to a single PPO.

High volume is the key to profitability for PPOs. Physicians are not employees of the PPO as they are of the HMO; therefore, they can continue to provide service under the traditional fee-for-service arrangement.

Independent Practice Association

An independent practice association (IPA) is similar to an HMO. IPAs consist of a group of physicians who serve the IPA's members. The doctors maintain their own offices and may have contracts with more than one IPA, as well as having some private patients. The IPA pays an agreed-upon fee to the doctor for each IPA patient whom the doctor treats.

FIGURE 1-3 Three most common types of managed competition

ters may have direct contact with patients, as in research hospitals, or they may do laboratory research with body tissue, cells, organs, and fluids to provide answers to health questions.

Frequently, the work of research centers is experimental, and many decades may pass before an answer is found that remedies a public health problem. For example, after decades of scientific study, physicians and scientists in major research centers have told us that cigarette smoking may contribute to lung cancer. Laws have been enacted forcing tobacco companies to add a warning to cigarette advertising, and in the last decade many public buildings have become smoke-free.

The Centers for Disease Control and Prevention (CDC) in Atlanta, Georgia is a government agency that employs 4,000 people and provides research in a wide range of programs (Figure 1-4). Its primary responsibility is to safeguard health by preventing and controlling disease. For example, each year, scientists at the CDC announce the results of the previous year's study of influenza outbreaks internationally and predict how that will affect U.S. citizens during the next flu season. The CDC identifies the group (for example, the aged) that will be most affected by future outbreaks and recommends proper preventives. Recently, the CDC has publicized research findings concerning AIDS, genetic mapping, and the development of a blood test to detect breast cancer in women.

Laboratories

A medical laboratory is a room or building equipped for scientific experimentation, research, testing, or clinical study of materials, fluids, or tissues obtained from patients. An experimental laboratory is a component of almost all research facilities, except for those that study only medical records. In addition to doing research, independent laboratories provide the routine analysis of patient materials, fluids, and tissues. When a patient has a routine blood test, the analysis is conducted by a physician's office laboratory or by an independent laboratory. Using the modern laboratory's sophisticated technology, a technician or physician can determine the cause of a patient's medical problem and follow through with the proper treatment.

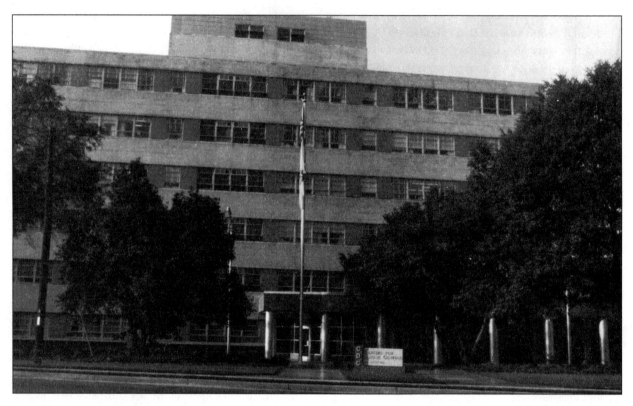

FIGURE 1-4 The best-known research center in the United States is the Centers for Disease Control and Prevention in Atlanta, Georgia. (Courtesy of Centers for Disease Control and Prevention)

Laboratories provide a valuable service in treating disease by focusing years of experimentation on a specific problem. A laboratory researcher is like a detective seeking a clue in a baffling case. Answers to some of our most challenging medical questions have been found through laboratory experimentation. Recently the National Institutes of Health released the result of a ten-year diabetes study, which supports the American Diabetes Association's position that "tight control" of the patient's condition is an important way to delay the onset and dramatically slow the progression of complications from diabetes. The results of this landmark research will probably affect the treatment of millions of people with diabetes.

Nursing Homes

Contemporary nursing homes offer many services to all age groups. Some nursing homes act as rehabilitation units for the physically disabled and for accident victims, while others offer services for the aged. The care may be short term, with the nursing home acting as a temporary therapy facility after a patient's hospitalization, or it may involve long-term assisted living.

Specialized Care Centers

Specialized care centers have received attention in recent years, primarily from the publicity surrounding several drug treatment centers. For example, the Betty Ford Drug Treatment Center in California has become widely known because of famous people who seek treatment there; however, this type of medical institution is not a new phenomenon. Specialized care centers for the treatment of polio, tuberculosis, malaria, and similar diseases affecting large numbers of people have been available since the beginning of modern medicine. Today, in addition to the traditional specialized care centers, newer centers specialize in psychiatric care, rehabilitation care, situations such as head trauma, and out-patient surgical care.

Hospitals

Hospitals provide medical care and surgery for the sick and injured. Private physicians serve on the staff of one or more hospitals and refer their patients to the hospitals they serve. Physicians may also have "visiting physician" privileges at other hospitals, though they may not routinely admit their patients to them.

A hospital's size is measured by the number of rooms and beds it provides. Some hospitals are small; others may have hundreds of rooms. Hospitals may be categorized as general hospitals, teaching hospitals, or research hospitals. General hospitals may be found in almost every town, and several general hospitals may serve the population in large cities. They provide the community with both routine and special health care services. A teaching hospital is usually affiliated with a medical school, and medical students participate in treating patients under the supervision of staff physicians. A research hospital, as the name implies, is an institution with twin goals of treating patients and performing research. A research hospital may also be a teaching hospital.

Hospitals are licensed by state or local licensing groups. Each state may license hospitals as it chooses. One cannot assume that a hospital licensed in one state meets the same health care standards as a similar hospital in another state. Federal hospitals, such as Veterans' Administration hospitals, are regulated by the federal government.

IN YOUR OPINION

1. What are the advantages and disadvantages, economic and otherwise, of practicing alone or in a group?
2. As a medical assistant, how will "managed care" affect your work in a solo practice, a group practice, an ambulatory center, a hospital, or one of the other facilities named? Why?
3. How does working in a laboratory compare with working in a well-baby clinic?

The Language Of Medicine

Case histories, consulting reports, doctor's notes, and other medical documents contain many words that, if spelled or used incorrectly, could result in improper diagnosis and treatment of a patient. Therefore, you as a medical assistant must thoroughly understand medical terminology in order to produce accurate reports. A brief explanation of medical terminology is given in this section. However, a complete understanding requires one or more courses in anatomy and physiology, medical terminology, the language of medicine, or similar courses.

ROOT WORDS, PREFIXES, AND SUFFIXES

Many medical words are formed by combining a root, or basic word, and a prefix or suffix. For example, the root **neur-** refers to the nervous system, and the root **orth-** means "straight" or "in proper order." When these roots are used with a prefix or suffix, they form medical words. Therefore, **neurology** means the branch of medicine that deals with the nervous system, and **orthopedics** means the branch of medicine that deals with disorders that require restructure, such as setting a broken leg. A combining form, usually the vowel "o," is added to root words to aid in pronunciation. A sample of root words with prefixes or suffixes is shown in this chart:

Prefix	Root Word	Suffix	Meaning
	cardi- (heart)	-ology (study of)	study of the heart
	cardi- (heart)	-ologist (specialist)	a specialist who studies the heart
contra- (against)	indicated (point out)		points out inappropriate form of treatment
	derma- (skin)	-(t)ology (study of)	study of the skin
ex- (out)	-cise (cut)		cut out
	gastro- (stomach)	-scopy (look)	look in the stomach (with a medical instrument)
peri- (around)	cardium (heart)		fibrous sac enclosing the heart

ABBREVIATIONS

Abbreviations for laboratory tests, chemical elements, measurements, medications, dosages, and names of organizations often replace medical words in reports. A sample of common abbreviations is given in the following chart. Refer to a medical dictionary for a complete list of abbreviations.

Abbreviation	Complete Word or Name
b.i.d.	twice a day
CAT	computerized axial tomography scan
CPE	complete physical exam
EEG	electroencephalogram
EENT	eye, ear, nose, throat
EKG	electrocardiogram
EMG	electromyogram
h.s.	at bedtime
IV	intravenous
mg.	milligram
mm.	millimeter
p.r.n.	as needed
q.h.	every hour
q.2h.	every two hours
q.i.d.	four times a day
RBC	red blood count
segs	segmented neutrophiles (white blood cells)
T3, T4, T7	thyroid profile
t.i.d.	three times a day
UA	urinalysis
VA	visual acuity
WBC	white blood count

BODY SYSTEMS

An understanding of human anatomy helps the medical assistant determine whether words are correct in a medical report, especially if the dictation is garbled or the handwriting difficult to decipher. Body systems are discussed briefly in this section.

Circulatory System

The circulatory system consists primarily of the heart, the blood vessels, the blood, and the lymphatic system. The heart pumps blood that travels through blood vessels to organs of the body. It cleanses the organs of waste and provides them with oxygen and food. Cardiologists, vascular surgeons, and hematologists study and treat the circulatory system.

Digestive System

All the organs and glands associated with ingestion and digestion of food make up the digestive system, including the mouth, pharynx, esophagus, stomach, small intestine, appendix, and large intestine. The digestive system breaks down food into simple substances that the cells can use, absorbs food as needed, and eliminates leftovers in the forms of wastes. Gastroenterology is the study of the digestive system.

Endocrine System

The glands that regulate body functions are a part of the endocrine system, and specialists who diagnose and treat these glands are called endocrinologists. The endocrine system plays a major role in regulating growth, in the reproductive process, and in the way the body uses food. The primary endocrine glands include the adrenal glands, pituitary gland, parathyroid glands, thyroid gland, and sex glands.

Integumentary System

The organ system that refers to the skin and related appendages, including nails and hair, is called the integumentary system. The skin is the largest organ of the body and measures about 20 square feet on a 150-pound person. The outer layer of the skin is made up of dead cells and is called the epidermis. The middle layer of skin, the dermis, maintains an even temperature. The innermost layer of skin, the subcutaneous layer, helps retain body heat, cushions the tissues against blows, and provides extra fuel for the body. The study of the skin is called dermatology.

Muscular System

The body has more than 600 muscles that contract and pull tissue to create body movement. Skeletal muscles move the bones that allow us to walk, throw a ball, or make other voluntary movements. Smooth muscles, which are found in the internal organs, move food through the digestive system. They also control the width of the blood vessels and the size of the breathing passages. The study of the muscular system is called rheumatology.

Nervous System

The nervous system regulates and coordinates the activities of all the other systems of the body. It enables the body to adjust to changes that occur within itself and its surroundings. The central nervous system, which is made up of the brain and spinal cord, receives messages from the senses and sends instructions. A neurologist is the specialist in the study of the nervous system. A neurosurgeon specializes in the surgical treatment of the nervous system.

Respiratory .System

The organs that allow breathing make up the respiratory system. They include the nose, mouth, pharynx, larynx, trachea, bronchi, and lungs. The primary jobs of the respiratory organs are to provide the body with oxygen and to rid it of carbon dioxide. Breathing allows humans to inhale air as the lungs expand and to exhale as the lungs push air out. Physicians who treat respiratory diseases are called pulmonary specialists.

Reproductive System

The organs of the reproductive system enable men and women to have children. The male reproductive organs are the testicles, scrotum, and penis. Physicians who diagnose and treat problems with these organs are called urologists. The female reproductive organs are the ovaries, fallopian tubes, uterus, and vagina. Physicians who specialize in the treatment of female reproductive problems are called gynecologists. Physicians who treat women during pregnancy and childbirth are called obstetricians.

Skeletal system

The skeleton of an adult consists of about 200 bones that support and protect the body. The skull protects the brain, the ribs protect the heart and lungs, and the spinal column protects the spinal cord. The skeletal system and muscles together allow the body to move. The study of the skeletal system is called orthopedics.

Urinary system

The urinary system, made up primarily of the two kidneys, filters various wastes from the blood and flushes them from the body in a fluid called urine. About 1,700 quarts of blood flow through the kidneys each day. Physicians who treat the urinary system are called urologists. Physicians who treat only diseases of the kidneys are called nephrologists.

Medical Specialties, Subspecialties, and Dental Specialties

The complexity of the body's structure and the way it functions calls for a thorough understanding of the body systems and a knowledge of the effect that each system has on the healthy or diseased body. That is the reason most physicians today choose to specialize or subspecialize.

MEDICAL SPECIALTIES

Specialists are physicians who concentrate on certain body systems, specific age groups, or complex scientific techniques developed to diagnose or treat certain disorders. Medical specialties developed originally because of the rapidly expanding body of knowledge about health and illness and the constantly evolving new treatments for disease. Today, no one physician can hope to master the total field of medical knowledge or to maintain the skills necessary for all diagnostic tests, treatments, and procedures.

A specialist's training begins after the physician receives an M.D. degree from a medical school. This first year of residency in the past was called an internship. Resident physicians dedicate themselves to a period of three to seven years of full-time experience in a hospital or ambulatory center, caring for patients under the supervision of experienced teaching specialists. Educational conferences and research experience are also part of the training.

Specialty boards certify that physicians have met published standards, including testing. Twenty-four specialty boards are recognized by the American Board of Medical Specialties (ABMS). To be certified as a medical specialist by one of these boards, a physician must complete its requirements. Not all physicians choose to become certified.

MEDICAL SUBSPECIALTIES

A subspecialist is a physician who, after completing training in a general medical specialty, takes additional training in a more specific sub-area of that specialty. This training increases the specialist's depth of knowledge in the specialty field. For example, cardiology is a subspecialty of internal medicine; pediatric surgery is a subspecialty of surgery; and child psychiatry is a subspecialty of psychiatry. The training of a sub-specialist requires an additional one or more years of full-time education in a program called a fellowship.

A brief description of the specialties and subspecialties recognized by the American Board of Medical Specialties (ABMS) is given in Figure 1-5.

DENTAL SPECIALTIES

The practice of dentistry has changed in the last ten years. This can be attributed to differing dental care needs of the population, greater use of support personnel, and technological advances that affect the materials and techniques

---

Specialties and Subspecialties

Allergy and immunology Evaluates, diagnoses, and manages disorders involving the immune system, such as asthma, eczema, and adverse reactions to drugs, foods, and insect bites.

Anesthesiology Provides pain relief and maintenance of a stable condition during a surgical, obstetric, or diagnostic procedure.

Colon and rectal surgery Diagnoses and treats diseases of the intestinal tract, rectum, and anus, including such conditions as hemorrhoids, polyps, cancer, colitis, and diverticulosis.

Dermatology Prevents, diagnoses, and treats benign and malignant disorders of the skin and related mouth tissues, external genitalia, hair, and nails.

Emergency medicine Manages immediate intervention to prevent death or further disability, usually based in an emergency department or trauma center.

Family practice Treats the general health of the individual and the family.

Internal medicine Provides care for nonsurgical illnesses of adolescents and adults.

    Cardiovascular medicine Manages complex diseases of the heart, lungs, and blood vessels.

    Critical care medicine Manages acute, life-threatening disorders such as shock, coma, heart failure, and drug overdoses in intensive care and other settings.

    Diagnostic laboratory immunology Uses laboratory tests to diagnose and treat disorders of the body's immune system.

    Endocrinology Concentrates on disorders of the endocrine glands, such as the thyroid and adrenal glands.

    Gastroenterology Treats the digestive organs, including the stomach, bowels, liver, and gallbladder.

    Hematology Diagnoses and treats diseases of the blood, spleen, and lymph glands, such as anemia, clotting disorders, sickle cell disease, and leukemia.

    Infectious diseases Deals with infectious diseases of all types and in all organs.

    Medical oncology Diagnoses and treats benign and malignant tumors.

    Nephrology Treats disorders of the kidneys.

    Pulmonary diseases Manages diseases of the lungs and other chest tissues, including conditions such as bronchitis and emphysema.

    Rheumatology Focuses on diseases of the joints, muscles, bones, and tendons.

FIGURE 1-5 Specialties and subspecialties

Neurological surgery Evaluates and treats diseases of the brain, spinal cord, and nerves.

Neurology Treats all categories of disease involving the central, peripheral, and autonomous nervous system.

Nuclear medicine Employs the nuclear properties of radioactive and stable nuclides to evaluate conditions of the body.

Obstetrics and gynecology Cares for disorders of the female reproductive system, the fetus, or the newborn.

    Gynecologic oncology Treats cancer of the female reproductive system.

    Maternal–fetal medicine Cares for patients during high-risk pregnancies.

Ophthalmology Provides comprehensive care of the eyes.

Orthopedic surgery Preserves and restores the extremities, spine, and associated body structures.

Otolaryngology Treats disorders of the ears, respiratory, and upper alimentary systems, medically and surgically.

Pathology Diagnoses the causes of disease and predicts the course of disease.

    Blood banking Maintains an adequate, safe blood supply.

    Chemical pathology Uses understanding of the chemical systems of the body in diagnosing and monitoring diseases.

    Dermatopathology Diagnoses and monitors diseases of the skin.

    Forensic pathology Investigates and establishes the cause of death.

    Immunopathology Monitors the course of disease by applying immunological principles to the analysis of tissues, cells, and body fluids.

    Medical microbiology Isolates and identifies microbes that cause disease.

    Neuropathology Diagnoses diseases of the nervous system and skeletal muscles.

Pediatrics Treats the health of children from birth to young adulthood.

Physical medicine and rehabilitation Evaluates and restores patients with many types of disabilities.

Plastic surgery Repairs, replaces, and reconstructs defects of form and function of the skin and its underlying systems.

Preventive medicine Focuses on maintenance of healthful lifestyle habits that prevent disease.

Psychiatry Diagnoses and treats mental, emotional, and behavioral disorders.

Radiology Uses x-rays to picture, diagnose, and treat diseases.

    Therapeutic radiology Uses radiant energy to treat cancer.

    Diagnostic radiology Uses x-rays as a diagnostic tool.

    Nuclear radiology Uses other imaging techniques in diagnosis.

    Radiological physics Regulates safe radiological practices.

    Therapeutic radiological physics Treats diseases using x-rays and related sources.

    Diagnostic radiological physics Uses x-rays and related sources in diagnosis.

    Medical nuclear physics Uses radionuclides to diagnose and treat disease.

General surgery Provides surgical procedures.

    General vascular surgery Surgically treats disorders of the blood vessels, excluding those of the heart, lungs, and brain.

    Pediatric surgery Surgically treats infants, children, and adolescents.

    Surgical critical care Cares for critically ill patients and postoperative patients.

    Thoracic surgery Evaluates and surgically treats conditions within the chest, such as congenital defects and heart diseases.

Urology Treats disorders of the adrenal glands and of the genitourinary system.

FIGURE 1-5 Specialties and subspecialties (continued)

dentists employ. Because nine of ten dentists practice privately, they handle the business aspects of running an office as well as the diagnosis and treatment of dental disease. Dental assistants help the dentists with a variety of administrative tasks, from keeping the books to ordering supplies.

About 20 percent of all dentists practice in one of eight specialty areas listed below. Each is recognized by the American Dental Association.

- Orthodontist — Straightens and aligns teeth. This is the largest group of dental specialists
- Oral and maxillofacial surgeon — Operates on the mouth and jaws. This is the second largest group of dentists
- Pediatric dentist — Specializes in children's dentistry
- Periodontist — Treats gum diseases
- Prosthodontist — Develops artificial teeth or dentures
- Endodontist — Provides root canal therapy
- Public health dentist — Provides community dental health
- Oral pathologist — Treats diseases of the mouth

Computers in Contemporary Medicine

Computers are used for diagnosing and treating disease and for managing medical facilities. Computers can tell a physician whether a patient's vital signs are normal, track the course of the patient's health after surgery, and record the costs of the patient's treatment. The pattern of an illness can be traced by computer, and the appropriate test or procedure can be identified from the pattern.

COMPUTERS IN PRIVATE PRACTICE

In the past few years, the number of computers in private practice has tripled. Physicians are taking advantage of computerized patient accounting, billing, scheduling, payroll completion, word processing, and database management. Medical record management, tracking, diagnosis, and data referral are other important applications. Another reason for the increased use of computers by physicians is access by modem to on-line databases such as Medline and MEDIS that help the physician provide better treatment. The physician or medical assistant can retrieve the most recent and technical medical journals quickly and easily, including journals published abroad.

As a medical assistant preparing to enter the medical job market, you can expect to work with computers daily. You can also expect to continue your education by taking additional courses in your field. As technology develops, new applications will be added to your responsibilities, and you must continue learning.

COMPUTERS IN THE HOSPITAL

Computers are used in hospitals to maintain a record of each patient's health, handle administrative responsibilities, cross check drugs, and develop illness patterns. Nurses read physicians' instructions from a computerized database before giving medications. They enter notes

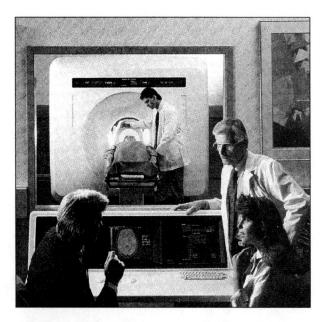

FIGURE 1-6 Magnetic resonance imaging system. The scan is shown on the computer screen on the console in the foreground. (Courtesy of GE Medical Systems)

about the patient's condition for the physician to read during hospital rounds.

Computers are involved in many aspects of high technology diagnoses. Magnetic resonance imaging (MRI) scans, for example, are used to produce a cross-sectional image of the head, back, knee or other body area. The patient rests inside a tube while a magnetic force rotates around the patient "taking pictures" from every angle, as shown in Figure 1-6. Computers can analyze and refine data from the image making machine.

IN YOUR OPINION

1. What do you think leads a physician to spend the additional time required to become a specialist?
2. What additional training and experience do you think is necessary for a medical assistant working in a subspecialty?
3. If the "paperwork hassle" involved in providing a health care service is eliminated under a national health care plan, do you believe computers will continue to be an important part of a physician's office? Explain your answer.

REFERENCES

American Board of Medical Specialties, Evanston, Illinois, "Approved Specialty Boards and Certificate Categories."

"Americans Don't Want a Health-Care Revolution," *Wall Street Journal,* June 17, 1993.

"The Clinton Cure," *Newsweek,* October 4, 1993, p. 39.

Eisenbert, Robert S. "Human Body," *The World Book Encyclopedia.* Vol. 9. 1983 ed.

Humphrey, Doris D. *Pediatric Associates, P.C.—The Medical Secretary.* Cincinnati, Ohio: South-Western Publishing Co., 1988.

"Ready to Operate," *Time,* September 20, 1993.

"Results of the 1991 AAMA Employment Survey," *The Professional Medical Assistant.* November/December 1991, pp. 23–26.

Sormunen, Carolee, and Marie Moisio. *Terminology for Allied Health Professionals.* Cincinnati, Ohio: South-Western Publishing Co., 1995*.

Thomas, Clayton L. ed. *Taber's Cyclopedic Medical Dictionary.* Philadelphia: F.A. Davis Company, 1989.

U.S. Department of Labor, Bureau of Labor Statistics. *Occupational Handbook,* 1992–1993 ed.

*Currently published by Delmar Publishers

Chapter Activities

PERFORMANCE BASED ACTIVITIES

1. Read two articles written on health care reform issues within the last three months. Select two important issues and create a short paper that supports the need for change. Support your position with facts and examples. Debate these issues with another student in the class. Use the chart below to prepare short paper notes for your debate.

Most important issues   *Facts*   *Examples*

1. _____

2. _____

3. _____

(DACUM 1.3, 2.6, 2.7, 2.10, 2.11)

2. Complete the following chart to communicate clearly the advantages and disadvantages of a managed care system for a medical practice.

Advantages and Disadvantages of Managed Care

Advantages   *Disadvantages*

1. _____

2. _____

3. _____

4. _____

5. _____

(DACUM 1.8, 2.10, 2.11)

3. Using the chart below, compare and contrast the responsibilities of an internal medical specialist and a cardiovascular subspecialist in treating the same patient.

Responsibilities of a Specialist and Subspecialist

Internist   *Cardiovascular Specialist*
Responsibilities   *Responsibilities*

1. _____

2. _____

3. _____

4. _____

4. What are the areas of overlapping responsibility? What is the value to the patient of having each specialist involved in treatment?

Overlapping Responsibilities   *Value of a Specialist*
      Plus a Subspecialist

1. _____

2. _____

Overlapping Responsibilities   *Value of a Specialist*
                                                   Plus a Subspecialist

3. _____

4. _____

5. _____

6. _____

(DACUM 2.6, 2.10, 2.11)

5. Using the Specialties and Subspecialties chart on pages 12 and 13 and the body systems identified in this chapter, associate each of the body systems to the appropriate medical specialty.

Body System Relationship to Specialty

Body System   *Specialty/Subspecialty*

1. _____

2. _____

3. _____

4. _____

5. _____

6. _____

7. _____

8. _____

9. _____

10. _____

(DACUM 2.7, 2.10)

EXPANDING YOUR THINKING

1. A friend who wishes to work in the medical field asks you for advice about different types of medical offices and medical institutions where jobs might be available. What might you tell your friend?

2. Your employer, who has agreed to talk to a group of college students about medical specialties and subspecialties, asks you to develop a brief outline for the talk. Include the following points in your outline:

   a. The difference between a medical specialty and a medical subspecialty

   b. The difference in training for a specialist and subspecialist

   c. Examples of specialties and their subspecialties

3. Describe the types of changes required when two practices merge into one. What do you think the advantages and disadvantages of merging with another group are?

Chapter 2

The Medical Staff

BOSTON, MASSACHUSETTS

This is my first week working for Women's Medical Associates. I recently graduated from an accredited medical assistant program and I'm ready to apply what I learned. Although I had opportunities to observe and even to intern at another practice, I never realized how fast the day would go here.

At our practice three MAs work with two doctors during office hours. One person is a CMA, which means she may use the certified medical assistant credential after her name. Since our practice believes in cross-training, we are all expected to perform a variety of duties, everything from greeting the patients to administering selected tests ordered by the doctors. We rotate, so one day I handle administrative functions and the next I assist the doctor! Let me give you some idea of what the first week was like.

On Monday, Wednesday, and Friday, Barbara and I worked the back office. With both doctors having office hours, we saw about forty patients each day. We prepared the treatment rooms and interviewed the patients about any changes since their last visit. Of course, we took vital signs and did urinalysis for each. Then we helped the physician with the exam. Although most patients are in for routine prenatal or annual checkups, sometimes things aren't so routine; that's when I'm glad I got the right training. One patient, a young mother-to-be, was recently diagnosed with breast cancer. She's facing several tough decisions regarding the impact of treatment options on her unborn baby. Another

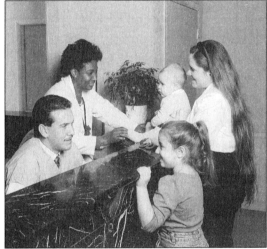

patient, an elderly woman brought in by her daughter, absolutely refused to cooperate. It took all of my interpersonal skills to resolve her concerns effectively.

Tuesday and Thursday were my days to handle the front office. Here, I greeted the patients and helped new patients fill out a questionnaire. It's my job to enter patient information into the computer. After the patients saw the doctors, I scheduled follow-up appointments. In between, I also helped answer the phone and made calls to insurance companies regarding outstanding claims. All in all, I would say it was a pretty good start. What do you think?

Carla Swan
Medical Assistant

PERFORMANCE BASED COMPETENCIES

After completing this chapter, you should be able to:

1. Compare and contrast the clinical and administrative responsibilities of a medical assistant. (DACUM 2.3, 2.10, 7.4)
2. Analyze and project the demand for medical assistants until the year 2000 in view of a changing health care environment. (DACUM 2.7, 5.7)
3. Identify and discuss interpersonal skills that nurture a team concept among the medical staff. (DACUM 1.5, 2.3, 2.5)
4. Make recommendations for education and credentialing that will enhance a medical office assistant's career. (DACUM 1.3, 5.6)

HEALTHSPEAK

Ambulatory care centers Twenty-four-hour medical centers that treat patients with minor illnesses or injuries.

CMA Certified Medical Assistant, a credential earned through the American Association of Medical Assistants.

CPT Current Procedural Terminology.

Credentialing Examination that certifies the medical assistant in administrative and clinical procedures.

DACUM Acronym for Developing A CUrriculuM.

Multi-functional medical assistant Medical assistant who is trained in both administrative and clinical duties.

OMA Ophthalmic Medical Assistant, a credential earned through the Joint Commission on Allied Health Personnel in Ophthalmology.

Physician extenders Paramedical staff trained to support the physician by performing some tasks previously performed only by the physician.

RMA Registered Medical Assistant, a credential earned through the American Medical Technologists.

The size of a medical practice determines the number of employees and the scope of their duties. A solo practice may require only a nurse and a multi-functional medical assistant, whereas a group practice may require several physicians, nurses, laboratory technicians, and medical assistants.

The role of the medical assistant is changing from a loosely defined support function to a professional, highly visible career. The demand for well-trained medical assistants possessing a wide range of human relations and technology skills grows each year.

The Medical Assistant

The term **medical assistant** refers to a broad category of medical office professionals. Receptionists, medical transcriptionists, appointment schedulers, billing clerks, examination assistants, and phlebotomists are all medical assistants. Sometimes several medical assistants are responsible for different tasks, or a multi-functional medical assistant may assume all of these responsibilities. Medical assistants work in a wide variety of specialties and subspecialties. Figure 2-1 illustrates where medical assistants are employed.

The medical assistant's job can be separated into two distinct categories: (1) administrative responsibilities, which include both routine and special office tasks, and (2) clinical responsibilities, which involve helping the physician examine and treat patients. In larger offices, medical assistants usually specialize in either the administrative or the clinical aspect of the job, while the multi-functional medical assistant frequently works in an ambulatory center or in a solo practice where fewer medical assistants are on duty at one time.

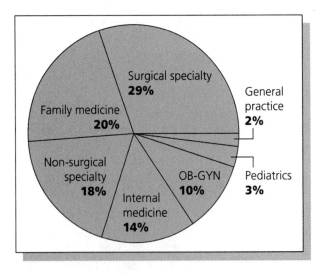

FIGURE 2-1 Medical assistant employment by type of practice

Medical assistants receive their education in community colleges, universities, and vocational schools, or through on-the-job training. Although there are no general licensing requirements for medical assistants, some states require the successful completion of a test or a short course as a prerequisite for performing procedures such as taking x-rays, drawing blood, or giving injections. Some employers prefer to hire either experienced workers or certified applicants.

Voluntary certification is offered through several professional organizations. Some of these include the American Association of Medical Assistants, which awards the Certified Medical Assistant (CMA) credential; the American Medical Technologists, which awards the Registered Medical Assistant (RMA) credential; and the Joint Commission on Allied Health Personnel in Ophthalmology, which awards the Ophthalmic Medical Assistant (OMA) credential.

You should seriously consider sitting for a credentialing examination and continuing education seminars or workshops after you begin work. A credentialed medical assistant is viewed as the "cream of the crop" and often can move into administrative and office management positions.

Employment of medical assistants is expected to grow faster than the average for all occupations through the year 2005 due to expansion of the health services industry. According to the 1994–1995 *Occupational Outlook Handbook,* employment growth will be spurred by the increasing number of group and health care practices that use support personnel. These outpatient settings are where medical assistants primarily work. Job openings will also be created because experienced medical assistants will leave the occupation by laddering to other health service careers or through retirement. In light of this high turnover and the preference for trained personnel, job prospects should be excellent for medical assistants with formal training or experience, particularly those with certification.

The current era of cost-containment in health service has provided an increased demand for generalist health care workers possessing basic skills in multiple areas. Medical assistants in the future will be expected to be broadly trained, both in administrative and clin-

ical tasks and in the use of computers and other technology. The medical assistant's responsibilities are varied, interesting, and rewarding. Anyone who likes to work with people, who has a desire to help others, and who is willing to learn will enjoy this challenging profession.

THE MULTI-FUNCTIONAL MEDICAL ASSISTANT

Competitive pressures on medical practices, hospitals, and other health care facilities have resulted in an emphasis on efficiency and reduction of idle time. Today's health care professionals handle a variety of administrative and clinical tasks. This trend is especially evident in the medical assisting profession where, in 1985, the broad CMA credential replaced the pediatric, administrative, and clinical specialties once available beyond the initial CMA credential. Medical assistants who were awarded the specialty credentials before 1985 may re-certify through continuing education units (CEUs).

Ambulatory care centers, often staffed twenty-four hours a day, seven days a week, are projected to grow at a rapid pace, and an increased need for multi-functional medical assistants will parallel this growth. Since it is not economical to staff a center with several different employees possessing specialized skills, the medical assistant with both administrative and clinical training will be in high demand.

RESPONSIBILITIES OF THE POSITION

Medical assistants perform a variety of administrative and clinical duties. Administrative duties include answering the telephone, greeting patients and other callers, recording and filing patient data and medical records, completing medical reports and insurance forms, handling correspondence, scheduling appointments, arranging for hospital admission and laboratory services, completing record keeping and billing, and transcribing dictation. Clinical duties include recording patient height, weight, temperature, and blood pressure; obtaining medical histories; performing basic laboratory tests; preparing patients for and assisting in examinations; sterilizing instruments; drawing blood; preparing patients for x-rays and EKGs; and applying dressings.

Computer use is an important part of both the administrative and clinical duties of a medical assistant's job. Any machine that shows a digital readout is computer based, and the number and kind of these machines are increasing. Patient temperature can be taken with a thermometer attached to a small hand-held device that shows a digital readout. Computers analyze blood and urine and do many other laboratory tests conducted in the medical office.

Computers have revitalized many boring, time-consuming administrative tasks traditionally completed by hand. If you had gone to work as a medical assistant ten years ago, you would probably have spent several days preparing the monthly billing manually and by typewriter. Now, patient billing is completed in a few hours by a computer programmed for the task (Figure 2-2).

THE DACUM ANALYSIS

In 1979, the American Association of Medical Assistants conducted an analysis of the medical assisting career to determine the responsibilities of people employed in the profession. Using a process called DACUM, which stands for Developing A CUrriculuM, the analysts developed a chart listing the skills performed daily by medical assistants. The DACUM analysis has undergone several revisions as major changes in medical science and in the health care delivery system have affected the medical assistant's re-

sponsibilities. The most recent update occurred in January, 1990.

The DACUM chart shown in Figure 2-3 (on pages 24 and 25) lists the responsibilities the analysts developed. It identifies eight general areas of competence and seventy-nine individual skills required of medical assistants. Sixty-five of the individual skills are considered entry-level skills, and fourteen are considered advanced-level skills. The advanced skills are denoted by an asterisk in the chart. General areas of competence are listed at the right and required skills are listed to the left. In reading each statement, you should precede it with the words, "The medical assistant should be able to…."

Review the DACUM chart carefully. The range of responsibilities is broad, from Listen and Observe, which is considered an entry-level skill, to Manage Personnel and Benefits, an advanced skill.

JOB TITLES AND JOB SITES

Medical assistant job titles often describe specific responsibilities. Typical titles include medical secretary, office manager, receptionist, word processing specialist, computer operator, billing clerk, bookkeeper, records manager, transcriptionist, and laboratory technician. According to *Occupational Outlook Handbook*, published by the U.S. Department of Labor, medical assistants held about 149,000 jobs across the United States in 1991.

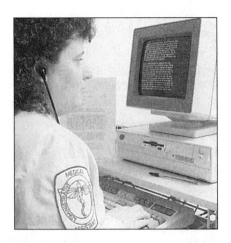

FIGURE 2-2 Computer billing can save a practice time and money. (Courtesy of Keir, Wise, and Krebs, *Medical Assisting, Administrative and Clinical Competencies,* copyright 1993, Delmar Publishers)

IN YOUR OPINION

1. Which medical assisting responsibilities do you think you will like best?
2. How can a medical assistant show interest in assuming extra responsibilities?
3. Why did you decide to pursue a career as a medical assistant?

The Roles of Medical Professionals

As a medical assistant, you will work with a variety of health care professionals who diagnose and treat diseases, help the disabled, provide laboratory services, advise patients on ways to maintain and improve their health, and attempt to prevent disease. The following section will help you understand how the methods, procedures, and technology differ among health care deliverers.

PHYSICIANS

Physicians perform medical examinations, diagnose illnesses, treat injuries and diseases, and advise patients. In the past, almost all medical practices were owned by a physician or a group of physicians; however, practice patterns have changed. Today, many younger physicians work in salaried positions in health maintenance organizations, ambulatory centers, government institutions, and other health care facilities.

PHYSICIAN EXTENDERS

During the 1960s physicians investigated other resources to extend their practices. The idea of physician extenders, identified as Physician Assistants (PAs), Certified Registered Nurse Practitioners (CRNPs), and Certified Midwives, was created to relieve doctors of some time-consuming tasks. Vietnam veteran medical corpsmen, nurses, and others with patient-care experience took advantage of additional training at medical teaching centers and hospitals.

Today, physician extenders perform a wide range of duties. Based on the licensure requirements of their states, they may interview patients, take medical histories, perform physical examinations, order laboratory tests, make tentative diagnoses, and prepare patients for treatment. They always work with a supervising physician. Physician extenders frequently work in long-term care institutions and rural settings where they fill a vacuum caused by a shortage of local physicians. Employment of physician extenders is expected to grow faster than the average for other medical occupations through the year 2000.

NURSES

Nurses are licensed professionals who observe, assess, and record symptoms, dispense medications, and aid in patients' convalescence and rehabilitation. They also provide instruction in proper care to patients and their families and help people understand the importance of diet, exercise, and daily habits to health improvement. Sometimes they perform routine laboratory and office work, especially in solo and small practices.

After completing years of education and training, including some of the same courses required for physicians, nurses are licensed to practice as registered nurses (RNs) or licensed practical nurses (LPNs or LVNs in some states). Registered nurses train from two to five years after high school, and they supervise licensed practical nurses, who usually train for one year after high school. An LPN/LVN may continue his or her education and eventually become licensed as a registered nurse.

In general, nurses see patients more often and spend more time with them than physicians. Physicians often pass directions for care and instructions for medication along to a nurse for administration.

MEDICAL TECHNOLOGISTS AND TECHNICIANS

As advanced diagnostic techniques, laboratory procedures, and treatment methods develop through medical technology, new jobs are created for people who operate the highly specialized equipment. Known as medical technologists and technicians, these people often carry titles associated with the equipment they use, for example, radiologic technologist, electrocardiograph technician, and dialysis technician. Others who test body fluids and tissues are called laboratory technologists or technicians. Projections indicate that 50 percent of the technology that will be used by today's eighth graders when they begin their careers has not yet been invented.

MEDICAL RECORDS PERSONNEL

Medical records employees manage an information system of patient records that meet medical, administrative, ethical, and legal requirements. **Medical records administrators** direct the activities of large departments, handling thousands of patient records yearly. Their job is to

1.0 Display Professionalism	1.1 Project a positive attitude	1.2 Perform within ethical boundaries	1.3 Practice within the scope of education, training, and personal capabilities	1.4 Maintain confidentiality	1.5 Work as a team member	1.6 Conduct oneself in a courteous and diplomatic manner	1.7 Adapt to change
2.0 Communicate	2.1 Listen and observe	2.2 Treat all patients with empathy and impartiality	2.3 Adapt communication to individuals' abilities to understand	2.4 Recognize and respond to verbal and non-verbal communication	2.5 Serve as liaison between physician and others	2.6 Evaluate understanding of communication	2.7 Receive, organize, prioritize, and transmit information
3.0 Perform Administrative Duties	3.1 Perform basic secretarial skills	3.2 Schedule and monitor appointments	3.3 Prepare and maintain medical records	3.4 Apply computer concepts for office procedures	3.5 Perform medical transcription	3.6 Locate resources and information for patients and employers	3.7 Manage physician's professional schedule and travel
4.0 Perform Clinical Duties	4.1 Apply principals of aseptic technique and infection control	4.2 Take vital signs	4.3 Recognize emergencies	4.4 Perform first aid and CPR	4.5 Prepare and maintain examination and treatment area	4.6 Interview and take patient history	4.7 Prepare patients for procedures
5.0 Apply Legal Concepts to Practice	5.1 Document accurately	5.2 Determine needs for documentation and reporting	5.3 Use appropriate guidelines when releasing records or information	5.4 Follow established policy in initiating or terminating medical treatment	5.5 Dispose of controlled substances in compliance with government regulations	5.6 Maintain licenses and accreditation	5.7 Monitor legislation related to current healthcare issues and practices
6.0 Manage the Office	6.1 Maintain the physical plant	6.2 Operate and maintain facilities and equipment safely	6.3 Inventory equipment and supplies	6.4 Evaluate and recommend equipment and supplies for a practice	6.5 Maintain liability coverage	6.6 Exercise efficient time management	*Supervise personnel
7.0 Provide Instruction	7.1 Orient patients to office policies and procedures	7.2 Instruct patients with special needs	7.3 Teach patients methods of health promotion and disease prevention	7.4 Orient and train personnel	*Provide health information for public use	*Supervise student practicums	*Conduct continuing education activities
8.0 Manage Practice Finances	8.1 Use manual bookkeeping systems	8.2 Implement current procedural terminology and ICD-9 coding	8.3 Analyze and use current third-party guidelines for reimbursement	8.4 Manage accounts receivable	8.5 Manage accounts payable	8.6 Maintain records for accounting and banking purposes	8.7 Process employee payroll

FIGURE 2-3 1990 DACUM analysis of the medical assisting profession (Reprinted with permission from the American Association of Medical Assistants, Inc.)

1.8 Show initiative and responsibility	**1.9** Promote the profession	*Enhance skills through continuing education				

2.8 Use proper telephone technique	**2.9** Interview effectively	**2.10** Use medical terminology appropriately	**2.11** Compose written communication using correct grammar, spelling, and format	*Develop and conduct public relations activities to market professional services		

4.8 Assist physician with examinations and treatments	**4.9** Use quality control	**4.10** Collect and process specimens	**4.11** Perform selected tests that assist with diagnosis and treatment	**4.12** Screen and follow-up patient test results	**4.13** Prepare and administer medications as directed by physician	**4.14** Maintain medication records	*Respond to medical emergencies

*Develop and maintain policy and procedure manuals	*Establish risk management protocol for the practice

*Develop job descriptions	*Interview and recommend new personnel	*Negotiate leases and prices for equipment and supply contracts

*Develop educational materials

> *Denotes advanced-level skills.
> *The medical assistant should be able to perform all other skills after completing a CAIIEA-accredited program and starting a first job.*

*Manage personnel benefits and records

Developed by:
The American Association of Medical Assistants, Inc.,
20 North Wacker Drive, Suite 1575,
Chicago, IL 60606.
312-899-1500;
toll-free 800-228-2262.
Consultants: Mary Lee Seibert, EdD, CMA, and Patricia A. Amos, MS

FIGURE 2-3 (continued)

develop systems for efficient documentation, storage, and retrieval of records. **Medical records technicians** compile, organize, and evaluate patients' records for completeness and accuracy (Figure 2-4). They use standard coding and classification systems such as ICD-9-CM, *International Classification of Disease, Ninth Edition, Clinical Modification,* and CPT-4, *Current Procedural Terminology,* Fourth Edition, to list symptoms, diseases, operations, procedures, therapies, and diagnoses on each patient's record. Physicians are primary users of patient records; however, nonconfidential information may also be supplied to insurance companies, government agencies, public health agencies, and other institutions.

The size of a medical facility determines the degree of responsibility of its medical records personnel. In private practices and small facilities, one person may be responsible for managing all aspects of record keeping, whereas in larger facilities an administrator and several technicians and clerks may be required. Credentialing for medical records personnel is available through the American Medical Record Association, which awards the Accredited Record Technician (ART) and the Registered Record Administrator (RRA) professional credential.

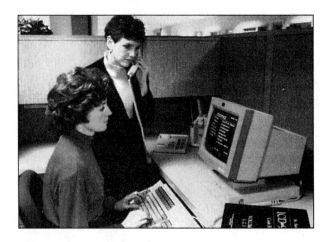

FIGURE 2-4 Medical records technician (Courtesy of Hinsdale Hospital, Hinsdale, IL)

fic for the physician, and preparing the bill before the patient leaves. If you have additional clinical responsibilities, you may prepare the treatment room, locate and retrieve supplies needed by the physician or nurse, apply bandages, and give injections.

As a member of the health care team, you must respect and support all your co-workers. This means you must understand the professional responsibilities of each person and provide the help he or she needs, recognizing that every task is important if the physician, nurse, or laboratory employee requires assistance in patient care.

Medical assistants often increase their value to a medical practice simply by being willing to assume extra responsibilities. With motivation, enthusiasm, the desire to work hard, good judgment, and good training, you can become very important to the success of a practice. You will determine whether you have a job or a career, and you can ensure your own success by becoming a valuable support employee for the physician and other professionals.

IN YOUR OPINION

1. Compare the medical assistant's duties to those of the physician's extenders. Which position do you think is most important to the future growth of a physician practice?

2. How do you think national health insurance will change the role of medical professionals?

3. What is the importance of a medical record employee's job?

Working with the Medical Professionals

In your role as medical assistant, you will work with all the health care professionals. Most of your work will be of a support nature, including registering the patient upon arrival, organizing patient records for the physician and nurse to review, maintaining an even flow of patient traf-

WORKING WITH THE PHYSICIAN AND THE HEALTH CARE TEAM

Physicians spend many years in training to treat the physical and mental ills of individuals in our society. Their study is intense, encouraging a fast-paced and demanding lifestyle that can carry over to the physician's private practice after formal education is completed. The nurses,

Honesty	Dishonesty
Correctly reporting daily work hours	Failing to report late arrival; "stretching" breaks and lunch hours; conducting personal business, such as phone calls and chores, during scheduled work hours
Taking responsibility for errors and omissions; correcting errors and planning ways to prevent errors in the future	Blaming others for errors, complaining, and being defensive
Properly accounting for money, office supplies, medical supplies, and drugs	"Borrowing" from petty cash, taking drug samples or supplies without permission, making personal telephone calls without logging them

FIGURE 2-5 Comparison of honesty and dishonesty

laboratory technologists, and medical assistants work under intense pressure at times. In order for this diverse team of professionals to use their efforts best, each must work at top efficiency and use good interpersonal skills. Several characteristics that add to a medical assistant's success are discussed in the next section.

Honesty

A medical assistant's honesty must be beyond reproach. Since the physician is responsible for employees actions, a dishonest employee can unknowingly involve a physician in a crime or malpractice lawsuit. A medical assistant who dishonestly alters a patient's record because of a mistake reflects on the physician and may cause a malpractice lawsuit; in the same way, a bookkeeper or accountant who reports dishonest tax information involves the physician in a crime.

Dishonesty does not always involve a crime. The person who lies about a minor infraction of office policy and the person who does not tell the whole truth are dishonest. Consider the situations in Figure 2-5; some may seem unimportant, but all are dishonest and can destroy a medical assistant's career.

Cooperation

"No man is an island unto himself" is a famous quotation that characterizes the necessity of cooperation among members of the medical office staff. Although each person has special responsibilities, all the responsibilities combine into one major effort to treat patients. When several people work toward a common goal, each must support all the others involved in the effort. One person who does not cooperate can spoil the success formula.

A cooperative person suppresses personal goals if these goals do not agree with the group goal. For example, as a medical assistant you will not be able to eat lunch each day at 11:30 A.M. if routine lunch hours are scheduled for 12:30 P.M. Your desire to answer the telephone and greet patients must be adjusted and the task given to someone else if the day's agenda calls for you to mail monthly statements.

Cooperation is pleasurable, and the rewards are both personal and financial. Personal reward comes through ego support and good will from colleagues, while monetary recognition results in salary increases. Cooperative people are well liked and their services are in demand. A list of suggested ways a medical assistant can show cooperation is given in Figure 2-6.

Assertiveness

Assertiveness refers to making a point positively or putting your views forward. Assertiveness is sometimes confused with aggressiveness; however, the two terms are not the same. Aggressiveness means pushiness or the desire to attack; it is considered a negative term when applied to relationships with others. On the other hand, assertiveness is a positive characteristic that means standing up for yourself or speaking when a comment is needed.

Problem	Cooperation Shown by
Fellow employee must leave fifteen minutes early to pick up child at daycare	Offer to cover for employee during absence
You dislike a co-worker	Be polite to all co-workers
You disagree with a decision	Explain why you disagree, then support the final decision
The day after the cleaning crew has cleaned the office, a child spills grape juice on the carpet	Quickly and quietly mop it up
Emergency situations	Do whatever is necessary to assist in the situation

FIGURE 2-6 Suggestions for cooperation

As a medical assistant, you should be assertive and offer new ideas when they improve office procedures or activities. If you have a personal concern or a complaint, such as a promised pay increase that you have not received, or if you feel resentment because long-time employees seem not to be sharing the work, you should discuss the problem with the physician or office manager. However, if you are a new employee you should understand fully why a chore or responsibility is handled in its particular way before offering a suggestion. You should allow plenty of time to pass before bringing up a personal concern. Embarrassment can occur if you are assertive without having all the facts.

The best approach is to delay making a move until you are absolutely satisfied that your question or remark is justified. It is a good idea to ask advice from someone you trust or a person who has been employed in a similar job before approaching the physician or office manager. Then, when you are confident you have waited long enough, use your most professional manner. State the problem or suggestion clearly, objectively, and without emotion. You may be slightly nervous; that is a natural feeling when you are discussing an important matter with a superior. However, once you have communicated your point, you will probably feel more confident. Be sure to use good oral skills to make your point and to read the feedback. If nonverbal feedback indicates that your point is not being well received, tactfully drop the subject and reconsider your position before speaking up again. You may want to consider submitting your idea or concern in writing. Be sure to sign and date your

Assertive	Aggressive
Thursday will be my six-month anniversary of employment. I would like to schedule a review with you at your convenience.	I work twice as hard as everyone else around here for less money. I thought I would get a raise by now.
I think it would be possible to shorten our billing cycle by combining steps.	Your billing system here is really Stone Age. I can't believe how much time you waste doing all those steps.
I will need to leave early tomorrow afternoon. Would you prefer that I stay late tonight, come in early tomorrow, or make up the time in some other way?	I'm leaving early today. I'll make it up.
I must complete this report for Dr. Joyce, but I'll be happy to help you when I'm finished.	How come I get stuck with all the work? I'm not supposed to do filing; you are.

FIGURE 2-7 Comparison of assertive and aggressive behavior

letter or memorandum. To clarify the differences between assertiveness and aggressiveness, several examples are given in Figure 2-7.

Dependability

In a busy medical office, employees must be able to depend on one another. As a medical assistant, you should know what needs to be done, when it needs to be done, and how to do it. The physician depends on the medical assistant to make the right decision or to ask questions as necessary with little direct supervision.

When you are dependable, you arrive at work on time each day and you finish your work without being reminded, even though you may have to stay after hours (Figure 2-8). You take sick leave only when you are sick, and you use only the allotted time for lunch. You tackle unpleasant tasks without complaint and without being asked or reminded. People who are undependable usually lose their jobs because they cannot be counted on when needed.

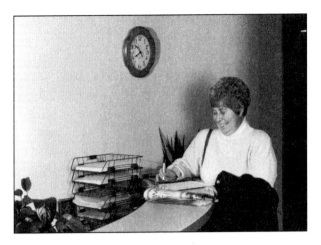

FIGURE 2-8 Arriving on or before time reflects a responsible attitude.

some people like to gossip, complain, or ask "nosy" questions. A loyal medical assistant remains silent or defends the practice when patients or other employees engage in negative conversation.

Compare the loyal and disloyal medical assistants quoted here:

UNDEPENDABLE MEDICAL ASSISTANT

8:30 A.M.:	I'm sorry, Dr. Richter, I won't be in today. My daughter has the day off from school.
Day preceding monthly billing:	We can't do the billing tomorrow, Dr. Richter, because I forgot to order return envelopes.
After lunch:	Gee, I'm sorry I'm late, Dr. Richter. The mall was having a great sale.
In conversation with another medical assistant:	Janie, I know I said I would work late for you tonight, but Rob just called to take me out.
In conversation with a patient:	Mrs. Cristini, I'm sorry I didn't mail the insurance forms. I just forgot.

Loyalty

The employees of a medical office must be loyal to the physician and to other staff members. Loyalty carries a responsibility to defend the physician and colleagues tactfully from unworthy remarks from patients, outsiders, and other employees.

When a person works with the public, many opportunities exist for disloyal words and acts. A medical assistant who is in close contact with many different people during the day learns that

---

**LOYAL MEDICAL ASSISTANT
SITUATION ONE**

(Listens to patient's question about the physician's recent divorce): "Dr. Levine doesn't tell us about his personal life, so I don't know where his children are living."

SITUATION TWO

(Listens to a fellow employee complain about delay of the lunch hour): "I'm hungry, too, but I don't think it's Dr. Levine's fault that we're behind. Two patients were very late for their appointments."

**DISLOYAL MEDICAL ASSISTANT
SITUATION ONE**

(Listens to fellow employee complain about the physician's irritability): "I agree. Dr. Levine has been a real pain lately, and I don't like it at all."

SITUATION TWO

(Listens to a sales representative's insult about the office furniture): "Yes, we do have old-fashioned furniture, but between you and me, we'll probably have it another five years. Dr. Levine is a real penny pincher."

COORDINATING WITH THE HOSPITAL STAFF

Hospital employees you will work with most often include business office personnel regarding fees and codes, scheduling personnel who admit patients, and laboratory technicians who process samples. When working with hospital staff, your communication, cooperation, and assertiveness skills are important. As a representative of the physician, you must make sure the interests of your patients are carefully considered; however, the degree of urgency and the availability of hospital personnel to perform services may at times appear to be at odds with the patient's needs.

Patients being admitted to a hospital present a challenge in terms of coordination, and it is the medical assistant who is primarily responsible for making the arrangements. Since hospitals sometimes have a limited number of beds available and can admit only a specified number of patients, the admittance scheduler may have to determine which patients are admitted first. You must learn to discriminate between the patient's need for hospitalization and the hospital's limited access to beds. If you find yourself pushing for a faster hospitalization than the scheduler wishes to provide, review the patient's needs with the physician to determine if you have any flexibility in scheduling. You should possess the human relations skills to reach a solution that satisfies everyone.

When you work with a hospital's billing department, you may be asked to contribute information that helps in coding procedures, treatments, and services. This is an important responsibility that requires diligence, attention to detail, and desire to provide the best information. The hospital and the doctor's remuneration depends on the responsible handling of billing matters between the medical assistant and the hospital billing assistant.

Coordinating with the hospital staff should be viewed as an opportunity to create and build a good working relationship. An adversarial relationship can develop when the medical assistant and the hospital personnel do not understand the limitations imposed by the systems within which they work. You should guard your relationship carefully as you and the hospital staff are mutually dependent.

INTERACTING WITH OTHER OUTSIDE PROFESSIONALS

As a representative of the practice, the medical assistant has a responsibility to offer a positive image. Rescue teams, independent laboratories, and other allied health units call the medical office for instructions, information, and questions. Often, their first and last contact is the medical assistant, and any opinion they form will be based on this encounter. By using interpersonal skills and good communication, you can make a good first and last impression.

Be courteous, helpful, and cooperative with outside professionals, and they will respond in a like manner. Because you will request the services of these deliverers often and regularly, you should treat them as allies. Although they do not work in a salaried position for the physician, personnel from outside agencies play an important role in the day-to-day activities of the practice. The practice can be adversely affected if related units do not experience cooperation with the medical office assistant.

IN YOUR OPINION

1. What personal characteristics do you think are most important in the medical office?
2. Do you think your being undependable may result in injury or harm to a patient?
3. How would you handle working with a person who is aggressive?

REFERENCES

"The DACUM Revisited: The 1990 Update on the Profession of Medical Assisting," *The Professional Medical Assistant.* May/June 1990.

"Synergy in the Medical Office," *The Professional Medical Assistant.* May/June 1990.

Bamberg, Richard, Jean Keenon, and Keith D. Blayney. "Multi-skilled Medical Assistants in Physician Practices," *The Professional Medical Assistant.* November/December 1990.

U.S. Department of Labor, Bureau of Labor Statistics. *Occupational Outlook Handbook,* 1992–93 ed.

Chapter Activities

PERFORMANCE BASED ACTIVITIES

1. Summarize the differences between a multi-functional medical assistant and a medical assistant who handles only clinical or administrative medical responsibilities. Using correct grammar and format, compose a short paper expressing your opinion of the best career path between these two approaches. Give reasons for making this choice. (DACUM 2.6, 2.11)

2. On the following chart, contrast the duties of a medical assistant who works in a solo physician practice to one who works in a large group clinic. What are the advantages and disadvantages of each?

   Solo Practice   *Clinic*

   Advantages

   1. _____

   2. _____

   3. _____

   Disadvantages

   1. _____

   2. _____

   3. _____

   (DACUM 2.7)

3. Evaluate the advantages of credentialing in terms of securing and maintaining a position as a medical assistant.

   Advantages of Credentials

   Getting a job

   1. _____

   2. _____

   3. _____

   Advancing in a career

   1. _____

   2. _____

   3. _____

   Advancing on the career ladder

   1. _____

   2. _____

   3. _____

   (DACUM 2.6, 5.6)

4. On the following lines, list the personal characteristics of a medical assistant that improve relationships with patients and other staff members. Compare the list with your own traits and develop a plan for improving your relationship characteristics.

Improving Relations

Personal Characteristics Needed   *Do I Possess These Traits? (Yes or No)*

1. _____

2. _____

3. _____

4. _____

5. _____

6. _____

My personal plan for improvement

Goal:

When:

How will I achieve my goal?

1. _____

2. _____

3. _____

4. _____

(DACUM 1.1, 1.5, 1.6)

5. Read a recent article on health care reform or use one of the articles you read in Chapter 1. Project changes in health care that might influence the number or types of jobs available to medical assistants between now and the year 2000.

*Characteristics of Health Care Reform That Might Influence the
Number and Type of Medical Assisting Jobs Available in the Future*

Fee-for-Service System   *Managed Care*

(DACUM 2.7, 2.11)

EXPANDING YOUR THINKING

1. Describe how you would handle a fellow employee who is showing negative personal characteristics. How would such behavior adversely affect the general morale and productivity of the medical office?

2. What would you do if:

   a. a patient complains because she has been waiting for fifteen minutes to see the doctor.

   b. a patient tells you he heard that the physician and his wife are getting a divorce.

   c. a young mother whose six-week-old baby is ill brings her two-year-old child with her to the medical office. The two-year-old causes problems in the reception area.

   d. an elderly patient tells you that the medicine the physician gave her at her last visit made her sicker.

   e. another medical assistant, the receptionist, complains to you that the physician took too long with a patient, thus delaying the schedule and causing patients to be impatient with the receptionist.

   f. one of the nurses confides in you that she is pregnant and unmarried.

   g. you overhear two physician partners talking about a staff member they plan to replace because the person is tardy too often.

Chapter 3

Medical Ethics

PHILADELPHIA, PENNSYLVANIA

Over the past five years, our patients who are enrolled in an HMO, PPO, or IPA have increased by 50 percent. Today, about one third of our total patients participate in some type of plan. This requires Drs. Tobin and Wallace, the primary care doctors, to give authorization before diagnostic tests or additional services can be provided by a specialist. Since our patients really like Dr. Tobin and Dr. Wallace as their family doctors, they are usually cooperative about seeing us first before they go to a specialist. Every now and then we have a problem case like Tommy Wilson's.

For about ten days, Tommy has been running a fever and getting severe headaches. The doctors have seen him at least four times and prescribed antibiotics. But Mrs. Wilson, who is frustrated and worried, insists on a referral to a neurologist. Tommy has missed several days of school and Mrs. Wilson doesn't want to just "wait around" for the headaches to go away. She's extremely concerned that Tommy's symptoms indicate something serious, like a brain tumor. Although the doctors are quite certain that Tommy has the latest strain of flu, they told me to go ahead and process the referral to a neurologist. I am sure this is an unnecessary cost; but I have to wonder, what if Tommy were my child?

I've been thinking a lot about ethics lately.

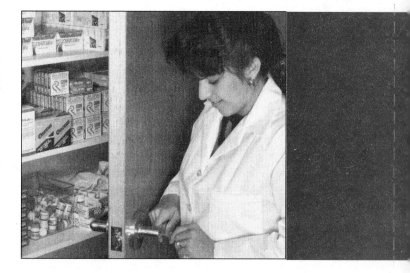

Yesterday, a team of surgeons operated on conjoined twins at the hospital across the street. The surgery was expensive, and care will continue to be extremely costly, perhaps for their whole lives. Everyone in the hospital cafeteria has been discussing whether it was right to operate. In thinking about the issues we faced in Tommy's case, I'm really concerned that health care will be rationed because of money. Doctors, patients, and legislators may have tough choices to make in the next several years.

Jordon Bensinger
Medical Assistant

PERFORMANCE BASED COMPETENCIES

After completing this chapter, you should be able to:

1. Identify five important social policy issues related to medicine and discuss the ethical implications of each. (DACUM 5.7)
2. Outline procedures for maintaining the confidentiality of computerized records. (DACUM 1.4, 3.4)
3. Create examples of ethical dilemmas that might involve a medical assistant, and discuss different ways of resolving them. (DACUM 1.2)
4. Compare the value of improved medical technology with the ethical problems that may result. (DACUM 1.8)

HEALTHSPEAK

Bioethics Branch of medical ethics concerned with moral issues resulting from high technology and sophisticated medical research. Social issues such as abortion, fetal research, artificial insemination, and euthanasia are important bioethical questions.

DNR Do Not Resuscitate order permits the patient to die without cardiopulmonary resuscitation. This order is commonly used in treating terminally ill or elderly patients.

Durable power of attorney Document that provides broad powers of medical authority to an individual, often either a family member or an attorney, who is given legal power to decide what extraordinary measures should be taken with a patient when the patient is too sick to decide. A durable power of attorney usually accompanies a DNR in the patient's hospital record.

Genetic counseling Counseling related to gene disorders. Prospective parents often receive genetic counseling regarding the likelihood of bearing a child with genetic disorders.

Genetic engineering Advanced, complex, and often controversial means of isolating and replacing part or all of a "mutant" gene to reduce or eliminate the chances that a person will develop a particular disease.

Genetics Study of genes and their role in illness and disease. Gene therapy is an exciting, emerging field of medical study because it promises a cure for some illnesses now considered terminal.

Living will Legal document, signed by an individual, that provides precise instructions about the amount of extraordinary care to be delivered in the event of a life-threatening medical situation.

Medical ethics Term applied to the principles governing medical conduct. Medical ethics deals with the relationship of the physician to the patient, the patient's family, fellow physicians, and society.

Medical law Standards set by elected officials in the state and nation. An illegal act is always unethical, according to the American Medical Association's Principles of Medical Ethics, but an unethical act may not be illegal.

Patient's Bill of Rights Established by the American Hospital Association in 1972, the Patient's Bill of Rights provides basic guidelines for the care of hospitalized patients.

Patient Self-Determination Act Federal law requiring all hospitals and nursing homes to explain in detail the extraordinary care their state permits. These facilities must alert patients of their right to execute living wills or appoint a health care proxy through a durable power of attorney.

Medical Ethics and the Law

Medical ethics refers to moral conduct or to what is right or wrong, based on religious teachings from the Judeo-Christian, Buddhist, Islamic, and other religious traditions, and the Hippocratic Oath (Figure 3-1). Medical ethics are often stricter than standards set by law, but they are never less strict. Ethical dilemmas in medicine occur when (1) legal enforcement does not appear to provide justice; (2) there is no obvious right or wrong behavior; (3) right behavior appears to have the wrong outcome; and (4) personal sacrifice is the consequence of following one's ideals.

One of the most pressing issues in modern medicine is the question, "What is ethical conduct?" Abortions are legal, but are they ethical? Should extraordinary measures be used to prolong life in a mentally and physically deficient newborn likely to survive only a short time? Will the current experimentation in genetic engineering lead to other experimentation that may

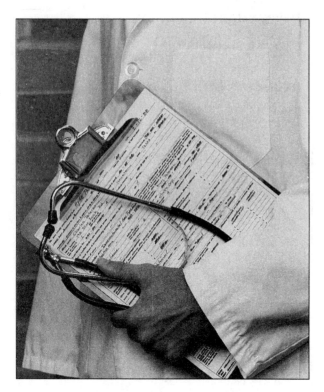

FIGURE 3-1 Medical ethics refers to moral conduct. Codes of ethics remind medical professional of proper conduct, and of their duty to patients

be unethical? Should extraordinary measures be used for a patient in the last stages of a terminal illness? The greatest minds in the legal and medical professions today are struggling with these and other complex ethical questions.

IN YOUR OPINION

1. Who makes the ultimate decision about the type of care a patient receives? For example, when do you think that a daughter or son has a right to decide what level of care is appropriate for an elderly parent?
2. What are some of the risks of establishing policy statements about patient treatments?
3. How do you feel about physician-assisted suicides?

Ethics Statements of the Medical Associations

The system by which a profession sets standards of right and wrong behavior for its members is called its code of ethics. Through these codes, the professions attempt to maintain high stan-

dards of competence, to strengthen the relationship among members, and to promote the welfare of the whole community.

Medical professionals, including physicians, nurses, medical assistants, laboratory employees, and others may join an organization in their career field that establishes a statement of ethics or a professional code for its members. Although an organization cannot guarantee that its members will abide by the code, it serves as a reminder of proper conduct. Members who ignore the code and who are reported may be expelled from the organization. Membership does not exempt a member from being charged with a crime if the conduct is both unethical and illegal.

The earliest written code of medical ethics, called the **Code of Hammurabi**, was conceived by the Babylonians around 2000 B.C. It was so specific and detailed that it probably would not be applicable today. The Oath of Hippocrates, written by a Greek physician around 400 B.C., is a better-known statement of ethical principles that has been accepted throughout history as a standard of behavior for physicians.

The Oath of Hippocrates does not impose authority over or prescribe punishment for a physician, but it does give the medical profession a sense of duty to humankind. The oath (1) protects the rights of the patient, (2) appeals to the inner and finer instincts of the physician, and (3) includes rules for the relationship between a doctor and a patient. Many medical students still take the Oath of Hippocrates before graduation and display it in their offices once they begin to practice medicine.

AMA PRINCIPLES OF MEDICAL ETHICS

The American Medical Association (AMA) assumes leadership in the United States for setting standards of ethical medical behavior for physicians. In 1847, the AMA adopted its first ethical guidelines, based on a **Code of Medical Ethics** written by Thomas Percival, an English physician, philosopher, and writer. The current text, **Principles of Medical Ethics**, was revised by the AMA in 1980 in an attempt to clarify and update the language, eliminate reference to gender, and find a balance between ethical standards for physicians and changing legal standards.

Ethical behavior, according to the AMA Judicial Council, refers to (1) moral principles and practices, (2) the customs and usage of the medical profession, and (3) matters of medical policy. The word **unethical** is used to describe behavior that fails to conform to ethical standards. When a physician is accused of unethical conduct, the AMA Judicial Council has the authority to dismiss the accusation, issue a warning or criticism, or expel the physician from membership in the Association. However, the AMA does not have the authority to bring legal action against a member for unethical behavior.

The **1992** revision of the **Principles of Medical Ethics** is given in Figure 3-2. These principles speak of human dignity, honesty, responsibility to society, confidentiality, continued study, freedom of choice, and responsibility to an improved community.

AMERICAN HOSPITAL ASSOCIATION

In recent years, patients have become better informed about medical services. Startling medical breakthroughs are publicized by the media, including daily reports on the progress and prognosis of patients undergoing experimental procedures. Media attention to medicine advises us of many previously unknown options in health care, and an important patient's rights movement has grown out of this newfound knowledge. In the past, the patient rarely questioned a physician's diagnosis, procedure, or treatment, but today's educated patient is not as accepting. By joining together, private citizens have brought significant pressure on the medical community to protect patients' rights. As a result, patients and their families are more actively involved in treatment and in decisions involving surgery than in the past.

This change in patients' attitudes is apparent in the 1993 case of the Lakeberg twins. The twins, conjoined at the chest and sharing a single six-chamber heart, were born in Chicago. Their doctors decided against surgery. However, the parents, Kenny and Reitha Lakeberg, persisted in seeking medical intervention and transferred their daughters to Children's Hospital in Philadelphia. One twin died in surgery, as the

Preamble:

The medical profession has long subscribed to a body of ethical statements developed primarily for the benefit of the patient. As a member or this profession, a physician must recognize responsibility not only to patients, but also to society, to other health professionals, and to self. The following Principles adopted by the American Medical Association are not laws, but standards of conduct which define the essentials of honorable behavior for the physician.

I. A physician shall be dedicated to providing competent medical service with compassion and respect for human dignity.

II. A physician shall deal honestly with patients and colleagues, and strive to expose those physicians deficient in character or competence, or who engage in fraud or deception.

III. A physician shall respect the law and also recognize a responsibility to seek changes in those requirements which are contrary to the best interests of the patient.

IV. A physician shall respect the rights of patients, of colleagues, and of other health professionals, and shall safeguard patient confidences within the constraints of the law.

V. A physician shall continue to study, apply and advance scientific knowledge, make relevant information available to patients, colleagues, and the public, obtain consultation, and use the talents of other health professionals when indicated.

VI. A physician shall, in the provision of appropriate patient care, except in emergencies, be free to choose whom to serve, with whom to associate, and the environment in which to provide medical services.

VII. A physician shall recognize a responsibility to participate in activities contributing to an improved community.

FIGURE 3-2 Principles of Medical Ethics. (Reprinted with permission from *Code of Medical Ethics: Current Opinions of the Council on Ethical and Judicial Affairs* of the American Medical Association, copyright 1992.)

medical team knew she would. Doctors estimated a survival of only a few months or years for the second twin. Great public controversy erupted over this case. Should the one million dollars spent for an almost hopeless operation have been used on medical care for other sick babies, or for preventive prenatal care for other patients?

Treatment decisions about a parent, spouse, child, or other family member are often difficult to make, considering the technological advances available to prolong life. Medical ethicists are now trying to come to grips with how to help patients better control their own destinies. Living wills and durable powers of attorney are other means for patients to make their wishes known.

A living will gives patients the opportunity to state in advance, while they are capable of doing so, what type of medical treatment they would consent to or refuse in the future. Also, known as "advance directives," a living will generally follows a set format of "if/then" statements. The "if" refers to the patient's condition; for example, "if I am terminally ill." The "then" statement involves the treatments the patient would want withheld or withdrawn, for example, "then I direct my attending physician to withhold or withdraw life-sustaining treatment that serves only to prolong the process of dying." A durable power of attorney allows patients to designate a responsible person to make decisions on their behalf. Often a family member or trusted friend is designated. Living wills and durable powers of attorney are discussed further in Chapter 4.

In 1972 the American Hospital Association established a **Statement on a Patient's Bill of Rights**, as shown in Figure 3-3, which has become the standard for the medical community. The focus of the statement is on the patient's right to know and participate in decisions about treatment, including the right to accept or reject treatment. A new federal law, the **Patient Self-Determination Act**, went into effect on December 1, 1991. This law requires all hospitals, nursing homes, and health maintenance organizations to ask on admission whether a patient has a living will or a proxy and, if so, to note its provisions in the patient's chart.

AMERICAN ASSOCIATION OF MEDICAL ASSISTANTS

Although medical assistants usually are not involved in life-and-death ethical decisions, you will probably confront ethical dilemmas that will cause frustration, anxiety, guilt, and a great deal of soul searching. Should you, for example, allow the mayor or school principal to see the physician ahead of other patients who have been waiting longer? Should you keep silent about foul language another employee uses in front of patients? Should you break a promise to work late when a more appealing option becomes available?

The American Association of Medical Assistants (AAMA) is an association of medical secretaries, receptionists, medical office managers, and back office medical assistants who work with physicians. Recognizing that its members face ethical dilemmas every day, the Association has established a standard of ethics to guide them through their daily activities. The AAMA **Code of Ethics**, a part of the organization's bylaws, enumerates responsibilities of service, confidentiality, honor, improving knowledge, and improving the community. The AAMA Code of Ethics is shown in Figure 3-4.

IN YOUR OPINION

1. What are the advantages and disadvantages for family members when a loved one prepares a living will?
2. Should patients with health insurance be scheduled before uninsured patients? Defend your answer.
3. Is scheduling of medical office employees an ethical question? Should the newest medical assistant be required to work all weekends or should the responsibility be shared, even though employees with seniority have previously "put in their time" on weekends? Why or why not?

Social Policy Issues

The term **social policy** refers to rules or guidelines that make the world a better place in which to live. Each nation develops its own social policy by taking into consideration the religion(s) of the people, its culture, history,

Bill of Rights

1. The patient has the right to considerate and respectful care.

2. The patient has the right to obtain from his physician complete current information concerning his diagnosis, treatment, and prognosis in terms the patient can be reasonably expected to understand. When it is not medically advisable to give such information to the patient, the information should be made available to an appropriate person in his behalf. He has the right to know, by name, the physician responsible for coordinating his care.

3. The patient has the right to receive from his physician information necessary to give informed consent prior to the start of any procedure and/or treatment. Except in emergencies, such information for informed consent should include but not necessarily be limited to the specific procedure and/or treatment, the medically-significant risks involved, and the probable duration of incapacitation. Where medically-significant alternatives for care or treatment exist, or when the patient requests information concerning medical alternatives, the patient has the right to such information. The patient also has the right to know the name of the person responsible for the procedures and/or treatment.

4. The patient has the right to refuse treatment to the extent permitted by law and to be informed of the medical consequences of his action.

5. The patient has the right to every consideration of his privacy concerning his own medical care program. Case discussion, consultation, examination, and treatment are confidential and should be conducted discreetly. Those not directly involved in his care must have the permission of the patient to be present

6. The patient has the right to expect that all communications and records pertaining to his care should be treated as confidential.

7. The patient has the right to expect that, within its capacity, a hospital must make reasonable response to the request of a patient for services. The hospital must provide evaluation, service and/or referral as indicated by the urgency of the case. When medically permissible, a patient may be transferred to another facility only after he has received complete information and explanation concerning the needs for and alternatives to such a transfer. The institution to which the patient is to be transferred must first have accepted the patient for transfer.

8. The patient has the right to obtain information as to any relationship of his hospital to other health care and educational institutions insofar as his care is concerned. The patient has the right to obtain information as to the existence of any professional relationships among individuals, by name, who are treating him.

9. The patient has the right to be advised if the hospital proposes to engage in or perform human experimentation affecting his care or treatment. The patient has the right to refuse to participate in such research projects.

10. The patient has the right to expect reasonable continuity of care. He has the right to know, in advance, what appointment times and physicians are available and where. The patient has the right to expect that the hospital will provide a mechanism whereby he is informed by his physician or a delegate of the physician of the patient's continuing health care requirements following discharge.

11. The patient has the right to examine and receive an explanation of his bill, regardless of source of payment.

12. The patient has the right to know what hospital rules and regulations apply to his conduct as a patient.

FIGURE 3-3   A Patient's Bill of Rights. (Reprinted with permission of the American Hospital Association, copyright 1992.)

Code of Ethics

The Code of Ethics of AAMA shall set forth principles of ethical and moral conduct as they relate to the medical profession and the particular practice of medical assisting.

Members of AAMA dedicated to the conscientious pursuit of their profession, and thus desiring to merit the high regard of the entire medical profession and the respect of the general public which they serve, do pledge themselves to strive always to:

A. render service with full respect for the dignity of humanity;

B. respect confidential information obtained through employment unless legally authorized or required by responsible performance of duty to divulge such information;

C. uphold the honor and high principles of the profession and accept its disciplines;

D. seek to continually improve the knowledge and skills of medical assistants for the benefit of patients and professional colleagues;

E. participate in additional service activities aimed toward improving the health and well-being of the community.

Creed

I believe in the principles and purposes of the profession of medical assisting.

I endeavor to be more effective.

I aspire to render greater service.

I protect the confidence entrusted to me.

I am dedicated to the care and well-being of all patients.

I am loyal to my physician-employer.

I am true to the ethics of my profession.

I am strengthened by compassion, courage and faith.

FIGURE 3-4   AAMA Code of Ethics. (Copyright by the American Association of Medical Assistants, Inc. Revised December 1992. Reprinted with permission.)

technology, demographics, ethics, and other related issues. In Hindu societies, for instance, women are required to cover their faces and assume a secondary role, whereas women in the United States play prominent roles in all spheres, with laws protecting their equal status and treatment. Each society must develop its own social policy from the values, customs, and constraints of its circumstances.

Some of the most difficult social policy issues in the United States concern medical ethics. To illustrate, consider these questions: Is artificial insemination by an anonymous donor ethical? Is releasing medical information about some patients ethical, for example, patients who have AIDS and may have infected others in the community? Are prescribing birth control devices for teenagers or performing abortions without their parents' permission ethical decisions for a physician? The answers to these questions are complex and cannot be answered simply. Leaders of the medical profession refer to the ethics codes of their profession, legal statutes, and historical precedents as they try to set guidelines for the future.

In 1984, the Judicial Council of the American Medical Association published an interpretation of the AMA Principles of Medical Ethics called *Current Opinions of the Judicial Council of the American Medical Association.* Revised periodically to address current thinking or new issues, *Current Opinions* provides direction for physicians about responsible professional behavior. Although *Current Opinions* is not the only guide to ethical professional behavior, it provides a basis for understanding what is considered ethical and unethical in our society. Individual physicians' opinions about social issues may differ from those expressed in *Current Opinions* and are explored in the next section.

ABORTION

Today the term **abortion** is commonly used to mean **induced** abortion, the intentional and deliberate ending of a pregnancy. Actually, abortion may be spontaneous or nondeliberate and result from natural causes. The term is properly used to describe any termination of pregnancy during the first three months. Whether induced or spontaneous, abortion results in the death of the embryo or fetus.

Abortion is a controversial subject. Churches have spoken out on this issue; many women's rights groups have taken a strong position in favor of abortion; and others concerned with the moral questions surrounding abortion have debated the issue both publicly and privately. The controversy involves two important questions: (1) Should a woman be permitted to have an abortion by law and under what circumstances? (2) To what extent should the law protect the unborn child's right to life?

The term **pro-choice** describes the position of a person who thinks that abortion is proper under some circumstances and that it should be a matter of personal choice. Pro-choice advocates believe that abortion is acceptable if a woman's life or health will be endangered by pregnancy or if there is evidence that the child will be born with a serious mental or physical defect. They also approve of abortion when pregnancy results from rape.

The terms **pro-life** and anti-abortion describe the position of a person who thinks that abortion is always wrong. Groups who are anti-abortion believe that abortion is an unjustified killing of an unborn child, based on the idea that life begins when sperm fertilizes an egg. They argue that legal abortion will increase the incidence of irresponsible sex and lead to disrespect for human life. Anti-abortion activists often picket abortion clinics and are seen on the news for their activities. Physicians and their staffs have been wounded and even murdered by individuals opposed to abortion.

In 1973 the United States Supreme Court legalized abortion performed during the first three months of pregnancy. Provision was made for individual states to regulate abortion to protect the mother's health after the first three months. Physicians are not prohibited from performing an abortion in accordance with good medical practice and under circumstances that do not violate the law. Although you as a medical assistant will not be directly involved in decisions involving abortions for patients, you should be aware of the stress and concern faced by patients and physicians, especially if you work for an obstetrician/gynecologist or a surgeon. You should be supportive, understanding, nonjudgmental, and noncritical of their decisions.

ABUSE OF CHILDREN, ELDERLY PERSONS, AND OTHERS AT RISK

Physicians *are required by law* to report suspected cases of child abuse and abuse of elderly persons or others. This may represent a dilemma for the doctor because the abused person may deny being harmed in order to protect the abuser. Fearful of losing their parents, children may say their injuries came from a fall or another accident, and, afraid of the repercussions if they confide in the physician, elderly people may deny that their injuries were inflicted by someone else.

The incidence of physical violence is increasing, with many cases going unreported. The law clearly says that suspected cases of abuse must be reported, obligating the physician and medical staff to protect the patient even though the patient may not wish to cooperate.

ALLOCATION OF HEALTH RESOURCES

The health care environment is constantly changing because of the introduction of new technologies and treatments. A few years ago, individuals with rare heart, lung, or liver disorders were poor candidates for transplant surgery. Now, new anti-rejection drugs make transplants a more feasible option.

Because a shortage of donor organs exists, the decision to allocate limited health care resources must be made fairly. According to *Current Opinions*, limited health care resources should be given to patients who are most likely to be treated successfully or who will have long-term benefits. A patient's social worth or relative worth to society should not determine whether the patient is denied or given preference in receiving scarce health care treatment or resources.

Although regional and state organ banks have protocols to determine who is next in line for available organs, controversy still occurs. In 1993, Pennsylvania's Governor Robert Casey received a heart–liver transplant after being on a waiting list for less than twenty-four hours. Many people, including other potential transplant patients who had been waiting for over a year, questioned whether priority treatment had been given to the governor. The medical center that performed the transplant said no priority was accorded the governor, indicating that Casey's was the first name on a special list for *dual organ* transplant patients. Dual organ transplants routinely were performed before single organ transplants at this facility.

The question of rationing health care based on age or overwhelming odds against survival surfaces in such diverse cases as Baby Faye, an infant who received a baboon's heart transplant, and Mrs. Helga Wanglie, an elderly woman with irreversible brain damage. Baby Faye did not live, and Mrs. Wanglie was hospitalized for two years at a cost of $800,000, when the hospital filed suit to terminate her care. As technology continues to advance and the elderly population of the United States grows, physicians are faced with many legal and ethical questions regarding the allocation of resources and the division of responsibility among individuals, medical institutions, and the government (Figure 3-5).

ARTIFICIAL INSEMINATION AND ARTIFICIAL INSEMINATION BY DONOR

Artificial insemination is a procedure whereby a physician takes live sperm from a husband or donor and places it by syringe injection at the entrance to the cervix of a woman's uterus. In the case of husband and wife, the informed consent of both parties is necessary. The physician should inform both parents that any child conceived by artificial insemination has the same rights as a child conceived naturally.

Artificial insemination by donor is a far more controversial issue. Since the recipient is usually not provided with the donor's identity, the physician has a responsibility to use the most sophisticated tests available in screening and selecting donors and recipients. Otherwise, the risk of a poor match exists, with undesirable genetic and biological consequences. In addition, a physician has an ethical responsibility to avoid the frequent use of semen from the same sources.

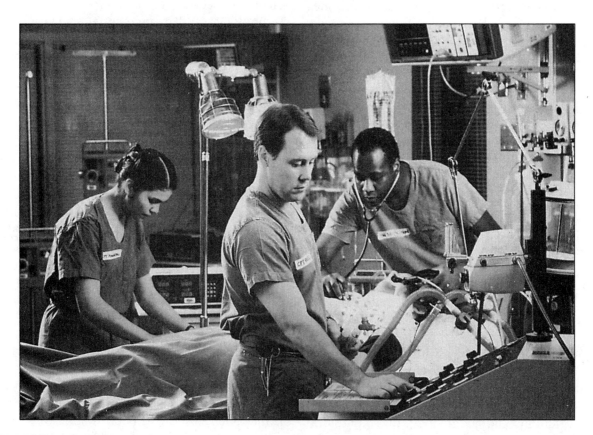

FIGURE 3-5 Because health care resources are limited, ethical questions arise as to who should receive these resources. (*"Be All You Can Be"* Courtesy U.S. Government, as represented by the Secretary of the Army)

Surrogate motherhood is a form of artificial insemination that has received a great deal of publicity. In surrogate motherhood, the father's semen is artificially inseminated into a female who has signed a contract with the father to bear a child. The surrogate mother agrees that, if she is impregnated, she will give the child to the father. Sometimes the surrogate mother is paid a fee for her services.

Both ethical and legal questions have arisen over the issue of surrogate motherhood. Is selling babies ethical? Will the contract stand if the mother decides she does not want to give up the baby? In a custody battle between a father and surrogate mother, what are the baby's rights? In the 1987 New Jersey "Baby M" case, Stern vs. Whitehead, the judge decided that the baby should remain with the father and his wife rather than with Whitehead, the surrogate mother. In early 1988 the New Jersey Supreme Court ruled that surrogate motherhood is now illegal in that state. However, it also allowed Whitehead visitation rights.

Although artificial insemination offers parents who cannot conceive the opportunity to have a child, many people feel that adoption is preferable. They argue that as long as large numbers of unwanted and uncared for children are available, bringing additional children into the world through expensive and artificial means is irresponsible.

IN VITRO FERTILIZATION

In vitro fertilization, or fertilization "in glass," is a recent scientific development in which an egg and sperm unite in an artificial environment outside the woman's body. The embryo is then transferred to the mother's reproductive system to develop normally. In vitro fertilization allows couples to conceive and bear a child even though they have previously been unable to do so. The few children conceived to date in vitro are sometimes called "test tube babies."

Ethical issues surround in vitro fertilization. For example, in 1991, Mrs. Arlette Schweitzer gave birth to twins fertilized in vitro with her daughter's eggs and her son-in-law's sperm. The daughter had been born without a uterus, and the mother volunteered to carry her daughter's

babies to birth. The physician who participates in this method of reproduction is bound by the highest ethical standards and must follow the Principles of Medical Ethics strictly.

CAPITAL PUNISHMENT

A physician may have an opinion as an individual about whether capital punishment is right or wrong. However, as a member of a profession dedicated to preserving life, a physician should not participate in an execution although it may be legally authorized by the court system.

CLINICAL INVESTIGATION

New medical procedures and drugs for treating disease are introduced only after many years of clinical research and experimentation on animals. After a procedure or drug is deemed safe for humans, the Federal Food and Drug Administration may approve clinical investigation and experimentation of these procedures or drugs on people. With the hope of controlling the AIDS epidemic, many new drugs and treatment protocols have been approved more rapidly than usual.

A physician may participate in clinical investigation and experimentation only if the study is scientifically valid. The physician has a responsibility to keep the patient's interests above the need for research and must not perform any procedures without the consent of the patient or the patient's representative. Participation is considered coercive and involuntary if the participant is pressured into the activity.

FETAL RESEARCH GUIDELINES

Research on fetuses is acceptable when the research is part of a valid scientific study, when it has been preceded by research on animals, and when it involves no monetary payment for fetal material. While President George Bush was in office, a limited ban was placed on fetal research, but the ban was lifted shortly after President Bill Clinton took office. The issue of using fetal tissue is often clouded by the abortion issue, rather than viewed as a separate concern. Fetal research has received a great deal of attention in recent years due to the development of a treatment for Parkinson's disease that requires fetal tissue. The physician should demonstrate the same degree of care for the fetus in research as for any other fetus in a nonresearch setting. This includes arranging for the proper consent of the mother or the fetus's representative. In treating a fetus, the physician must use the simplest and safest treatment.

GENETIC COUNSELING AND GENETIC ENGINEERING

Genetics is the study of genes and their role in illness and disease. Over 2,000 genetically related disorders have been identified, including Down syndrome, sickle cell anemia, and multiple sclerosis. Researchers at the National Institutes of Health are currently participating in a worldwide study to map genes. Mapping will assist researchers in determining which specific gene is missing or damaged in certain diseases and disorders.

Genetic Counseling

Prospective parents may request screening before conception to predict the likelihood of bearing a child with a gene disorder. After conception, **in utero** gene testing is performed on the fetus through ultrasound, amniocentesis, and fetoscopy to determine the fetus's condition.

Genetic counseling is available to individuals who may be at risk of having certain illnesses or diseases. In March 1993, Dr. Nancy Wexler, a Columbia University researcher, successfully located the gene that causes Huntington's disease. Wexler's efforts started in 1968, when her mother was diagnosed with Huntington's disease. Wexler learned she had a 50 percent chance of inheriting the illness, which leads to severe brain damage and death. Due largely to Wexler's global research effort, tests are now available to determine whether or not individuals carry the disease.

Physicians engaged in genetic counseling have an ethical responsibility to provide parents with complete information for making a decision about childbearing. This presents a dilemma for physicians who oppose contraception, sterilization, or abortion, since the parents faced with a genetic defect in the fetus may request an abortion based on their own beliefs. In such cases, the physicians may decide to refer the parents to another doctor.

Genetic Engineering

Genetic engineering, or altering of genes, is one of the most advanced, complex, and controversial of all contemporary social issues. In genetic engineering, a gene is isolated and replaced, or its components are rearranged to form a mutant gene that may reduce or eliminate the chances of a person's developing a particular disease. Currently, for example, researchers are trying to isolate a gene that appears in people with Alzheimer disease, which affects approximately 2.5 million people in the United States. If this gene can be identified, it may help scientists find a cure for this disease.

Scientists have found the approximate location of this gene. They have also mapped the approximate location of the genes responsible for manic depression, which afflicts two million Americans; neurofibromatosis, or elephant man's disease, which affects 100,000; and cystic fibrosis, the most common genetic killer of young people, which afflicts 30,000. Other diseases, such as heart disease, arteriosclerosis, diabetes, and cancer, which are strongly influenced by hereditary or genetic factors, are drawing attention, and many of the mysteries surrounding these diseases will surely be illuminated through genetic study during the next several years.

One of the most exciting breakthroughs came in July, 1987, when scientists finally identified the gene responsible for muscular dystrophy, which affects 50,000 Americans. After the initial discovery, it took only nine months, until March, 1988, for scientists to discover the protein missing in Duchenne, the most common childhood dystrophy. Following these discoveries, there is hope that muscular dystrophy patients will be cured in the future. For the present, the rate of deterioration caused by the disease will be slowed. During the 1970s, researchers were able to engineer bacteria that produced small quantities of human insulin, a hormone used to treat diabetes, and human interferon, a protein that fights viral infections. If researchers can produce hormones and proteins in large quantities, they may provide an inexpensive means of treatment for these diseases.

If and when genetic engineering allows gene replacement to treat human disorders, physicians must make certain that Judicial Council guidelines on clinical investigation are followed, along with the usual and customary standards of medical practice. The full procedure should be discussed with the patient and written consent obtained. The procedure must be in conformance with other standards outlined in the Judicial Council.

ORGAN TRANSPLANTATION GUIDELINES

Transplants of the heart, lungs, kidney, and liver offer patients with organ disorders a chance at life that was not possible only a few years ago. Yet in any organ transplant procedure, the physician must protect the rights of both the donor and the recipient. This means disclosing all known risks and possible hazards to both parties. The physician's interest in advancing scientific knowledge must always be secondary to his or her concern for the patient. A transplant should be performed only if other therapy has been ineffective. When a vital organ is transplanted, the donor's death must be certified by a physician other than the recipient's physician. Because few organs are available and the waiting list is long, tissue matches may identify several patients who are eligible for a transplant. Ethical guidelines with clear priority standards must be established.

QUALITY OF LIFE

The physician's primary responsibility always is to do what is best for the patient. Therefore, quality of life becomes an important factor in determining the treatment for seriously deformed newborns, critically injured accident victims, and patients suffering from terminal illnesses. If prolonging life would result in inhumane or unconscionable treatment, withholding or removing life support systems is ethical. Normal care of the patient should be continued after removing life support systems.

Withholding treatment is such a controversial social issue that physicians and hospitals are reluctant sometimes to remove life support sys-

tems. Faced with the threat of a medical malpractice lawsuit, a hospital or physician may take a less controversial course and continue extraordinary treatment although the patient is living in a vegetative state. In recent years, families of permanently comatose patients have gone to court to force hospitals or physicians to withhold treatment. These cases usually take years to settle in court and cost the family a great deal in legal fees and personal agony. Even so, the outcome may be to continue treatment.

One such case in Massachusetts was Brophy vs. New England Sinai Hospital. The patient, Brophy, who was in an irreversible coma after suffering an aneurysm remained alive only because a feeding tube was surgically implanted in his stomach. The family asked the hospital to remove the tube and let Brophy die; however, the hospital refused, even though the court ruled that this was acceptable procedure. The court acknowledged the hospital's right and allowed the family to move the patient to another facility that eventually granted the family's request.

Society seems to have grown more comfortable with allowing terminally ill patients to die. In March 1986, the AMA stated that discontinuing or withholding life-prolonging medical treatment, including food and water, for the terminally ill is not unethical (Figure 3-6). In June 1987, the New Jersey Supreme Court made three landmark decisions that allowed patients who were in a near-vegetative state to refuse life-sustaining medical treatment, even though they were neither terminally ill nor elderly. In each case, the patient's request to be allowed to die was granted. State laws vary on providing nutrition to a comatose patient, therefore, court rulings in one state may not apply in other states.

TERMINAL ILLNESS

Physicians are bound to prolong life and relieve suffering. When one conflicts with the other, the physician, patient, and family together may resolve the matter. The physician may not intentionally cause death; but with informed consent, the physician may cause or omit treatment to allow a terminally ill patient to die. Do Not

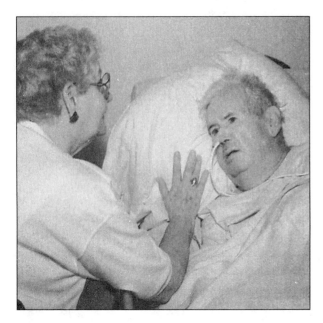

FIGURE 3-6 The issue of quality of life is an important factor in determining treatment for a critically ill or injured person. (From Hegner and Caldwell, *Nursing Assistant,* 7th ed., copyright 1995, Delmar Publishers)

Resuscitate (DNR) orders are common in facilities that treat elderly patients. These orders clearly state that when the lungs or heart stop the patient will not be subjected to an aggressive attempt to restart them. No matter what the age of the patient, the physician is ethically bound to alleviate severe pain for the comfort of the patient. In the past few years, a few doctors have gained notoriety by assisting in suicides of terminally ill patients. This type of assistance is viewed as unethical by most medical professionals, although assisted suicide has been decriminalized in the Netherlands.

HIV TESTING

The threat of AIDS has resulted in a requirement that individuals be tested for the human immunodeficiency virus (HIV) before joining the military and as a prerequisite for some jobs. Physicians must ensure that HIV testing is conducted in a way that respects the patient's rights and ensures patient confidentiality. Therefore, they should secure the patient's informed consent before testing for HIV. Because of the need for pretest counseling and the potential consequences of an HIV test on an individual's job,

housing, insurability, and social relationships, the consent should be specific for HIV testing. In addition to protecting patients' rights, health care workers also have the responsibility of self-protection. It is recommended that universal precautions and body fluid precautions be used for all patients, especially when the infection status of the patient is unknown.

DRUG AND SUBSTANCE ABUSE

Drug abuse is one of the major factors in the rise in health care costs because physicians and hospitals must provide long-term care not only to drug addicts, but also to those injured during drug-related crime, the battered spouses of addicts, and babies born to drug-addicted mothers. Drug users are also susceptible to many serious infections, including hepatitis and HIV. Often, other complications develop, requiring surgery. Although drug users are more likely to be infected with HIV and to place the surgical team at great risk, it is considered unethical to deny treatment to a known drug user. In some states, however, denial of treatment may not be illegal.

Physicians are required to follow established standards and should not be influenced by financial considerations in prescribing drugs. Although doctors may dispense drugs from their offices, patients have the right to obtain and fill prescriptions wherever they wish. Physicians must be alert, however, to the patient who is attempting to obtain legal drugs for resale, or other illegal use.

As physicians and their staffs have access to drug and prescription forms, care must be exercised to prevent abuse within the office. Proper inventory control is important in preventing improper usage. Physicians, because of their easy access, are in a tempting position to abuse drugs. Physicians cannot ethically or legally practice medicine while under the influence of a controlled substance, alcohol, or other chemical agent. If, as a medical assistant, you become aware of a substance abuse problem in your office, you must bring the problem to the attention of your employer. If your employer is the abuser, seek advice from an individual whose judgment you respect on how to report the abuse. Many local or state medical societies have resources to assist an impaired physician in receiving help to overcome a substance abuse problem.

COSTS

Concern for the patient's care should be the physician's primary consideration, with cost of treatment being a secondary consideration. Nevertheless, the physician may participate in policy-making decisions concerning health care costs, either as a member of a professional group or as a private citizen. Health care reforms are being discussed widely by physicians who anticipate that their incomes will be affected.

UNNECESSARY SERVICES AND WORTHLESS SERVICES

Physicians cannot ethically provide or prescribe unnecessary services or treatments in unnecessary facilities. The physician is compelled to ask privately: "Is this additional diagnostic test (which adds to my practice's income) necessary for my patient's treatment?" "Does this patient really need to be rechecked in two weeks (when I will receive an additional fee)?" "Should I transfer this patient to the nursing home (which I partially own) or is treatment at home sufficient?" Furthermore, a physician should not provide services that reputable physicians would regard as worthless. These services might include knee surgery for a patient whose knee will heal if left alone or eye surgery for a patient who has no hope of recovering sight.

As a medical assistant, usually you will not have the medical background or knowledge to determine when a physician is supplying unnecessary or worthless services. However, if clear-cut patterns of unethical service exist, you probably can detect them. For example, the physician who routinely sends patients for a second opinion to a relative who is also a physician may be crossing the boundaries of ethical behavior. A physician who recalls patients several times for minor medical problems may be increasing the practice's income at the patients' expense.

Providing unnecessary services is not only unethical but also may be illegal. The federal government is concerned about the amount of fraud and abuse in the health care system. According to a General Accounting Office report, fraud and abuse account for over $10 billion a year. Under the False Claims Act, it is illegal to bill for services not provided, overbill for the care provided, or bill for "assembly line" care, such as performing a urinalysis for every patient. Under the anti-kickback statute, physicians cannot legally receive any type of payment, in cash or in kind, for the referral of a patient. In the past, the physician usually was the only person held responsible for fraud or abuse. Today, the medical assistant who knowingly and willingly participates in providing unnecessary services is also at risk to be prosecuted.

IN YOUR OPINION

1. After freezing the husband's sperm, a couple decides to divorce. The wife sues to maintain the sperm, as she would like to become pregnant in the future. The husband countersues to destroy the sperm, citing legal and financial obligations. Who do you think is right? Why?
2. A wealthy person creates an infomercial for cable TV to plead for a liver transplant for his small son. Parents in another city offer to donate the liver of their child who has been killed in an automobile accident. Should the child of the wealthy parents receive the liver ahead of other children who may need it more?
3. Under what circumstances do you think patients should be tested for HIV?

Computers and Ethics

Computer technologies allow medical information to be accumulated in large quantities and retrieved quickly; however, the potential for access to patient information is greater with a computerized system than with traditional paper systems. Protection of patient confidentiality is a concern as computers proliferate in medical offices and other health care facilities (Figure 3-7).

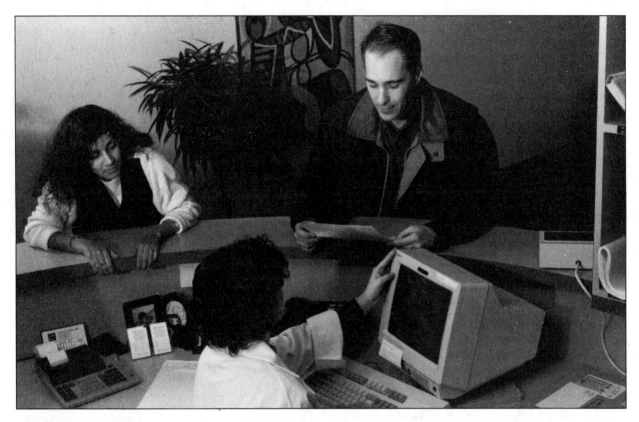

FIGURE 3-7 Unless medical records are kept secure, computer technology can pose a real threat to patient confidentiality.

CONFIDENTIALITY AND COMPUTERS

Although computer technology represents outstanding opportunities for efficiency and record keeping, it poses a threat to patient confidentiality unless medical records are properly secured. Computer "hackers," or people with the ability to break into a computer's files from a remote location, have invaded the central storage of some of the country's most sophisticated computer installations. Although many of these hackers are amateurs testing their ability to break into a computer's code, their activities are illegal and should be reported when discovered. When a hospital computer is invaded and the hacker looks at medical records, patient privacy is violated. Because medical records show personal as well as medical information, a hacker can gain a variety of confidential information. This kind of crime is not yet widespread; however, computer piracy offers some fairly dramatic opportunities for the hacker with a vivid imagination. Consider the criminal who wishes to use negative or potentially injurious medical information to bribe a judge undergoing treat-

ment for alcoholism or to bribe a political candidate who had psychiatric treatment in the past.

If you are working in a large computer center and you discover suspicious activity within patient records or accounts, you must report your suspicions immediately to the person in authority. After you have worked in a medical facility for several months, you will learn the charges for certain procedures and treatments. An account that has been changed to reflect lower charges will catch your attention and should be reported. For example, several incorrect charges in the same patient's account over a period of time should raise your suspicions. On a simpler note, patient confidentiality is threatened when a medical secretary leaves the desk but allows the computer screen to remain visible to patients or office visitors.

AMA POSITION ON COMPUTER SECURITY

The AMA has adopted guidelines for patient records in computer databases. Although these guidelines focus on computer services, many are relevant for private practices as well. AMA guidelines are given in Figure 3-8.

The Medical Assistant's Role in Ethical Issues

Medical assistants who suspect a physician of unethical behavior face a difficult dilemma. To accuse the physician will almost certainly result job termination, and the accusation may be inappropriate and unfair, especially if it is based on a difference in philosophy of what is ethical. After you begin work as a medical assistant you should not make negative statements about a physician's ethics unless you have verifiable evidence of unethical behavior. If you and the physician disagree on what is ethical, you should look for employment with another practice. If, however, you possess information that conclusively shows unethical behavior, you should report your concerns to another physician who knows the local customs for policing physicians' ethics. Because you can destroy the reputation of a physician by assuming knowledge you do not have or interpreting medical situations incorrectly, you should allow another professional with the appropriate medical background to pursue the matter.

You will also be faced with ethical issues not directly related to the social issues discussed in this chapter. For example, physicians often charge patients for long-distance telephone calls related to a case, such as a consultation with a physician in another city or a return call to a patient who is out of town. You must make sure that nonpatient-related long-distance calls are not charged to patient accounts.

Physicians' fees represent another ethical area involving the medical assistant. Most physicians charge for office visits based on the amount of time spent with the patient. Some physicians identify the type of visit on the patient's charge slip, but others expect the medical assistant to complete this information based on the reason for the visit and the medical assistant's knowledge of the physician's procedures. You may face ethical dilemmas from time to time about the correct charge. If so, make sure that both the patient and the practice are treated fairly.

Ethical issues that are harder to describe but just as important to the medical assistant involve sensitivity to people's feelings. Courteous behavior toward elderly, handicapped, or anxious patients; honesty with other staff members; respect for patients' privacy when undressing; and related issues occur almost daily. No one can tell you how to act in each situation; however, your personal sense of ethics and service to your profession can help you act responsibly. A medical assistant's ethics must be impeccable because nothing can destroy a career faster than the appearance of unethical behavior.

REFERENCES

American Association of Medical Assistants Bylaws. Chicago: American Association of Medical Assistants.

American Association for Medical Transcription Bylaws. Modesto, California: American Association for Medical Transcription.

Current Opinions of the Judicial Council of the American Medical Association. Chicago: American Medical Association, 1992.

DeBlakey, Michael, Dr., "The Era of the Gene Points the Way to Treatment, Even Cures," *Parade Magazine,* September 5, 1993.

Derricks, Joette P. "Claim Review and the Audit Process," Pennsylvania Medical Assistants Association, October, 1993.

Dubler, Nancy, and David Nimmons. *Ethics on Call,* Harmony Books, 1992.

Flight, Myrtle R. "Medical Ethics—Reach Out and Touch Everyone." *The Professional Office Assistant.* November/December 1987, pp. 20–24.

Humphrey, Doris, and Kathie Sigler. *The Modern Medical Office: A Reference Manual.* Cincinnati, Ohio: South-Western Publishing Co., 1990.*

"In Genetics, Hope for Muscular Dystrophy—and More." *The Philadelphia Inquirer,* March 20, 1988, p. IA.

Kempler, Vickie and Peter Montgomery, "Milking Medicare," *Common Cause Magazine,* January/February, 1991.

A Patient's Bill of Rights. Chicago, Illinois: American Hospital Association, 1992.

Schmitt, Richard B., "It Can Pay to Be Whistle-Blower in Health Fraud," *The Wall Street Journal,* September 2, 1993.

"The Twins and Choices in Revising Health Care," *The Philadelphia Inquirer,* August 29, 1993.

"Wexler Receives Award," *The Associated Press,* September 30, 1993.

*Currently published by Delmar Publishers.

Confidentiality: Computers.

The utmost effort and care must be taken to protect the confidentiality of all medical records. This ethical principle applies to computerized medical records as it applies to any other medical records.

The confidentiality of physician–patient communications is desirable to assure free and open disclosure by the patient to the physician of all information needed to establish a proper diagnosis and attain the most desirable clinical outcome possible. Protecting the confidentiality of the personal and medical information in such medical records is also necessary to prevent humiliation, embarrassment, or discomfort of patients. At the same time, patients may have legitimate desires to have medical information concerning their care and treatment forwarded others.

Both the protection of confidentiality and the appropriate release of information in records is the rightful expectation of the patient. A physician should respect the patient's expectations of confidentiality concerning medical records that involve the patient's care and treatment, but the physician should also respect the patient's authorization to provide information from the medical record to those whom the patient authorizes to inspect all or part of it for legitimate purposes.

Computer technology permits the accumulation, storage, and analysis of an unlimited quantum of medical information. The possibility of access to information is greater with a computerized data system than with information stored in the traditional written form in a physician's office. Accordingly, the guidelines below are offered to assist physicians and computer service organizations in maintaining the confidentiality of information in medical records when that information is stored in computerized data bases. It should be recognized that specific procedures adapted from application of these concepts may vary depending upon the nature of the organization processing the data as well as the appropriate and authorized use of the stored data.

Guidelines on a computerized data base:

(1) Confidential medical information entered into the computerized data base should be verified as to authenticity of source.

(2) The patient and physician should be advised about the existence of computerized data bases in which medical information concerning the patient is stored. Such information should be communicated to the physician and patient prior the physician's release of the medical information. All individuals and organizations with some form of access to the computerized data bank, and the level of access permitted, should be specifically identified in advance.

(3) The physician and patient should be notified of the distribution of all reports reflecting identifiable patient data prior to distribution of the reports by the computer facility. There should be approval by the physician and patient prior to the release of patient-identifiable clinical and administrative data to individuals or organizations external to the medical care environment, and such information should not be released without the express permission of the physician and the patient.

(4) The dissemination of confidential medical data should be limited to only those individuals or agencies with a bona fide use for the data. Release of confidential medical information from the data base should be confined to the specific purpose for which the information is requested and limited to the specific time frame requested. All such organizations or individuals should be advised that authorized release of data to them does not authorize their further release of the data to additional individuals or organizations.

(5) Procedures for adding to or changing data on the computerized data base should indicate individuals authorized to make changes, time periods in which changes take place, and those individuals who will be informed about changes in the data from the medical records.

(6) Procedures for purging the computerized data base or archaic or inaccurate data should be established and the patient and physician should be notified before and after the data has been purged. There should be no commingling of a physician's computerized patient records with those of other computer service bureau clients. In addition, procedures should be developed to protect against inadvertent mixing of individual reports or segments thereof.

(7) The computerized medical data base should be on-line to the computer terminal only when authorized computer programs requiring the medical data are being used. Individuals and organizations external to the clinical facility should not be provided on-line access to a computerized data base containing identifiable data from medical records concerning patients.

(8) Security:

A. Stringent security procedures for entry into the immediate environment in which the computerized medical data base is stored and/or processed or for otherwise having access to confidential medical information should be developed and strictly enforced so as to prevent access to the computer facility by unauthorized personnel. Personnel audit procedures should be developed to establish a record in the event of unauthorized disclosure of medical data. A roster of past and present service bureau personnel with specified levels of access to the medical data base should be maintained. Specific administrative sanctions should exist to prevent employee breaches of confidentiality and security procedures.

B. All terminated or former employees in the data processing environment should have no access to data from the medical records concerning patients.

C. Involuntarily terminated employees working in the data processing environment in which data from medical records concerning patients are processed should immediately upon termination be removed from the computerized medical environment.

D. Upon termination of computer service bureau services for a physician, those computer files maintained for the physician should be physically turned over to the physician, or destroyed (erased). In the event of file erasure, the computer service bureau should verify in writing that the erasure has taken place. (IV)

FIGURE 3-8 AMA position on computer security. (Reprinted with permission from *Code of Medial Ethics: Current Opinions of the Council on Ethical and Judicial Affairs* of the American Medical Association, copyright 1992.)

Chapter Activities

PERFORMANCE BASED ACTIVITIES

1. Choose a social policy issue you believe will probably become more important in the future. Debate the issue with another member of the class. Name the point of view you will debate, either pro or con, and list in the chart below the points you will make.

Ethical Issues Debate

Position Statement
"I believe…

Points To Be Made
"Why…

1. _____
2. _____
3. _____
4. _____
5. _____
6. _____

(DACUM 1.8, 5.7)

2. Study a report on genetic engineering research from a general news periodical published within the last two years. Summarize the research and discuss the social, ethical, and medical implications.

Genetic Engineering Research

Name of Report _____

Publication_____ Date_____ Page_____

Research Summary

Implications

Social

Ethical

Medical

(DACUM 1.2, 1.3, 2.7)

3. Develop a plan to protect the confidentiality of patient records in a medical office that has just purchased a computer. Call two experienced medical assistants who handle computerized records for their office. Use their advice plus your own recommendations to create a chart showing what will be done and who will be responsible for each phase:

Computer Security

Methods for Protecting Confidentiality

Method   *Responsible Person*

_____

_____

_____

_____

_____

(DACUM 1.4, 1.7, 3.3, 5.1)

4. Develop an ethical situation in which a medical assistant might become involved, and role-play the scene with another class member. (DACUM 1.1, 1.5)

EXPANDING YOUR THINKING

1. In what situations do you think violating patient confidentiality is the ethical choice?

2. In a recent New Jersey case, a prison psychiatrist informed the police chief of a parolee's home town that she thought the parolee represented a danger to society. Do you agree with this action? Why or why not?

3. In what ways might your professional ethics conflict with your personal beliefs?

4. A member of the medical staff is an avid gambler and has been known to incur large gambling debts. In what ways might this situation create a professional dilemma?

5. A neighbor of yours is a patient of your practice. A mutual friend has noticed that this person has recently lost a great deal of weight and asks you if this person has AIDS. What do you reply?

Chapter 4

Medical Law

BIRMINGHAM, ALABAMA

Ten years ago, it was much simpler for a physician to practice medicine. Every time I open the mail these days it seems I get something about a change in the laws or about medical malpractice. No wonder Dr. London continues to send me to conferences on legal issues in the medical office. He can't practice medicine and keep up with all the legal questions, too.

My job has become more complex because of the records required to keep a doctor out of court. The trust between physician and patient just isn't as strong as it used to be. Patients are more likely to blame the doctor when they experience complications and sue when they aren't satisfied. I guess it's because we live in such a mobile society. People don't form the close relationships with their physicians that were so common in the past.

Now, I make sure patients sign a consent form for every procedure. I also double-check all licensing requirements and renewal dates for Dr. London and the nurses. Beyond that, I check insurance forms for the patient's permission to release information and prepare physician-withdrawal letters the minute Dr. London tells me he is withdrawing from a patient's case. Handling all this preventive paperwork takes a lot of time, but it's necessary if we are to reduce legal claims against the doctor and the practice.

Last year I got a real scare! A legal summons was hand delivered to me for the doctor about

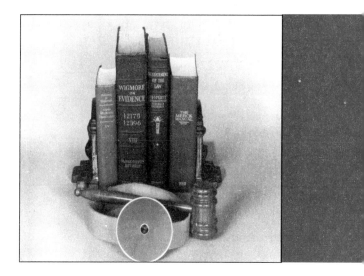

the same time an emergency patient appeared. I took the papers, laid them on my desk, and, though I'm embarrassed to admit it, they were misplaced during the crisis. I had to call Dr. London's attorney, who traced them back to the local court. Dr. London had been issued a summons in a malpractice suit; and if he had not answered the summons by the required date, he would have been held in default. I've learned that I just cannot ignore anything having to do with the legal system. It's too important to a physician and the medical practice.

Basil Ohlsen
Medical Office Manager

After completing this chapter, you should be able to:

1. Determine needs for documentation and report and document accurately. (DACUM 5.1, 5.2)
2. Advise patients on their rights regarding advance directives. (DACUM 5.2, 5.3)
3. Trace a malpractice claim from its inception through settlement or trial. (DACUM 5.1, 5.4, 5.7)
4. Use appropriate guidelines when releasing records or information. (DACUM 5.3)
5. Follow policy in disposing of controlled substances. (DACUM 5.5)
6. Use appropriate guidelines in terminating medical treatment by means of a withdrawal letter. (DACUM 5.4)

HEALTHSPEAK

Advance directives Patient's wishes regarding future treatment if the patient is incapacitated.

Civil law Rights and obligations that people have toward one another, usually concerned with a wrong or injury one person inflicts upon another.

Criminal law Rights and obligations people have toward society.

Drug schedules Categories of drugs divided according to their potential for abuse.

Good Samaritan laws Laws that protect the physician and other health care professionals who assist people in unusual emergency situations.

Informed consent Law that states a patient must be given medical information about risk before undergoing a procedure.

Medical law is becoming increasingly complicated and controversial as technology advances. Physicians today can offer treatments that only five years ago were considered impossible. We learn of organ transplants, experimental drugs, and newly developed medical procedures almost daily. But, because all medical breakthroughs are not in humanity's best interests, standards of acceptable practice must be established and legally enforced to protect patients. Genetic engineering, for example, is considered by many experts to be a positive step toward finding cures for many diseases; in the

wrong hands, however, gene mutations could cause great damage to the human race. As evidence of this, during World War II Adolf Hitler tried to create a super race of people through genetic engineering. Fortunately, Nazi scientists did not have the ability to design their perfect human being, nor do we have this capability today. Researchers can, however, alter a gene's characteristics. Therefore, we need laws to control potentially dangerous genetic engineering experimentation. We also need laws to protect us from negligent or unscrupulous physicians.

State Medical Practice Acts

Medicine, nursing, dentistry, and other professional health care occupations are regulated by laws in the fifty states. These laws, known collectively as the Medical Practice Acts, specify the training, set standards of competence, identify the tasks, and stipulate the category of patients that doctors, nurses, and others may treat. Licensure, license renewal, and license revocation or suspension are also established by the states. Because each state sets its own laws, the standards vary from state to state. As a medical assistant, you need to know about the laws of the state in which your practice is located, so you can coordinate the license renewals for the professionals with whom you work. For example, if you previously worked as a medical assistant in California and then moved to Iowa, you cannot assume that licensing requirements for physicians are the same in both states. Your employer will rely on you to be knowledgeable about the laws of your state.

LICENSURE

Physicians, nurses, dentists, pharmacists, and certain other health care professionals must be licensed to practice their professions (Figure 4-1). Two primary reasons exist for licensing: (1) to protect the public, and (2) to protect the profession. A license means that the practitioner has met some minimum standard and is qualified and capable of providing medical service to the public. Bogus or phony physicians are uncommon; however, occasionally we hear stories about physicians who have continued to

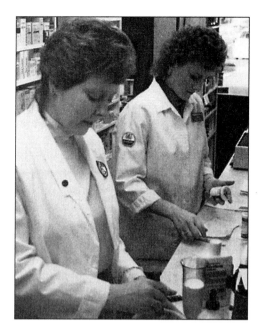

FIGURE 4-1 Pharmacists are among the health care professionals who must be licensed to practice their profession. (Courtesy of the Michigan Pharmacists Association and the Michigan Society of Pharmacy Technicians)

practice medicine after losing their licenses. When these people are caught, they are charged with a crime and are usually fined and jailed. Reputable physicians usually frame their licenses and display them prominently in their offices.

Because licensing is a matter of state law, requirements are not uniform across the country. However, typical requirements for physicians include graduation from an accredited medical school, completed residency, good moral character, and successful completion of the Federal Licensing Examination. Each state's medical board sets licensing requirements, approves and administers the written examination, and issues licenses to physicians, nurses, dentists, pharmacists, and others specified by the board. To practice in another state, a medical practitioner must meet its requirements and be granted a license. Reciprocity agreements between states with the same licensing requirements allow licenses to be granted to residents who move from one state to the other. Licensing is not required for medical assistants.

Medical practitioners who work for a federal government medical unit are not required to obtain a license from the state in which they practice. For example, an Army, Navy, or Air Force physician who practices in many different states during the course of a military career does not need a license from each state. Nor is a license required for a research physician who does not practice medicine.

RENEWAL OF LICENSE

Periodic renewal of a practitioner's license is required by all states. For physicians, successfully completing a minimum amount of continuing education is necessary before a license can be renewed. Continuing education requirements may be met through course work, professional reading, teaching, and self-instruction.

A physician may ask the medical assistant to maintain a file that documents the necessary professional activity for license renewal. This continuing education file should be current and well organized. If this is your responsibility as a medical assistant, you should be sure that all certificates, receipts, and other documents related to professional activity are clearly identified and stored together.

REVOCATION OR SUSPENSION OF LICENSE

The privilege of practicing medicine may be taken away from a physician who (1) is convicted of a crime, (2) engages in unprofessional conduct, or (3) is repeatedly negligent because of personal or professional incapacity. Crimes committed by unethical physicians include overprescribing or abusing narcotic drugs, sexually abusing patients, and engaging in other illegal activities. In a recent Pennsylvania case, a physician was charged with repeatedly fondling female patients while they were under mild anesthesia. After the first patient made a charge against the physician, others stepped forward to make the same claim. The case was proved, and the physician was fined, imprisoned, and his license suspended.

Physicians who practice obstetrics and gynecology are especially vulnerable to charges of sexual misconduct, and they take preventive measures so that their examinations cannot be misinterpreted or misrepresented. There are two reasons an obstetrician/gynecologist (OB/GYN), either male or female, calls a female nurse to the examining room during a woman's pelvic examination: (1) The patient is less likely to be embarrassed with another female in the room, and

(2) The patient will have difficulty proving sexual misconduct by the physician if a witness was present.

Unprofessional conduct refers to falsification of records, splitting fees with another physician for patient referrals, accepting gifts from pharmacies for referring patients, and engaging in advertising that misleads the patient; for example, advertising cosmetic surgery that promises certain results. A physician may be incapacitated personally or professionally because of alcohol or drug abuse, a physical injury, mental instability, or insanity. As a medical assistant, you are responsible for reporting to the licensing agency any physician who cannot function because of drug or alcohol addiction or any other problem that affects his or her competency.

A physician's license cannot be revoked or suspended without due process of law. This means that the state board bringing the charge must give the physician adequate notice of the charge, provide sound evidence for the charge, and allow a hearing at which the physician may be represented by legal counsel. The board then investigates and dismisses the charge or prosecutes the physician and makes a judgment.

Because nurses, medical assistants, and other allied health professionals, unlike physicians, are usually full-time employees, they do not have the same rights of due process as physicians unless specified in an employment contract. If no employment contract exists, they may be discharged for "good cause," "bad cause," or "no cause at all." Their employment is "at will," which means that the person can be terminated by the employer without reason. An employee who thinks that his or her termination is due to race or sex discrimination can file a complaint with the appropriate state or federal agency.

IN YOUR OPINION

1. What improprieties or crimes committed by your employer would cause you to bring charges?
2. What are the advantages and disadvantages of individual states developing their own licensing guidelines?
3. What conflicts of emotion do you think a medical assistant working for an alcoholic or drug-addicted physician might experience?

The Physician and the Law

Litigation has become an increasingly popular method of resolving conflicts between patients and their physicians. Physicians in high-risk specialties are either quitting their practices or reducing their patient load to guard against the possibility of being sued.

Physicians must be concerned about a variety of legal matters. As a medical assistant, you can assist the physician by (1) becoming familiar with the laws of your state; (2) compiling a file of all due dates for federal, state, and local forms, including license renewal; (3) maintaining complete and up-to-date patient records; and (4) keeping a proper inventory of all drugs received and dispensed (Figure 4-2).

Federal, state, and local law establishes the rules by which a society is governed. The law outlines a person's rights and obligations and sets penalties for those who violate the rules. The law is divided into two parts: (1) private or civil law, which is concerned with the rights and obligations people have toward one another, for example, a physician's responsibility to treat

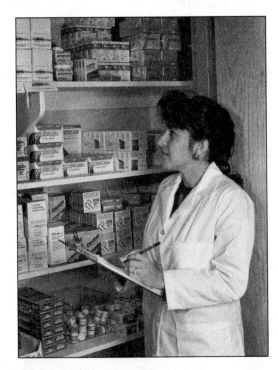

FIGURE 4-2 A medical assistant or medical office manager may be responsible for documenting the drugs received and dispensed for the physician and for maintaining the drug inventory.

patients according to accepted procedures; and (2) public or criminal law, which refers to the rights and obligations people have to live within the laws of society.

CIVIL LAW

Most legal cases involving physicians are based on civil law. The branch of civil law that usually applies to medical cases is called **tort law**. It is concerned with a wrong or injury one person inflicts on another.

A physician who is suspected of violating the law is subject to civil or criminal prosecution or both. If the physician is found guilty in a civil case, the physician or the physician's insurance company will likely have to pay monetary damages. For a criminal offense, the physician may be imprisoned.

Medical Malpractice/Professional Liability Insurance

A patient who thinks that a physician was negligent in diagnosing or treating an illness or accident may file a medical malpractice claim and, if the case is proved, recover monetary damages from the physician or the physician's insurance carrier. The number of malpractice, or professional liability, suits against physicians has risen dramatically since the 1960s, especially for those in high-risk specialties. The number of claims has risen almost 100 percent in the last decade.

Large monetary damages awarded in some cases have driven up the cost of malpractice insurance for physicians. The cost of insurance coverage at $10,000 to $100,000 per year is so prohibitive that some physicians have changed their specialty to one with a lower risk of being sued. Other doctors have become self-insured, meaning they cover their own malpractice court awards. This is highly risky. Obstetricians and gynecologists, for example, are often the target of malpractice lawsuits, and some have stopped delivering babies. Many insurance companies now refuse to offer medical malpractice coverage because of the large payments they are required to make when a jury has decided against the insured physician.

Medical professional liability is estimated to account for more than 15 percent of total ex-

penditures for physicians' services. These costs include professional liability insurance premiums, costs of defensive medicine, such as additional x-rays, and losses not covered by liability insurance. Ultimately, these costs must be passed along to the patient in the form of higher fees for physicians' services. Figure 4-3 shows the percentage of physicians who have incurred malpractice claims at some time in their career.

A survey of physicians by the American Medical Association (AMA) found that one third of U.S. physicians identify professional liability as medicine's primary problem. Physicians are practicing **defensive medicine** in an attempt to prevent lawsuits. In cases where one laboratory or diagnostic test might have been required previously, a physician may now ask for additional tests to confirm a diagnosis or treatment (Figure 4-4). A physician may ask a patient to return for additional visits to follow the progress of recovery. Each additional test, return visit, or other defensive measure increases the patient's medical costs. The AMA, along with local medical associations, private physicians, and other groups concerned about the spiraling cost of medical care, are seeking solutions to the problem of professional liability.

Percent of Physicians Incurring Professional Liability Claims at Some Time During Their Career, as of 1991	
	Percent
All physicians	39.0
Specialty	
General/family practice	37.2
Internal medicine	33.6
Surgery	49.4
Pediatrics	28.6
Obstetrics/gynecology	65.2
Radiology	36.4
Psychiatry	21.0
Anesthesiology	35.4
Pathology	27.4
Other	41.1

FIGURE 4-3 Percent of physicians incurring malpractice claims. (Source: Socioeconomic Environment of Medicine, Reprinted with permission American Medical Association 1994.)

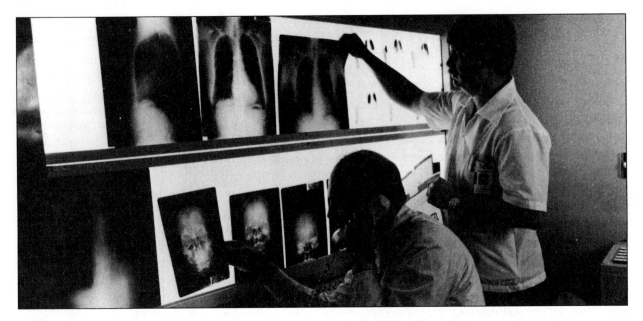

FIGURE 4-4 Because of professional liability, physicians are practicing defensive medicine by requesting more tests to confirm their diagnosis or treatment.

Medical Malpractice Claims

The concept of **negligence** is basic to any medical malpractice claim. The patient or other plaintiff must prove that the plaintiff was harmed in some way by the physician's or other health practitioner's failure to act. The plaintiff must prove failure to meet two standards of care: (1) what is considered normal care in the patient's geographic area, and (2) the care that another physician or health care professional would have shown in the same circumstances.

Negligence may be claimed when an incorrect procedure is performed, when a mistaken diagnosis is made, or when an improper treatment has been used. A patient may also claim negligence when a condition calls for treatment that the physician failed to provide; for example, when a medical condition is serious enough to warrant a specialist's advice which the primary care physician failed to get. The following cases are examples of negligence.

> Dr. Sanchez, a radiologist, fails to see a tumor on a patient's liver while reading the patient's ultrasound. He reports to the primary care physician that the ultrasound shows no irregularities. When the patient continues to complain of pain, the primary care physician conducts further tests that reveal a tumor. Even after surgery, the patient does not regain his health and dies two years later. The family, which was harmed by the death, has legal grounds for a malpractice (tort) claim against Dr. Sanchez.

> Holly David, a high school star basketball player, breaks her arm in a fall during a game. Dr. Chung, an orthopedist, sets the arm and puts it in a cast. When the cast is removed, Holly discovers that she can no longer shoot baskets successfully. An x-ray reveals that the break healed improperly because Dr. Chung did not set the arm correctly. Holly is harmed because she can no longer qualify for a four-year basketball scholarship to a major university. She has grounds for a malpractice suit against Dr. Chung.

Malpractice by the Physician's Staff

Physicians are liable and can be sued for the actions of their medical employees while the employees are on duty. For this reason, most physicians carry, as a part of their professional liability insurance, additional coverage for the clinical and office staff. The following case illustrates an employee's action for which the physician would be held responsible.

A patient, Mr. Senker, comes to the office for treatment of a gash in his forehead. The physician treats the head and instructs the medical assistant to give the patient a sample of a particular ointment. The medical assistant picks up the wrong sample and gives it to Mr. Senker who uses the sample on his head for two weeks. Mr. Senker's head becomes inflamed and infected. When he returns to the physician in great pain, the medical assistant's mistake is discovered. As a result of the error, Mr. Senker undergoes plastic surgery and several weeks of additional pain. He has a tort claim against the physician because he suffered a wrong or injury as a result of the medical assistant's mistake. The medical assistant can also be sued, but since the physician's assets and insurance coverage are likely to be greater than the medical assistant's, the physician will bear the brunt of the suit.

A medical assistant or other employee of a medical office should never rely fully upon the physician's insurance to provide for professional liability coverage because all employees are held responsible for their own professional conduct. A medical assistant, nurse, laboratory technician, medical technologist, or other employee can be held personally or jointly liable with the physician for medical malpractice. An especially dangerous situation exists when an employee is charged with practicing medicine without a license. This can happen innocently when an employee, who desires to be helpful, suggests medication or treatment for a patient. If the patient becomes ill or harmed as a result of the advice, the employee can be sued, both as an employee of the physician and as an individual. It is important, therefore, that you as a medical assistant never give the impression you are recommending a treatment or a medication. The following example illustrates a case in which a well-meaning medical assistant can be sued for practicing medicine without a license.

A young, inexperienced mother calls the pediatrician's office to ask the doctor about her son's high fever following the flu. When she discovers the physician is out of the office, she asks the medical assistant who answers the telephone what she should do. The medical assistant, who knows the physician usually prescribes aspirin or acetaminophen to reduce fever, suggests that the mother give one of the two medications to her son. When the mother asks if either medication will be all right, the medical assistant replies, "Yes." A week later the mother calls the office crying that her son is experiencing a seizure following severe vomiting in the morning. After giving the child emergency treatment, the physician diagnoses Reye's syndrome, a condition sometimes attributed to taking aspirin following the flu. The medical assistant and the physician can be sued because the medical assistant practiced medicine without a license by recommending that the child be given aspirin.

To be fully protected for professional liability, you should purchase a professional liability insurance policy as soon as you become employed in a medical office. This insurance can be purchased from the American Association of Medical Assistants (AAMA) for approximately $75 annually; the alternative, no protection, can cost thousands of dollars if you are sued.

Preventing Malpractice Claims
The best way to protect against medical malpractice lawsuits is to avoid situations that can lead to malpractice charges. The physician, nurses, medical assistant, and other medical staff should understand the two primary methods of reducing malpractice claims: informed consent and accurate medical records.

Informed Consent
A patient may consent to procedures for diagnosis and treatment, which relieves the physician of liability if the procedure fails or causes damage. A patient's consent may be oral, written, or implied by the actions of the patient, although most physicians and hospitals require the patient to sign a consent form before undergoing procedures that are considered risky in any way.

Informed consent, as created by the courts, is a doctrine stating that before consenting to undergo a procedure, a patient must be told (1) the reason for the procedure, (2) how the procedure will be performed, (3) the risks to the patient, including the possibility of bodily harm or death, (4) the benefits of the procedure, and (5) possible problems after recovery. The assumption is that before a patient can consent to a procedure, its implications must be clear. There are four reasons that a patient's informed consent is necessary:

1. Patients are not knowledgeable about medical science.
2. An adult of sound mind has the right to determine whether or not to submit to medical treatment.
3. To be effective, the patient's consent must be informed consent.
4. The patient depends on the physician for information to make a reasoned decision about treatment (Annas, 89).

A physician is legally required to disclose risks that might occur during a procedure. The modern legal interpretation is that informed consent is a duty of health practitioners and that the lack of informed consent is negligence. The courts use the term **material risk** to establish what risks should be disclosed; meaning that a risk should be explained if a reasonable person would consider it important. For example, the risk of death or injury during a cardiac catheterization should be disclosed; however, the risks associated with stitching a cut finger are not considered serious enough to merit a physician's disclosing them. Informed consent is given before surgery, experimental procedures, the administration of experimental drugs, or other treatments involving risk to the patient. For example, if you awoke one morning with a severe pain in your right side and, after visiting the physician, learned you required an emergency appendectomy, the surgery would not be performed unless you (assuming you are of legal age) or your parent or guardian signed a consent form.

Consent forms signed by the patient prior to receiving a treatment or procedure document that the patient has been fully informed of potential risk. Physicians and hospitals routinely require consent forms as a means of protecting themselves from claims. The consent form should be specific and provide enough detail

for the patient to understand fully what he or she is signing.

The physician will rely on you as a medical assistant to organize and coordinate the signing of all consent forms. This is an important responsibility, as these forms would be required as documentation in a lawsuit. Although a missing form might never be noticed, a multi-million dollar malpractice lawsuit could hinge upon evidence of a patient's informed consent.

To compile the necessary consent forms, the medical assistant must understand the procedures and treatments the patient will undergo. The physician usually supplies the names of the procedures and treatments; then the medical assistant determines which forms will be needed. If any question exists about the necessity for a form, the medical assistant should consult the physician. Refer to Figure 4-5 for an example of an informed consent form.

Even routine forms in the patient's medical records are important if a malpractice claim is filed. The patient's record is evidence that a physician tested and treated a patient thoroughly. Because no physician or medical assistant's memory can recall the circumstances of all treatments, only the documentation is valid proof that the physician followed the standard of care considered normal in the circumstances and, therefore, was not negligent in treating the patient.

Follow these procedures to assure that informed consent is always obtained:

1. Keep an adequate supply of consent forms.
2. Compile consent forms for each patient as needed before the patient arrives at the office.
3. Type a list of all consent forms needed and ask the physician to check the list for accuracy. Leave a blank line for the physician's check mark (✓).
4. Put all consent forms for an individual patient in a folder.
5. Review the forms with the patient, explaining the purpose of each form fully.
6. Ask the patient to sign and date all forms; then check the forms to be sure they are completed in full.
7. File the forms in the patient's medical record.

Acknowledgment of Informed Consent
for Surgical or Medical Procedures

I hereby indicate that I have given consent to _____Dr. Erin McDonald_____ (insert doctor's name), with associates or assistants of her choice, to perform the following surgical, diagnostic, and or medical procedure (including without limit anesthesia, x-rays, or laboratory tests on ~~myself~~ _____Albert Edwards_____ my _____son_____ (cross out inappropriate description of patient):

tonsillectomy _____

_____

_____

Name of Procedure(s)

I hereby indicate that in giving this consent the nature and purpose of the procedure; what the procedure is expected to accomplish; alternate means of therapy, if any; and reasonably known risks, complications, and discomfort have been explained to me by the above named doctor.

I understand that during the course of the above described procedure, unforeseen conditions may be revealed that make advisable an extension of this procedure or the use of a different procedure. I hereby authorize the above named doctor(s) to carry out any extension or to perform any other procedure that in the doctor's judgment is advisable for my well-being if circumstances make it impossible or, in the doctor's opinion, medically undesirable, to obtain my specific consent to such extension or other procedure. The authority granted under this paragraph shall extend to treating all conditions that require treatment and are not known to the above named doctors at the time the procedure is commenced.

I am aware that the practice of medicine and surgery is not an exact science and that the possibility and nature of results or complications cannot be anticipated with complete accuracy. I acknowledge that no guarantees, express or implied, have been made as to the results of the above described procedure or any cure.

I consent to the admittance of observers and to the photographing or televising of the surgical, diagnostic, and or medical procedure to be performed, including appropriate portions of my body provided my name or identity is not revealed by the pictures or by the descriptive texts accompanying them.

Date ____September 10, 19—____

Time ____8:00____ (A.M.) P.M.

_____
SIGNATURE OF PATIENT

Anthony Edwards
SIGNATURE OF PARENT (WHERE REQUIRED)

____*Pat Devani*____
WITNESS

_____
SIGNATURE OF OTHER PERSON WITH LEGAL
AUTHORITY (WHERE REQUIRED)

FIGURE 4-5 Consent form signed by patient

Medical Records

Besides informed consent, the most valuable preventive measure in reducing malpractice claims is maintaining documented medical records for each patient. Because medical records can be used as evidence during a malpractice court case, they should be complete, accurate, and up to date at all times. They should include (1) consent forms for procedures or treatments the physician has performed; (2) copies of all medical histories, laboratory reports, the physician's notes, and consulting physicians' reports; (3) a list of all medications prescribed and dispensed from the office; (4) permission forms authorizing the physician to release information about the patient; (5) miscellaneous medical information; and (6) records from any government-funded program, such as Medicare or Medicaid, in which the patient participates.

If the physician withdraws from the case for any reason, a **physician-withdrawal letter** should be sent to the patient, and a copy of the letter should be stored in the patient's file. A common reason physicians withdraw from cases is the patient's failure to cooperate with treatment; for example, a refusal to take a prescribed drug. Other reasons include a patient's move to another geographic area or a patient's doctor shopping; that is, going back and forth to a series of doctors for the same symptoms. Figure 4-6 shows examples of physician-withdrawal letters. (*Note:* This letter should be sent by registered or certified mail with return receipt requested.)

Advance Directives

Federal law requires all states and most health care facilities to give information to patients about their rights to make decisions about their health care. The law, known as the Patient Self-Determination Act, is intended to make sure that all adult patients know what their rights are in controlling their health care decisions and understand how to use so-called advance directives to protect those rights.

Advance directives are any expression of a person's wishes about the health care to be received at some time in the future, when the person may not be able to make personal decisions because of illness or accident. Written advance directives state a person's choices for

Form 1a

> Date: _____
>
> Dear _____:
>
> I will no longer be able to provide medical care to (you/your children). If you require medical care within the next _____ days I will be available, but in no event longer than _____ days.
>
> To assist you in continuing to receive medical care for (you/your children), we will make records available to a new physician as soon as you authorize us to send them to that physician.
>
> Sincerely,
>
> _____, M.D.

Form 1b

> Date: _____
>
> Dear _____:
>
> I find it necessary to inform you that I am withdrawing from further professional attendance upon you since you have persisted in refusing to follow my medical advice and treatment. Since your condition requires medical attention, I suggest that you place yourself under the care of another physician without delay. If you desire, I shall be available to attend you for a reasonable time after you receive this letter, but in no event for more than _____ days.
>
> This should give you ample time to select a physician of your choice from the many competent practitioners in this city. With your authorization, I will make available to this physician your case history and information regarding the diagnosis and treatment you have received from me.
>
> Very truly yours,
>
> _____, M.D.

FIGURE 4-6 AMA medicological forms with legal analysis (American Medical Association, copyright 1991)

health care or name someone to make those choices if the person is unable to make decisions. Written directives are usually either a living will or a durable power of attorney for health care.

Most hospitals provide advance directive forms, eliminating the necessity of having an attorney draw up the document. However, patients may want to discuss advance directives with an attorney.

Living Wills A living will is a simple document in which a person explains what kind of life-prolonging medical care is acceptable if the person is terminally ill or unable to make a decision.

Durable Power of Attorney A durable power of attorney for health care is a document in which an individual names another person to make medical decisions if the patient is unable to personally make the decision because of illness or injury. Instructions can be given about any treatment wanted or to be avoided. Unlike a living will, a durable power of attorney may apply when a patient has any serious medical condition, not only a terminal illness. Refer to Chapter 3 for additional information on a durable power of attorney as an ethical issue. A durable power of attorney is shown in Figure 4-7.

CRIMINAL LAW

Criminal law involves a wrong to society and is usually punishable by imprisonment, perhaps combined with a fine. A physician found guilty of a criminal offense is usually censured by or expelled from membership in the AMA or the local medical society. On the other hand, a physician who is acquitted by a court of law may still face disciplinary action from a medical society.

Illegal Acts by a Physician
In an imperfect world, physicians can be guilty of wrongdoing. Because physicians are faced with many temptations, some slip into criminal activities for which they must be prosecuted. The physician who evades taxes, dispenses illegal drugs, abuses drugs, or sexually assaults or physically harms a patient will be convicted of the crime if discovered. Physicians can also be involved in other crimes.

The Medical Assistant's Responsibility for Reporting Crimes
Most physicians and other medical professionals are moral people who never commit a crime. However, if, as a medical assistant, you learn that a physician or other office employee has committed a crime, you must report the crime to the authorities. A medical assistant who does not report a crime can be prosecuted as an accessory.

IN YOUR OPINION

1. Under what circumstances do you think it is fair for a patient to bring a malpractice suit?
2. In settings in which nurses, doctors, medical assistants, medical technologists, and other staff have access to patient records, who should be held accountable for missing documents?
3. Is the monthly premium for professional liability insurance for a new medical assistant a worthwhile expense or a waste of money? Explain.

Confidentiality

The law protects the patient's right of confidentiality, which means that employees of medical offices, hospitals, and other health care facilities are legally bound to keep all patient information confidential unless the law requires disclosure. The patient should feel free to provide complete information to the doctor without fearing that it will be revealed to others.

Certain news is a matter of public record, and the physician must report this information immediately. Information of this kind includes births, deaths, accidents, and police cases.

PATIENT–PHYSICIAN RELATIONSHIP

The legal concept of **privilege of patient confidentiality** guarantees that the medical information a patient gives a physician will be held in greatest confidence, by both the physician and the physician's employees (Figure 4-8).

Health Care Declaration and Power of Attorney of

_____

A. Health Care Declaration

I, _____, of _____ County, Pennsylvania, being of sound mind, willfully and voluntarily make this declaration to be followed if I become incompetent. This declaration reflects my firm and settled commitment to refuse life-sustaining treatment under the circumstances indicated below.

1. If I should be in a terminal condition or in a state of permanent unconsciousness, I direct my attending physician to withhold or withdraw life-sustaining treatment that serves only to prolong the process of my dying.

2. If I am in the condition described above, I direct that treatment be limited to measures to keep me comfortable and to relieve pain, including any pain that might occur by withholding or withdrawing life-sustaining treatment.

In addition, if I am in the condition described above, I feel especially strongly about the following forms of treatment:

I ( ) do ( ) do not want cardiac resuscitation.

I ( ) do ( ) do not want mechanical respiration.

I ( ) do ( ) do not want tube feeding or any other invasive form of nutrition (food) or hydration (water).

I ( ) do ( ) do not want blood or blood products.

I ( ) do ( ) do not want any form of surgery or invasive diagnostic tests.

I ( ) do ( ) do not want kidney dialysis.

I ( ) do ( ) do not want antibiotics.

I realize that if I do not specifically indicate my preference regarding any of the forms of treatment listed above, I may receive that form of treatment.

Other Instructions:

I hereby designate _____ [name and address of surrogate]

(Tel. No. _____) as my surrogate to make medical treatment decisions for me if I should be incompetent and in a terminal condition or in a state of permanent unconsciousness.

If the surrogate designated above is, for any reason, unable to serve, I designate as substitute surrogate to serve: [name and address]

(Telephone No. _____)

My surrogate or substitute surrogate ( ) is ( ) is not authorized to withhold tube feeding or any other artificial or invasive form of nutrition (food) or hydration (water).

FIGURE 4-7 Health care declaration and power of attorney

B. Power of Attorney:

In addition to the declaration and appointments made above, I, _____,
hereby appoint the surrogate and substitute surrogate named above, in the order listed, my attorney-in-fact for health care for me and in my name to:

1. Authorize my admission to a medical, nursing, residential, or similar facility; enter into agreements for my care, and authorize medical and surgical procedures; consent to, withhold consent from, waive, and terminate any and all medical and surgical procedures on my behalf, including, without limitation, the administration of drugs and the withholding of tube feeding of any other artificial or invasive form of nutrition (food) or hydration (water).

2. Have access and to authorize access for others to any and all medical information and records of mine and all related information concerning me.

3. Authorize the payment of all bills for my health and medical care, to have access to and complete insurance and other health record forms, applications, certifications, and other documentation.

4. Make all medical treatment decisions for me if I should be incompetent or unable to make them or to communicate such medical decisions for myself.

This Health Care Declaration and Power of Attorney shall not be affected by my subsequent disability or incapacity.

Should any specific direction in this Health Care Declaration and Power of Attorney be held to be invalid, such invalidity shall not offset other directions of this document which can be effected without the invalid direction.

I made this declaration on the _____ day of _____ 19___.

Declarant's signature: _____
                                                    NAME

Declarant's address:

The declarant (or the person who on behalf of and at the direction of the declarant) knowingly and voluntarily signed this writing by signature or mark in my presence.

Witness's signature: _____

Witness's printed name: _____

Witness's address:

Witness's signature: _____

Witness's printed name: _____

Witness's address:

FIGURE 4-7 (continued)

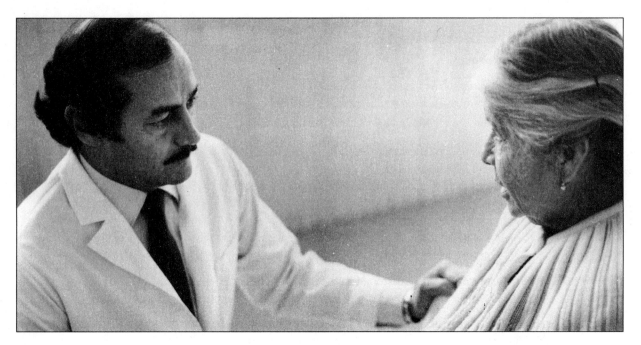

FIGURE 4-8 The legal concept of privilege of patient confidentiality guarantees that physicians and their employees will hold patients' medical information in strictest confidence. (Courtesy of Abbott Laboratories)

The contents of the medical records must also be safeguarded and held in complete confidentiality. The privilege of releasing information belongs to the patient, not to the physician.

The privilege of patient confidentiality assures patients that their records will be kept in complete privacy, even in court, unless they give written permission. However, if the patient waives the privilege of confidentiality, the physician may be required to testify in a court case. If the patient consents, the physician may discuss the patient's history, diagnosis, treatment, and prognosis with the patient's lawyer. Here is an illustration of the way the privilege of patient confidentiality works:

Alexander Onegin reveals his past alcoholism to his physician during an examination for an injury suffered while on the job. When Mr. Onegin files a worker's compensation claim, the employer suspects alcohol as a factor in the injury. The employer contacts Mr. Onegin's physician and asks about the patient's drinking habits. The privilege of patient confidentiality protects Mr. Onegin's privacy, and the information cannot be shared. The physician may be expected to provide *medical* details regarding the accident on a worker's compensation claim form.

Exception to the Patient–Physician Privilege

The **exception to the physician–patient privilege** protects society against harmful acts by or against the patient. For example, if an angry patient threatens to stab another person and shows the physician the knife that will be used, the physician is ethically and legally required to report the threat to authorities.

Physicians are also required to report gunshot wounds, rapes, stabbings, and other crimes against patients and to provide information that they believe will be helpful in solving the crime. However, only the physician may provide this information.

The medical assistant and other medical office employees are responsible for reporting to the physician any unusual cases that may involve a crime. These include suspected cases of child abuse, abuse against the elderly, and related crimes. If a parent waiting with a child in the lobby is verbally and physically abusive, as a medical assistant you should report this information to the physician immediately. If a patient who is bleeding profusely is brought to the office by another person who disappears, you should inform the physician so that the patient can be questioned about the circumstances of the injury. Here is another example of a situation that the medical assistant should report:

The medical assistant sees an elderly patient being brought into the office by a person who is apparently a relative. The patient is crying, and the relative is talking in a harsh manner. When the patient reaches up to touch the relative, the patient is given a sharp slap on the hand and shoved into a seat. This pattern of behavior, which the medical assistant considers abusive, continues until the relative accompanies the patient into the examining room. The relative is "all smiles" during the physician's examination of the elderly patient. The medical assistant has an ethical responsibility to call the doctor aside and report the behavior seen in the reception area.

The news media may ask for information about patients involved in accidents or about patients who are in the public eye, for example, movie stars, sports stars, politicians, community leaders, and others. A physician may not discuss a patient's medical condition, disease, or illness with the press without the patient's permission. However, information in the public domain, such as the patient's name, address, age, sex, and race, can be provided without the patient's consent, as can general information about an accident, such as the body part involved. Internal injuries and the patient's state of consciousness when brought to the hospital may be reported, but the physician may not state that a patient attempted suicide, that a patient was intoxicated or using drugs, or that a moral wrong was involved. The physician may make a general statement about the patient's condition. Furthermore, only the attending physician may make a statement about a patient's diagnosis or prognosis. As a medical assistant, you should refer all questions of this nature to the physician.

(Telephone rings)

Caller: This is CNN calling. We've just heard that the senator's son took a drug overdose and has been brought to your office. Is that true?

Medical Assistant: I can't answer any questions about private patients.

Caller: Just tell me if the senator's son is in your office now, so I can come take some pictures.

Medical Assistant: I can't release that information. I will not be able to help you.

PATIENT CONFIDENTIALITY AND INSURANCE COMPANIES

History, diagnosis, prognosis, treatment or service, and fee information acquired during the physician–patient relationship may be disclosed to an insurance company only if the patient provides written consent. Insurance companies generally include a statement of permission on their claim forms that the patient signs, granting the medical office the authority to release information to the insurance company. Without full documentation of diagnosis, treatment, and service, the insurance company will not pay benefits on a claim. Hospitals must also have written permission before releasing information about a patient.

Item 12 of the insurance claim form illustrated in Figure 4-9 shows the patient's signature giving permission to release medical information to the insurance carrier.

MEDICAL ASSISTANT'S RESPONSIBILITY FOR CONFIDENTIALITY

Except for insurance forms, which the medical assistant completes with the physician's permission, any information released about a patient should come only from the physician. Many doctors consider confidentiality to be the most desirable character trait that a medical assistant can possess. In addition to moral concerns for confidentiality, physicians are legally responsible for the actions of their employees during the course of duty. A physician can be sued if an employee releases confidential information. Consider this situation:

A medical assistant tells a friend who works for a Fortune 500 company that the company CEO is being treated by the physician, a psychiatrist, for alcoholism. The friend, unable to keep this information to himself, tells another person at work. Soon the grapevine has passed the story along to many employees, and someone leaks it to the news media. The negative publicity seriously reduces the value of a new stock offering. The Fortune 500 company traces the source of the story to the medical assistant, who loses his job as a result. The president has grounds for a lawsuit against the physician and the medical assistant.

APPROVED OMB-0938-0008

CARRIER

HEALTH INSURANCE CLAIM FORM

| | PICA | | | | | | PICA | |

1. MEDICARE	MEDICAID	CHAMPUS	CHAMPVA	GROUP HEALTH PLAN	FECA BLK LUNG	OTHER	1a. INSURED'S I.D. NUMBER	(FOR PROGRAM IN ITEM 1)
(Medicare #)	(Medicaid #)	(Sponsor's SSN)	(VA File #)	[X] (SSN or ID)	(SSN)	(ID)	331-26-9648	

2. PATIENT'S NAME (Last Name, First Name, Middle Initial)	3. PATIENT'S BIRTH DATE	SEX	4. INSURED'S NAME (Last Name, First Name, Middle Initial)
Stoner, Jay G.	MM 04 DD 03 YY —	M [X] F	Stoner, James B.

5. PATIENT'S ADDRESS (No., Street)	6. PATIENT RELATIONSHIP TO INSURED	7. INSURED'S ADDRESS (No., Street)
401 N. Broad Street	Self [ ] Spouse [ ] Child [X] Other [ ]	same as Item 5

CITY	STATE	8. PATIENT STATUS	CITY	STATE
Rockford	IL	Single [ ] Married [ ] Other [ ]		

ZIP CODE	TELEPHONE (Include Area Code)		ZIP CODE	TELEPHONE (INCLUDE AREA CODE)
61111-0136	(312) 555-3894	Employed [ ] Full-Time Student [ ] Part-Time Student [X]		(312) 555-3894

9. OTHER INSURED'S NAME (Last Name, First Name, Middle Initial)	10. IS PATIENT'S CONDITION RELATED TO:	11. INSURED'S POLICY GROUP OR FECA NUMBER
DNA		4324-8965

a. OTHER INSURED'S POLICY OR GROUP NUMBER	a. EMPLOYMENT? (CURRENT OR PREVIOUS)	a. INSURED'S DATE OF BIRTH	SEX
DNA	[ ] YES [X] NO	MM 01 DD 15 YY —	M [X] F [ ]

b. OTHER INSURED'S DATE OF BIRTH	SEX	b. AUTO ACCIDENT?	PLACE (State)	b. EMPLOYER'S NAME OR SCHOOL NAME
MM DD YY	M [ ] F [ ]	[ ] YES [X] NO		Grayson Agency

c. EMPLOYER'S NAME OR SCHOOL NAME	c. OTHER ACCIDENT?	c. INSURANCE PLAN NAME OR PROGRAM NAME
	[ ] YES [X] NO	Statewide Insurance

d. INSURANCE PLAN NAME OR PROGRAM NAME	10d. RESERVED FOR LOCAL USE	d. IS THERE ANOTHER HEALTH BENEFIT PLAN?
		[ ] YES [X] NO *If yes*, return to and complete item 9 a-d.

READ BACK OF FORM BEFORE COMPLETING & SIGNING THIS FORM.

12. PATIENT'S OR AUTHORIZED PERSON'S SIGNATURE I authorize the release of any medical or other information necessary to process this claim. I also request payment of government benefits either to myself or to the party who accepts assignment below.	13. INSURED'S OR AUTHORIZED PERSON'S SIGNATURE I authorize payment of medical benefits to the undersigned physician or supplier for services described below.
SIGNED *James B. Stone* DATE 5/21/—	SIGNED *James B. Stone*

14. DATE OF CURRENT: ILLNESS (First symptom) OR INJURY (Accident) OR PREGNANCY(LMP) MM DD YY	15. IF PATIENT HAS HAD SAME OR SIMILAR ILLNESS. GIVE FIRST DATE MM DD YY	16. DATES PATIENT UNABLE TO WORK IN CURRENT OCCUPATION FROM MM DD YY TO MM DD YY

17. NAME OF REFERRING PHYSICIAN OR OTHER SOURCE	17a. I.D. NUMBER OF REFERRING PHYSICIAN	18. HOSPITALIZATION DATES RELATED TO CURRENT SERVICES FROM MM DD YY TO MM DD YY

19. RESERVED FOR LOCAL USE	20. OUTSIDE LAB? [ ] YES [ ] NO	$ CHARGES

21. DIAGNOSIS OR NATURE OF ILLNESS OR INJURY. (RELATE ITEMS 1,2,3 OR 4 TO ITEM 24E BY LINE)	22. MEDICAID RESUBMISSION CODE	ORIGINAL REF. NO.
1. L___.___ 3. L___.___	23. PRIOR AUTHORIZATION NUMBER	
2. L___.___ 4. L___.___		

24. A. DATE(S) OF SERVICE From MM DD YY To MM DD YY	B. Place of Service	C. Type of Service	D. PROCEDURES, SERVICES, OR SUPPLIES (Explain Unusual Circumstances) CPT/HCPCS MODIFIER	E. DIAGNOSIS CODE	F. $ CHARGES	G. DAYS OR UNITS	H. EPSDT Family Plan	I. EMG	J. COB	K. RESERVED FOR LOCAL USE
1										
2										
3										
4										
5										
6										

25. FEDERAL TAX I.D. NUMBER SSN EIN	26. PATIENT'S ACCOUNT NO.	27. ACCEPT ASSIGNMENT? (For govt. claims, see back) [ ] YES [ ] NO	28. TOTAL CHARGE $	29. AMOUNT PAID $	30. BALANCE DUE $

31. SIGNATURE OF PHYSICIAN OR SUPPLIER INCLUDING DEGREES OR CREDENTIALS (I certify that the statements on the reverse apply to this bill and are made a part thereof.) SIGNED DATE	32. NAME AND ADDRESS OF FACILITY WHERE SERVICES WERE RENDERED (If other than home or office)	33. PHYSICIAN'S, SUPPLIER'S BILLING NAME, ADDRESS, ZIP CODE & PHONE # PIN# GRP#

(APPROVED BY AMA COUNCIL ON MEDICAL SERVICE 8/88) ***PLEASE PRINT OR TYPE*** FORM HCFA-1500 (U2) (12-90) FORM OWCP-1500 FORM RRB-1500

PATIENT AND INSURED INFORMATION

PHYSICIAN OR SUPPLIER INFORMATION

FIGURE 4-9 Insurance form giving permission to release medical information

Personal information that patients supply is also confidential, even though it may not be of a medical nature, and should not be released or discussed with anyone outside the office. Information falling into this category includes a patient's age, number of marriages, number of children, and similar facts. Information can be released inadvertently if the medical office staff is not cautious. An employee who speaks too loudly while visitors are in the reception area may reveal confidential information. Similarly, an employee who tends to "talk too much" may divulge confidential information unintentionally. Carelessly released information can cause ethical and legal problems for the physician and for the employee who released it. A good rule to follow is: Never talk about patients except with the professional medical staff.

Sometimes a husband, wife, friend, child, or employer of a patient may ask about a patient's condition. Although these questions are legitimate expressions of concern, a medical assistant should not provide information about the patient. Instead, the inquiry should be referred to the physician, as in this example:

A man who accompanies his wife to the gynecologist's office waits in the reception area while his wife talks with the physician. The husband tells the medical assistant that he believes his wife is pregnant but that she won't confirm the pregnancy. As her husband, he feels it is his right to know whether he is going to be a father, and he asks the medical assistant to check his wife's medical record. A medical assistant must keep confidential all information about the patient. The fact that the concerned person is the patient's husband has no bearing on the patient's right to confidentiality.

IN YOUR OPINION

1. What can you as a medical assistant do to guard against inadvertently releasing information about a patient?
2. If a medical assistant and nurse in an open office discuss a patient's answers to medical questions, how might they break the rule of patient confidentiality?
3. What advice regarding confidentiality would you give a new medical assistant?

The Physician in Court

Physicians are usually called to court for one of two reasons: (1) as the defendant in a lawsuit or (2) as an expert witness in a case. These situations may involve a variety of circumstances.

PHYSICIAN AS DEFENDANT

When a malpractice claim is made against a physician or other health care professional, the person being sued files the claim with his or her professional liability insurance carrier. The carrier may decide that the claim is invalid and refuse to make any settlement, or it may offer the patient a sum of money to settle the claim out of court. The patient can accept the offer, try to negotiate a higher settlement figure or counter offer with the carrier, or file a lawsuit that ultimately will end in a trial if the carrier and the patient cannot agree on a figure.

Settlement of Claims

Many malpractice lawsuits never go to trial because the insurance company and the patient agree on damages. The insurance carrier pays the patient and the patient drops the case against the physician. Sometimes negotiations continue while a trial is in session; if the two parties agree to a settlement during the trial, the case is dropped.

When an agreement between the patient and insurance carrier cannot be reached, the carrier hires an attorney to defend the physician or health care professional (Figure 4-10). The attorney reviews the patient's medical record and talks with the physician, patient, medical assistant, and any other principals involved in the case. After thoroughly reviewing the facts, the attorney answers the charge through legal documents filed with the court.

Court Papers

The patient is the plaintiff in a malpractice lawsuit, and the physician is the defendant. The burden of proof is on the plaintiff to show that the physician was negligent; the physician must show that the plaintiff's accusation is false. Since the outcome of many malpractice lawsuits depends on the contents of the patient's medical record, complete and up-to-date records are crucial.

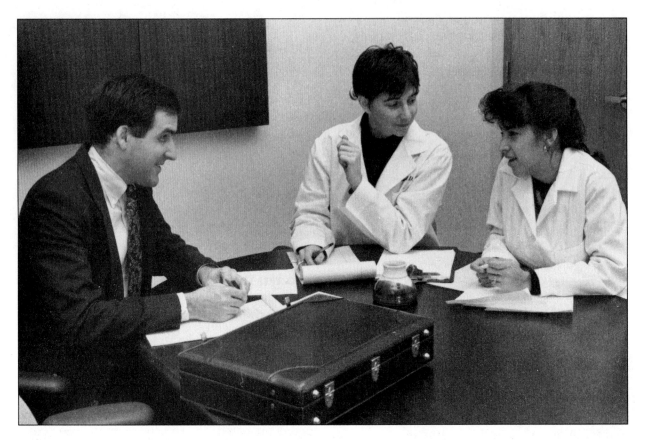

FIGURE 4-10 In some malpractice lawsuits, it becomes necessary for the insurance carrier to hire an attorney to defend the health care professional.

Summons and Complaint

If the physician is sued, a legal summons and complaint will be mailed or hand delivered to the physician by a member of the local sheriff's department. These documents may be left with the medical assistant if the physician is unavailable. They are extremely important and must be given to the physician immediately. Failure by the physician to answer the summons could result in a default judgment; that is, a judgment against the physician because no answer was made. Figure 4-11 illustrates a legal summons, and Figure 4-12 illustrates a complaint. You should become familiar with the appearance of these documents so you can recognize them if they are delivered to your office.

The physician notifies the attorney and insurance company at once if a summons and complaint are received. If the physician and the professional liability carrier believe that no malpractice was involved or if they cannot agree with the plaintiff on a settlement, the case goes to trial. During the trial, all parties involved in the lawsuit give evidence. Expert witnesses, including other physicians and related experts, may be called by the plaintiff to attest to the physician's negligence. The insurance carrier then presents expert witnesses to defend the physician's position.

After several days, weeks, or months of trial, during which negotiations for settlement may continue among the lawyers for the plaintiff and defendant, a judge or jury decides the physician's innocence or guilt. If the physician is found guilty, the judge or jury sets monetary damages, and the malpractice carrier pays the patient up to the limits set by the physician's insurance policy. The physician must personally pay any difference between the policy limits and the damages set by the judge or jury. The court may also dismiss the suit if the plaintiff fails to establish a cause of action against the doctor, or if the plaintiff's argument against the physician is not strong enough.

NAME AND ADDRESS OF ATTORNEY:	TELEPHONE NO:	FOR COURT USE ONLY
JUENGERT AND WATSON 1043 Peachtree Street Atlanta, GA 30033-4161 ATTORNEY FOR (Name) Plaintiff	(404) 555-4925	

Insert name of court, judicial district or branch court, if any, and Post Office and Street Address:

FULTON COUNTY DISTRICT COURT

Capitol Square, SW

Atlanta, GA 30334-4161

PLAINTIFF

    ARNOLD RIFKEN

    BERNICE RIFKIN

DEFENDANT

    ERROL DUPLESSIS, M.D.

    BEAU GIRARD, M.D.

SUMMONS	CASE NUMBER
NOTICE! You have been sued. The court may decide	**¡AVISO! Usted ha sido demandado. El tribunal puede**

FIGURE 4-11 Legal summons

PHYSICIAN AND MEDICAL ASSISTANT AS WITNESSES

Physicians may also be called as witnesses in court cases, either against themselves or as expert witnesses in other cases. Sometimes the physician must appear in the courtroom, or the physician may provide testimony through a **deposition**. A deposition is a sworn statement given by a party to a lawsuit before the suit goes to trial. During a deposition, which may be given in the attorney's office or in some other location, an attorney asks the witness questions. The witness's answers are recorded by a stenographer or court reporter who keyboards the proceedings in final form and notarizes it.

As a medical assistant, you may be asked to give a deposition. If this happens, tell the facts as you know them, without changing them in any way. When you are unsure of answers to any questions, say so. It is better to give no answer than to give an incorrect answer that might cause greater difficulty at a later time.

Good Samaritan Laws

Good Samaritan laws protect the physician and other health care professionals who help people in unusual emergency situations. This includes (1) the physician who stops at the scene of an automobile accident to offer aid; (2) the doctor who amputates the fingers of a man when he catches them in a boat motor; (3) the paramedic who treats a fire victim while off duty; and

NO. 430219.

PLAINTIFFS, Arnold Rifkin   I IN THE DISTRICT COURT

          Bernice Rifkin

vs.

DEFENDANTS, Errol DuPlessis, M.D.   I OF FULTON COUNTY, GEORGIA

          Beau Girard, M.D.   I 5th JUDICIAL DISTRICT

PLAINTIFFS' ORIGINAL PETITION

TO THE HONORABLE JUDGE OF SAID COURT:

COME NOW ARNOLD RIFKIN AND BERNICE RIFKIN, hereinafter styled Plaintiffs, complaining of ERROL DUPLESSIS, M.D. and BEAU GIRARD, M.D., hereinafter styled Defendants, and for cause of action would show to the Court as follows:

I.

This is a suit for wrongful death under Articles 4671 et. seq. of the Revised Civil Statutes of Georgia, and plaintiff BERNICE RIFKIN is the surviving mother of JEREMY RIFKIN deceased. Plaintiff, ARNOLD RIFKIN, is the father of JEREMY RIFKIN deceased. Said JEREMY RIFKIN, plaintiff's deceased 3-month old minor son, left no will and there was no administration on his estate and no necessity therefor. Plaintiffs are responsible for the debts of the estate of their deceased son, including funeral expenses.

II.

JEREMY RIFKIN was wrongfully killed as hereinafter described, but did not die instantly; he experienced conscious pain and suffering, for which he would have been entitled to recover damages; and the cause of action for damages of conscious pain and suffering prior to his death survived, and on his death accrued to his heirs at law under Article 5525 of the Revised Civil Statutes of the State of Georgia.

FIGURE 4-12 Legal complaint

(4) other medical practitioners who treat emergencies that would result in death if aid were not offered. Good Samaritan laws in all fifty states protect medical practitioners from fear of reprisal when they offer emergency care. Generally, these laws cover practitioners who provide treatment within their area of expertise. However, each state has different laws, so you should check the law in your state to determine the extent of liability for medical practitioners who assist people in an emergency.

The Physician and Controlled Substances

The Controlled Substances Act regulates the dispensing of drugs from medical offices. Physicians who dispense narcotic drugs are required to maintain complete and detailed records because of the potential for abuse. Less detail is required for nonnarcotic drugs. Generally, the medical assistant is responsible for keeping records of all drugs dispensed.

NARCOTIC DRUG RECORDS

Narcotic drugs that are dispensed from a medical office fall into a special category of importance. Since drug abuse has become a major problem today, all drugs must be monitored properly. Theft of drugs can be overlooked if the medical assistant does not follow strict recording procedures for the physician's drug file.

Procedures for Monitoring Dispensed Drugs

1. Record the date and time the drug was dispensed.
2. Record the name and address of the patient to whom the drug was dispensed.
3. Record the name and quantity of the drug dispensed.
4. Record the method of dispensing.
5. Explain the reason the drug was given.

An example of a narcotic record is shown in Figure 4-13.

DRUG SECURITY

Narcotic drugs should be secured in a locked cabinet at all times; the keys to the cabinet should be held only by the physician, and possibly the nurse. Prescription pads and drug samples should also be locked, so they cannot be stolen by visitors or disreputable staff members. The physician can be held liable if safe measures are not used to store narcotic drugs.

Federal drug enforcement officers have the right to inspect a physician's office and drug records if suspicion of dispensing abuse exists. If improper storage or record keeping is found, the physician may lose the right to dispense and prescribe drugs.

As a medical assistant, you must be sure that controlled substances are kept safely and disposed of in accordance with the law (Figure 4-14). If you have any concerns about the way drugs are stored, dispensed, or discarded, you should report them to the physician immediately.

Narcotic Record					
DATE	TIME	NAME OF PATIENT	DRUG	QUANTITY	EXPLANATION
4/6/—	2 p.m.	Pamela Ohlberg 202 W. 18th Street, Nashville, TN	Percodan	5.0 mgs	postoperative
4/10/—	10 a.m.	Erik Gladding 8504 Green Hills Pike, Nashville, TN	Ergostat	2 mg	migraine headaches

FIGURE 4-13 Narcotic record

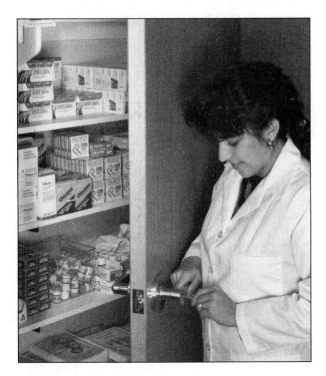

FIGURE 4-14 The medical assistant is responsible for ensuring that controlled substances are kept in a locked cabinet at all times.

Drug Schedules

Narcotic and nonnarcotic drugs are divided into five categories or schedules, depending on their potential for abuse. These schedules and some examples of drugs in each category are listed below.

SCHEDULE I

Drugs listed in Schedule I have a high potential for abuse. They are not legitimately used in the United States for treating patients; however, with special permission, Schedule I drugs may be used for research.

Examples: heroin, LSD, peyote, mescaline, and PCP

SCHEDULE II

Schedule II drugs have a high potential for abuse and may lead to psychological or physical dependence. Unlike Schedule I drugs, however, they have been accepted for medical use in the United States. Schedule II drugs can be dispensed only with a prescription signed by a physician; telephone prescriptions are not acceptable.

Examples: Percodan, morphine, codeine, Dilaudid, methadone, cocaine, Seconal, Nembutal, and Amytal

SCHEDULE III

The potential for abuse is lower with Schedule III drugs. Although use of the drugs is accepted in the United States, a moderate degree of physical or psychological dependence may result from abuse. Schedule III drugs can be dispensed with either a written or telephone prescription.

Examples: Tylenol No. 3 with codeine, Empirin No. 3 with codeine, Fiorinal, Phenobarbital, paregoric, Butisol, and Noludar

SCHEDULE IV

Schedule IV drugs have low potential for abuse and are accepted for medical use in the United States. Abuse may lead to limited physical or psychological dependence. Prescriptions for Schedule IV drugs may be written by a nurse or medical assistant as long as the physician signs the prescription. Refills can be approved by the medical assistant as long as the physician is consulted.

Examples: Valium, Librium, and Tranxene

SCHEDULE V

The potential for abuse of Schedule V drugs is low. These drugs are accepted for medical use in the United States and can be purchased without a prescription. Abuse may lead to a more limited physical or psychological dependence than will abuse of Schedule IV drugs.

Examples: Donnagel PG, Novahistine DH, and Novahistine Expectorant

IN YOUR OPINION

1. In giving a deposition, if a medical assistant has an opinion but no concrete proof of wrongdoing by a physician-employer, what should the medical assistant do?
2. Explain why Good Samaritan laws are necessary.
3. If a medical assistant discovers narcotic drugs missing from the office supply cabinet on several occasions and tells the physician, who does nothing, what steps should the medical assistant take?

REFERENCES

American Medical Association, Center for Health Policy Research. *Professional Liability Update,* February 1987. Chicago: Professional Liability Clearinghouse.

American Medical Association, Center for Health Policy Research. *Professional Liability Update,* June 1986. Chicago: Professional Liability Clearinghouse.

Annas, John D., and Nancy R. Rhoden. *Ethical Issues in Modern Medicine.* Mountain View, California: Mayfield Publishing Co., 1989.

Lewis, Marcia A., and Carol D. Warden. *Medical Law, Ethics, and Bioethics in the Medical Office,* 3rd ed. Philadelphia: F. A. Davis Company, 1993.

Chapter Activities

PERFORMANCE BASED ACTIVITIES

1. Create a dialogue with an elderly patient who has asked you to explain advance directives and their purpose. Print your dialogue. (DACUM 2.2, 2.3, 2.4, 5.3)

2. Make a chart tracing the development of a medical malpractice claim from its origination by the patient through trial.

Route of a Medical Malpractice Claim

1. _____

2. _____

3. _____

4. _____

5. _____

6. _____

7. _____

8. _____

(DACUM 5.1, 5.2)

3. Interview three medical assistants in your area. Ask what security procedures they follow for drugs kept in the office. Write a paper recommending what you consider to be the best procedure. (DACUM 2.9, 5.5)

EXPANDING YOUR THINKING

1. List at least three ways in which you can help yourself remember not to talk about patients outside of the office.

2. Do you think there should be a limit on the amount of damages a person suing for malpractice can be awarded? Why or why not?

3. What are some ways in which you as an assistant can prevent the wrong medication from being dispensed?

4. What record-keeping practices can help safeguard your office against malpractice claims?

5. Some well-respected authors believe that the availability of drugs should not be regulated by law. Do you agree? Why or why not?

Portfolio Assessment

DACUM 1.1–1.9, 2.1–2.11

Supplies
Portfolio or file folder
Printer paper
Tape recorder and tape, optional

1. Form a relationship with a medical practice in your town that will agree to serve as your mentoring practice during this course. The mentoring practice will provide a research and learning center as you analyze, compare, develop, and create materials.

   Call for the name of the managing physician or office manager and write a letter to this person making your request. Explain that the time required of the practice will be thirty minutes to two hours per week. Ask if one individual or mentor can be named to serve as your primary contact for questions or information. Provide a letter from your instructor confirming that this is a legitimate, required educational activity. Follow up with a phone call in one week to seek approval. You may need to ask several practices before you locate a mentoring practice. When you get a positive response, you will have begun a worthwhile relationship that can expand your learning far beyond the classroom. Store your requests and your responses in your portfolio.

2. Using the organization chart shown in Portfolio Figure PI-1 on the following page as a model, develop an organization chart for your mentoring practice. On a separate sheet, print the responsibilities of each position and the type and amount of training needed. Store the items in your portfolio.

Organization Chart

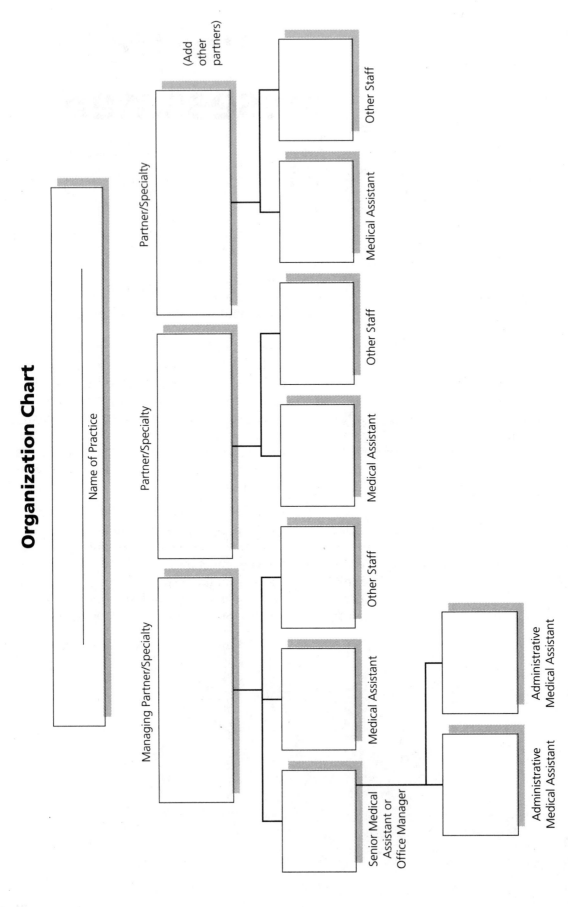

Name of Practice

Managing Partner/Specialty

Partner/Specialty

Partner/Specialty

(Add other partners)

Senior Medical Assistant or Office Manager

Medical Assistant

Other Staff

Medical Assistant

Other Staff

Medical Assistant

Other Staff

Administrative Medical Assistant

Administrative Medical Assistant

FIGURE PI-1 The staff positions identified on this chart may not exactly match the positions of your mentoring practice. Redraw the chart as necessary to accurately reflect the staff employed by your mentoring practice.

3. Arrange to spend one hour at your mentoring practice. Observe and record the activities and attitudes of the staff while you are present. Comment on what you learned about how the staff works.

Staff Member 1   Staff Member 2   Staff Member 3   Staff Member 4   Staff Member 5

Job: _____

Activities and attitudes observed:

1. _____
2. _____
3. _____
4. _____
5. _____
6. _____
7. _____
8. _____
9. _____
10. _____

What I learned from the staff:

1. _____
2. _____
3. _____
4. _____
5. _____
6. _____
7. _____
8. _____
9. _____

4. Interview the managing partner, asking the questions listed below. Audiotape the interview or prepare a one-page paper and deliver it to your class.

a. How will health care reform affect the practice?

b. What are the most difficult ethical issues the practice faces?

c. What malpractice issues occur in this type of specialty?
   Does the physician wish to offer an opinion about costs and issues involved in malpractice?

Store the printed and recorded portfolio items in your folder or portfolio.

Patient Relations

One of the greatest pleasures of the medical assistant's job is working with patients. The positive relationships you develop as a medical assistant will depend on your interpersonal skills, communication techniques, and confidence level. Remember that the success of the practice and your career is directly tied to high quality service and caring attitudes. Therefore, beginning with the patient's first visit and continuing during all successive appointments, you should put yourself in the patient's place. In addition to their physical discomforts, patients may be uncomfortable and anxious. They need to be shown empathy and a caring attitude.

Exciting developments in communication technology add a new dimension to interaction with patients. As a medical assistant, you will learn how to contact people and information sources all over the world with a single phone call. You must remember, however, to use technology to enhance your relationships with patients without allowing it to form a "technology barrier." The human touch supplemented by technological support is the balance you hope to achieve.

The next three chapters focus on your relationship with patients. The chapters on patient interaction, scheduling, and telephoning offer concrete suggestions for forming relationships with patients, coordinating patient visits, and for placing and taking telephone calls.

Chapter 5

Interacting with Patients

MCALLEN, TEXAS

I love my job, but some days it can really get to me. We are a small, family-oriented practice, and my three physicians see a lot of pediatric patients. First thing this morning, the waiting room was filled with babies scheduled for inoculations and routine checkups, as well as two children with suspected measles. I put the children with suspected measles in a private room away from the others. Then, suddenly the door burst open, and three big oilmen came in carrying a person with a head injury. What a commotion! All the babies started to cry at one time; blood was dripping on the carpet; and the men seemed to overpower the room. "Gentlemen," I said, almost as if I had expected them, "Come this way. The doctor will be right with you." I put them in one of the examining rooms and let the nurse know they were there. I went back to the waiting room with a damp cloth for the blood on the carpet. One of the pregnant mothers, Mrs. Kawang, had fainted. The babies were still crying, and the other mothers were gathered around Mrs. Kawang. I got the nurse for her, asked another mother to take the toddlers off to the play corner, handed out tissues and crackers and cleaned up the blood.

Luckily, we have a back entrance. When the ambulance came, I directed the paramedics to the back, so that the injured patient and his three compadres wouldn't disturb our smallest patients further.

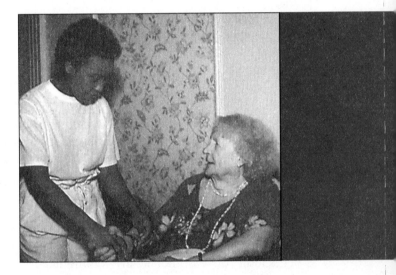

I needed all my verbal and nonverbal communication skills to maintain control in the waiting room. Working with patients is a challenge, and no two days are alike. With a day that started like this, I don't think I'll get my month-end report finished by 5:00.

Andres Munoz
Medical Assistant

PERFORMANCE BASED COMPETENCIES

After completing this chapter, you should be able to:
1. Compare and contrast appropriate and inappropriate behaviors for a medical assistant interacting with patients. (DACUM 1.6)

2. Demonstrate nonverbal behaviors you can use to show that you are listening to the patient. (DACUM 2.1, 2.4)

3. Prioritize interpersonal skills necessary for a medical assistant when dealing with patients. (DACUM 2.2, 2.3)

4. Analyze the effect of excessive paperwork and record keeping on a medical assistant's relationships with patients. (DACUM 1.5, 1.7, 2.7)

5. Establish guidelines for a well-managed reception area. (DACUM 6.1)

6. Compare and contrast the procedures for handling a walk-in emergency patient and a call-in emergency patient. (DACUM 4.3)

HEALTHSPEAK

Active listening Conscious attention to the speaker, asking open-ended questions that elicit additional information, and using verbal and nonverbal skills to provide feedback.

Empathy Mentally putting oneself in another's situation.

Feedback Responses that provide direction.

Interpersonal From one person to another.

Nonverbal communication The signals humans send out without speaking, including facial expressions, gestures, posture, and appearance.

Tact Diplomacy in handling difficult situations.

Have you ever been shopping in a grocery store, and felt that the checkout clerk did not even know that you were there? He or she was so busy having a personal conversation with another checker that the two of you didn't even make eye contact! How did that make you feel? On the other hand, have you ever had a shopping experience in which the salesperson gave you time and personal attention, and told you about your choices without patronizing or rushing you? How did that make you feel about that store and that purchase?

Patients are customers too—customers of medical goods and services. Sometimes they are anxious because they or their family members are ill. They can also be upset because of the confusing nature of medical terminology and baffling regulations about insurance procedures. As with any other customer, you want patients to feel confident they are receiving high quality service from caring people.

A medical assistant, often the receptionist who answers the telephone or greets visitors, provides the first impression of a medical office. Since the first impression sets the tone for future relationships, as a medical assistant your role is very important. You must make certain that the patient feels good about the first visit and will be comfortable about returning.

Interpersonal Communication

The term interpersonal communication refers to interaction among people. It is the way we relate to one another, the way we listen, and the way we look when we are listening. It is how we reassure and offer comfort in stressful situations and how we help people feel good about themselves. More people lose their jobs because of poor interpersonal skills than because of poor technical skills. A medical assistant who maintained an "A" average in school, knows the office routine perfectly, and possesses excellent technical skills will not succeed without good interpersonal skills.

Studies completed by the American Medical Association show that most medical malpractice suits could have been avoided if patients had felt they were listened to and that their questions were answered. Your attitude, speech and behavior are vital components of the caring, professional climate which is part of the service your office provides to its medical "customers."

This chapter discusses several behaviors necessary for good interpersonal relations in the medical office. Your employer hires not only your medical and office skills, but also your behavior while in the work place. As you read this chapter, think about words and atti-

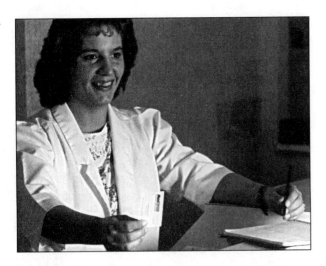

FIGURE 5-1 Smiling not only makes patient feel more comfortable but conveys a positive attitude. (From Krebs and Wise, *Medical Assisting, Clinical Competencies,* copyright 1994, Delmar Publishers)

tudes that will help you deserve your paycheck.

CONCERN FOR THE PATIENT

Most people are not in the doctor's office because they want to be there. They have no desire to be ill or injured; their normal routine is interrupted; and they are in an unfamiliar environment, which may make them feel out of control. To put patients at ease, greet them courteously and treat them with respect. Use the patient's full name, "Mrs. Stevenson" instead of "Mary," to show respect. A few words of greeting will also make them more comfortable.

Concern for people shows through your tone of voice, words, and actions. Since emotional sensitivity is higher when a person is sick, patients may be offended by an attitude, manner, or remark that would be completely normal in other circumstances, or they may read more into your words than you meant to communicate. You should choose your words carefully, use a soothing tone of voice, and display a professional manner. In the following examples, consider how the words and actions demonstrate that the medical assistant cares for the patient.

"Mrs. Guiterrez, how nice to see you today. I'm sorry it's so wet out. Would you like me to hang your raincoat in the hallway?"

Important Points: *(1) The medical assistant makes Mrs. Guiterrez feel that her comfort is important. (2) The medical assistant assumes partial responsibility for the coat and acknowledges that Mrs. Guiterrez has had to come out in bad weather, which establishes an "I am sorry for your inconvenience" attitude that will carry over to other aspects of the patient's care.*

"Good morning, Mr. Akkim. How is Elena's throat? The flu season has been very bad this year. She's still coughing a lot? The doctor will want to hear that."

Important Points: *(1) The medical assistant through words and tone of voice tells the patient, "I care about you." (2) The medical assistant remembers the patient's problem, which makes the person feel important. (3) The medical assistant reassures the patient about the care she will receive.*

"Hello, Ms. Costanzo. It's been a long time since we've seen you. You must have been taking good care of yourself! Has a year really passed since your last examination? I'm glad to see you again."

Important Points: *(1) The medical assistant pays Ms. Costanzo a compliment by suggesting that her good health is the result of her own actions. (2) The medical assistant implies "I like you" by saying "I am glad to see you again."*

LISTENING

Perhaps even more important than what you say to patients is how you listen to them. Listening shows respect for patients as human beings, not just as purchasers of medical service. You show patients that you are listening by facing them and making good eye contact, and by setting aside all other work while speaking with them. Have you ever tried to converse with someone who was looking at papers on a desk? Although the person said, "Go on, I'm listening," you probably didn't feel as though you had complete attention. Patients will know, too, when you are not listening attentively. A crowded waiting room is a very distracting environment, and you may find yourself unable to give patients your full attention right at the moment they arrive. When this is the case, acknowledge the patient's presence by saying, "Mr. Faust, we are very busy today. Please have a seat, and I will be with you as soon as I can."

EMPATHY

Empathy refers to understanding another's feelings and sensitively responding to those feelings. Empathy means putting yourself mentally in another's place. An empathetic medical assistant understands and offers comfort when a patient is anxious or in pain. Empathy is also important when dealing with relatives and friends of patients because they are worried, too. Consider the medical assistant's behavior in the two following situations. Does the medical assistant communicate empathy?

"Mrs. Robinette, I know how concerned you are about your mother's condition. The doctor will be able to tell you more about what you both can expect as she recovers."

Important Points: (1) The medical assistant tries to reassure the daughter. (2) The medical assistant doesn't make promises about the condition improving quickly.

(Interaction with a child.) "Don't worry, Raphael, if you can't give us a urine sample right now. You can try again before you leave the office. If that doesn't work, we'll give you a plastic container you can take home. Your mom can bring your sample back tomorrow."

Important Points: (1) The medical assistant tries to set the child at ease and does not embarrass him because he can't provide a urine sample immediately. (2) The medical assistant gives the child an alternative to providing a sample at the office, which relieves the child's stress.

You may not like every patient you meet, and you may not like some of the patients all of the time. But remember, you are paid to treat them courteously and professionally, not to like them.

TACT

Tact means taking an uncomfortable situation and turning it into a comfortable situation. A tactful person is diplomatic and uses good judgment when working with other people. Most of us would not say, "Are you pregnant, or have you just gained a lot of weight?," or "Simone seems awfully small for her age. Are you sure she's all right?" In a medical office, the situations requiring tact are less personal but just as important. The patient who owes the physician money must be tactfully reminded to pay; the person who disturbs the reception area by talking loudly should be asked to speak more quietly; and the child who enters the treatment area often to go to the bathroom should be requested to remain in the reception area.

Most people know the difference between tact and tactlessness and strive to be tactful. Unfortunately, medical assistants who don't understand the effect of tactless comments and actions may jeopardize their jobs. Consider this situation. Did the medical assistant handle the situation tactfully?

Patient:	These insurance companies are robber barons. I paid my insurance every month for thirty years, and now the company won't cover my wife's operation.
Medical Assistant:	It can be very frustrating when you are not used to the insurance paperwork. Is there anything about your coverage that you do not understand?

Important Points: (1) The medical assistant validates the patient's feelings by acknowledging them and offers to help explain the forms. (2) The medical assistant remains in control and does not make unprofessional remarks about insurance companies.

Here is another example.

"I'll leave the room while you undress, Miss Trollinger. Please remove your slacks and cover yourself from the waist down with this sheet (or gown). The doctor needs to check your abdomen and pelvis. You may wear your shirt."

Important Points: (1) The medical assistant, who is aware of the patient's modesty, leaves the room while the patient undresses. (2) The medical assistant provides explicit instructions about which clothes should be removed. (3) The medical assistant tells the patient the type of examination to expect.

PATIENCE

Perhaps no human relations skill is as important to a medical assistant as patience. Being patient means that you do not show anger or irritation, even when patients are angry and irritable. Patients do not want to be sick, they do not want to wait, they do not want to incur large expenses for health care; they do not want to be frustrated by confusing paperwork or worried by unfamiliar medical terminology. They are likely to be bothered by any or all of the above when you see them and, as a result, may sound as if they are being rude when actually they are frightened. You, as a medical assistant, cannot make them well, pay their bills, or take away all of their fears. What you can do is greet them calmly and courteously, listen attentively, and treat them with patience (Figure 5-2). Their anger is not directed at you, although it may seem so at times.

Patience often involves waiting—waiting for people to undress or dress, give you information, or pay their bill. You may want to hurry them, interrupt their sentences, or speed things up so you can move on to the next task. When you feel yourself becoming impatient, maintain your self-control, breathe deeply, smile, and look for realistic ways to remedy the problem. Consider these situations.

The reception area is crowded because an obstetrics patient in labor needed the physician at 4:00 a.m., and the doctor has not arrived at the office yet. Although waiting patients were understanding and gracious when they heard about the emergency, they are complaining to one another now about the delay, and several are irritable. One patient asks if she can be placed ahead of others.

"Mrs. Parella, I'm sorry you've been delayed. Only three people remain ahead of you; and they, too, want to leave. Your wait will not be much longer, at most thirty minutes. You may reschedule the appointment if you like, or if you have errands close by, perhaps you could do a few chores and come back in about thirty minutes."

Important Points: (1) The medical assistant recognizes that the patient's point is valid and that the wait has been long. (2) The medical assistant tries to give the patient a time frame for any additional wait and offers an alternative to waiting. (3) The medical assistant does not place this patient ahead of others.

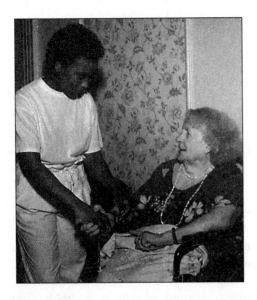

FIGURE 5-2 Patience is probably the most important human relations skill a medical assistant can possess. (From Hegner and Caldwell, *Nursing Assistant,* 7th Ed., copyright 1995, Delmar Publishers)

(Interaction with an elderly person.) "Mr. Nuyen, we'll take all the time you need to walk down this hall slowly; we're not in any hurry. Would you like to hold my arm?"

Important Points: (1) The medical assistant recognizes that the elderly patient has difficulty walking but attempts to put the patient at ease by implying, "It's all right to walk slowly." (2) The medical assistant gives the patient the option of an arm to hold but does not insist, recognizing that the patient may prefer to walk without help.

Efficiency and impatience should not be confused. Efficiency means making good use of available time, whereas impatience refers to being rushed or hurried. You may feel conflict as you try to complete your paperwork and office chores and still give patients the time and courtesy they require. Review the list in Figure 5-3 to determine whether you are susceptible to impatient behavior. If you are susceptible, work to reduce your impatience.

Importance of Oral and Nonverbal Communication

The words that come out of our mouths are known collectively as oral communication, but we all have many other ways of expressing our thoughts and feelings. Messages that aren't written and don't use spoken words are called nonverbal communication. Consider the following examples:

"I'm not angry," she says, but her mouth is tight, her shoulders tense, and she stalks out of the room. What nonverbal message does she deliver? Does it agree with her oral communication?

"You're such a bad boy," a father tells his infant, smiling tenderly and tickling the baby's tummy. Are you listening to the words or paying attention to the actions? What is the father's real message?

When working with patients, you must be careful that your oral and nonverbal communication sends the same message and that both forms are appropriate to the circumstances; otherwise, you may confuse, hurt, or offend someone. Consider the following situation. Do you think the medical assistant's verbal and nonverbal messages agree?

Impatient Behavior

Rushing patients

Finishing other people's sentences

Interrupting people

Feeling stressed

Feeling the urgency of time

Planning too far in advance

Skipping lunch or eating too fast at lunch

Looking at a clock often

Trying to do two things at once

Answering questions curtly

Taking on too many projects

FIGURE 5-3 Impatient behavior

The medical assistant is explaining office policy and procedures to a new patient. The assistant does not make eye contact with the patient, and her tone of voice is bored and flat.

"We strive to maintain a friendly, caring environment for all of our patients and want to hear your questions and concerns."

How likely is the new patient to have questions and concerns? Does the medical assistant's communication convey a real sense of caring?

ORAL COMMUNICATION

Oral communication refers to spoken messages and includes face-to-face encounters, announcements, questions, offhand remarks, telephone conversations, gossip, and other forms of communication. Successful communication depends on correct word choice and on the listener's understanding of what you say.

Many factors influence the communication process and affect understanding between communicators, including level of education, economic status, prior experiences, and cultural heritage (Figure 5-4). Because no universal meaning for words exists in people's minds, each person defines words based on his or her influencing factors. The greater the difference in backgrounds between communicators, the more

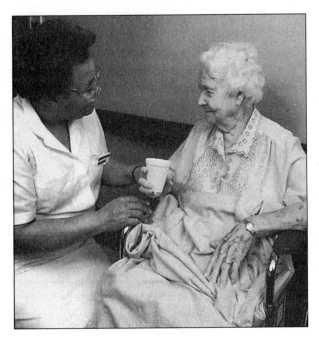

FIGURE 5-4 Many factors influence the process of verbal communication. What might some of those factors be in the face-to-face encounter shown here? (From Hegner and Caldwell, *Nursing Assistant,* 7th Ed., copyright 1995, Delmar Publishers)

difficulty they may encounter in understanding one another.

A patient who complains of a high fever may mean a temperature of 100 degrees, but the medical assistant may think of a "high" fever as anything above 102 degrees. If you advise a patient that the doctor is a "few minutes" behind schedule, your internal clock, the way you measure time, may be different from the patient's. The patient who expects to see the physician in ten or fifteen minutes may become angry at having to wait thirty or forty-five minutes. In each of these examples, you should be specific and avoid using general adjectives. You should ask the patient how high the temperature has been and provide an estimate of the length of the wait by saying, "Dr. Papastamou is about thirty minutes behind schedule."

As a medical assistant, you must be particularly careful about using technical or medical terms beyond the scope of the patient's understanding. Some people use technical words to impress the listener or to prove their superior knowledge. New employees or recent graduates, especially, may feel more important by using big words to show how smart they are. If you are confident of your education, you will recognize that use of medical words does not necessarily demonstrate knowledge, and you should not display your vocabulary at the expense of a patient's understanding or comfort. Consider this example.

"Mrs. Riser, here's a pamphlet on Lou Gehrig's disease that Dr. Valenti asked me to give you. It will help you understand your husband's illness. You'll notice from the pamphlet that weakness of the hand muscles is an early symptom."

This medical assistant knows that the patient will not understand medical language and uses layman's language to discuss the medical condition. A less informed medical assistant might have communicated in the following manner:

"Mrs. Riser, here's a pamphlet on amyotrophic lateral sclerosis that Dr. Valenti asked me to give you. The etiology of this disease is unknown; however, the pamphlet will help you understand your husband's illness. You'll notice from the pamphlet that atrophy of the hand muscles is an early symptom."

NONVERBAL COMMUNICATION

Nonverbal communication refers to messages sent without words or in addition to words. It includes facial expressions, touch, tone of voice, listening, eye contact, gestures, appearance, manner, time, body language, silence, and other nonverbal behavior (Figure 5-5). Every person sends and receives hundreds of nonverbal messages daily. They enhance the communication process and should be used by both the sender and the receiver to confirm verbal messages.

Nonverbal communication is important to any relationship, and this is especially true with people who are sick, uncomfortable, or anxious. If you are working with a diverse population, with patients from many different backgrounds and cultures, you will need to be especially sensitive and knowledgeable. In some cultures, touching the patient is not appropriate. This is a sign of disrespect. Your competence in using and interpreting nonverbal behavior will determine the degree of success you enjoy in your relationships with others. Several important nonverbal behaviors are explained in Figure 5-6.

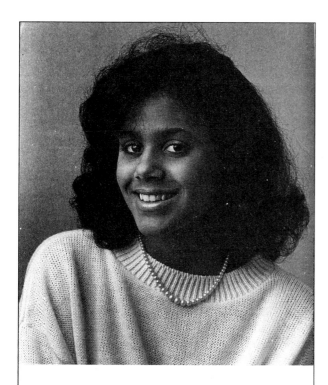

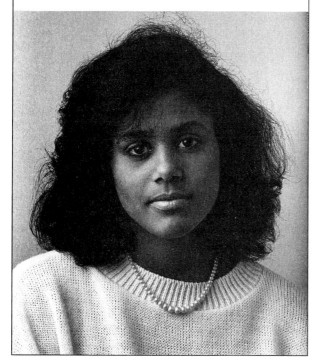

FIGURE 5-5 Facial expressions provide clues about how someone feels physically and emotionally.

Facial Expression
Appropriate Medical Assistant Facial Expression
- Responsive
- Alert
- Good eye contact
Revealing Patient Facial Expression
- Eyes looking away or down
- Frowning or sad expression
- Stare or unfocused look
- Thankful glance

Touch
Appropriate Medical Assistant Touch
- Firm handshake
- Light touch on arm or shoulder
- Guiding touch on elbow
Revealing Patient Touch
- Demanding grasp
- Grateful pat
- Attention-getting tap

Posture
Appropriate Medical Assistant Posture
- Upright
- Facing speaker
- "Open" posture; arms unfolded
- Relaxed, few distracting movements
Revealing Patient Posture
- Limping or otherwise showing pain
- "Closed" posture, feeling threatened
- Slumping, weary

Tone of Voice
Appropriate Tone of Voice for Medical Assistant
- Pleasant, clear
Revealing Patient Tone of Voice
- Sad
- Worried
- Fearful
- Bewildered

FIGURE 5-6 Nonverbal behavior

FEEDBACK

Feedback refers to responses to a communication; they may be verbal or nonverbal, positive or negative. Feedback is important when working with patients because it provides clues about the person's health that the patient may not articulate. As a medical assistant, you should be alert to patient feedback and use it to determine whether the patient's verbal and nonverbal messages agree. For example, the patient who replies, "Not really," and shrugs when the medical assistant asks, "Do you experience chest pains often?" may really mean "I experience chest pain enough that it bothers me, but I am frightened to talk about it." The answer, "Not really," therefore may mean "Yes." The shoulder shrug represents nonverbal feedback and should alert the medical assistant to ask additional questions: "When is the last time you experienced chest pain?", "How long did it last?", and "When was the time prior to the last time? Tell me about that time." The patient's posture, hand gestures, eye movement, and tone of voice are important clues to how the patient is feeling.

Computers and Relationships with Patients

Complex tasks involving mountains of data make computers indispensable in modern medical offices. Computers organize and maintain patient records, reduce appointment scheduling conflicts, bill patients, complete insurance forms, and perform a wide variety of other time-saving duties. The disadvantages occur when computerization reduces the interaction between the medical staff and patients or complicates interpersonal relationships.

You may get caught up in the task you are trying to complete on a computer and forget to make proper eye contact with patients (Figure 5-7). One good rule is to be out of sight of patients if you are busy with paperwork and record keeping, especially if the waiting area is full and many people are waiting in line. Speak with your office manager about such an arrangement.

As the use of computers in medical offices increases and takes over many of the clerical tasks assigned to medical assistants, you may work with patients on a one-to-one basis less frequently. You must continue to show empathy and understanding for each patient's individual problems. For example, the patient who questions a billing statement and insists that he mailed a check to cover a previous balance is rightly concerned about a possible lost check. As a medical assistant, you should review the

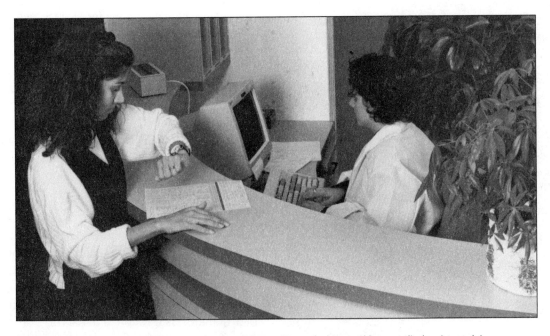

FIGURE 5-7 Patients who are waiting to be served do not like to feel ignored by a medical assistant doing record keeping.

patient's account immediately to determine whether a check was received and, if so, when it was received. Don't rely on the excuse of "computer error." The last thing a patient wants to hear about is your internal office problems.

In a medical office where patients' anxiety levels are related to a physical condition, computer errors become magnified and may cause extreme stress. You should be careful to avoid computer errors when possible and correct them if they do occur.

While you may spend much of your time at a computer keyboard, make sure that you always greet patients with a warm "hello" and spend a minute or so in a brief "good-bye" when the patient pays for the day's services. If you have time to chat with a patient, stand so you and the patient are on the same face-to-face level. Whether you are seated at your computer station or standing, maintain eye contact as you take part in each conversation.

Several danger signals for the medical assistant who uses computers are listed here. Can you add other Do Nots to this list?

1. *Do not* allow the computer to interfere with your relationships with patients.
2. *Do not* key data into a computer at the same time you talk with patients either in person or on the telephone.
3. *Do not* blame a computer for human errors.
4. *Do not* assume that mistakes will be eliminated when a computer is used. If computer input is flawed, a mistake will occur.
5. *Do not* allow patients to feel that they are merely accounts; they are people.
6. *Do not* refer to patients as numbers, for example, Patient No. 1602, or by their diagnosis; "the diabetic in 4."
7. *Do not* ask patients to wait several weeks for a computer correction of a billing or related problem.
8. *Do not* allow computerization to reduce your level of service to patients. If a patient makes a special request, follow up on it manually if the computer software does not allow the request; for example, typing a special billing for a particular month.
9. *Do not* send impersonal, computerized form letters to patients.

Managing Patient Activities

A medical assistant manages many different patient activities each day. The effectiveness with which you accomplish these tasks will depend on your organizational and interpersonal skills.

MANAGING THE RECEPTION AREA OR LOBBY

Managing the reception area or lobby is a constant challenge, especially during high traffic times. Since the reception area offers patients a comfortable place to rest while they wait to see the doctor and also provides the medical assistant with a means for monitoring patient traffic, you will be responsible for maintaining a gracious and tranquil environment. This means you must eliminate noisy play or running among children, ask patients to chat quietly, and remind smokers to move to the appropriate areas. Patients weeping or in obvious distress should be moved to a private office.

"Mr. Markham, you probably didn't notice our sign that this is a nonsmoking office. We've set aside a place just outside the reception area for our patients who like to smoke. You may go there and smoke if you like."

Important Points: *(1) The medical assistant suggests the patient did not see the sign. (2) The medical assistant suggests an alternative smoking area.*

Reception Area Appearance

Since the appearance of the reception area conveys a message about the organization of the medical office, it should be clean and inviting. Follow these procedures to create an attractive, pleasant place for patients to wait:

1. Arrange magazines in an orderly manner in a central location where they can be located easily. Discard magazines when they become outdated or tattered.
2. Discard dead or unattractive plants.
3. Reorganize children's toys several times during the day. Encourage children to keep toys within the area designated for play.
4. Arrange seating so that patients can chat, but make sure a few chairs provide privacy for patients who do not wish to socialize.
5. Use lighting to create a warm effect and provide good reading light near magazine stands and chairs.
6. Straighten crooked lamp shades.
7. Play soft and soothing music to create a relaxing atmosphere (Figure 5-8).

Orderly Flow of Patient Traffic

If possible, you should have an unobstructed view of the lobby entrance and the examining area entrance from your desk. Attach a bell or other device at the lobby entrance, if you cannot see it clearly, so you will know when a patient arrives. Check periodically to see that seating is available for everyone. Follow these procedures:

1. Answer the telephone before the third ring, if possible. An unanswered telephone is annoying both to patients waiting in the lobby and to the caller.
2. Complete the checkout procedure for patients who are ready to leave before registering new arrivals. (This procedure is discussed in detail in the following chapters.)
3. Ask arriving patients to sign the registration pad. Then suggest they take a seat until you have completed all checkouts. Call the patients back individually to the registration desk when other traffic has slowed.

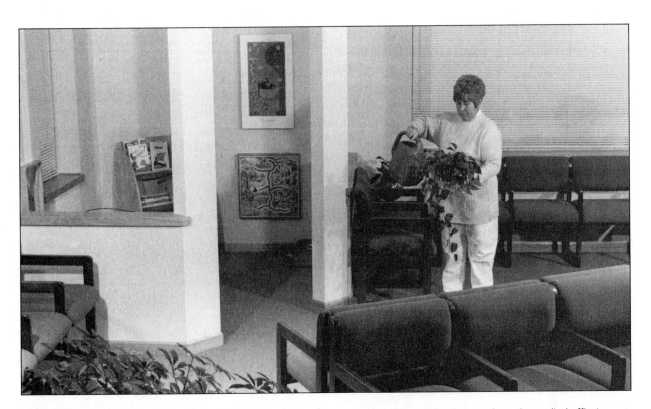

FIGURE 5-8 Both the physical appearance and the atmosphere of the reception area convey a message about the medical office's organization.

GREETING PATIENTS

Greet patients immediately when they walk into the office. If you are busy with a task that cannot be interrupted, stop long enough to say, "Hello, I'll be with you in just a minute." Finish your task quickly or find a logical stopping place; then give your full attention to the patient. If you are talking on the telephone, acknowledge the patient's arrival with a friendly nod and a smile. Finish your conversation as quickly as possible. Then help the arriving patient. Never wait more than one minute to greet a patient.

Medical assistant who is conducting a telephone conversation with another person gives a friendly smile and a welcoming nod when a patient arrives at the office. After finishing the telephone conversation, the medical assistant greets the patient:

"Good morning, Mr. Kapadia, how are you this morning? I hope you're feeling better."

Established Patients

Established patients know the office routine and usually sit and read or chat with other patients after checking in. They generally do not require a great deal of attention after they have registered with the receptionist; however, you should be alert to any special problems and help as needed. In this example an alert medical assistant makes the patient more comfortable.

An elderly patient on crutches is brought to the physician by her son, who must return to work. The patient looks confused and anxious as the lobby fills with other patients. The assistant asks,

"Mrs. Allenton, would you like to sit in Dr. Brader's office while you wait? I'll bring a magazine in for you to read, and you can call the nurses if you need anything. I think you may be more comfortable in the doctor's office."

Important Points: *(1) The medical assistant recognizes that the crowded lobby and the long wait may bother the patient. (2) The medical assistant tries to relieve the patient's stress by moving her away from other patients.*

New Patients

New patients require instruction in the registration procedure and office routine. Follow these procedures to orient new patients to the medical office:

1. Ask each new patient to sign the register; then give the person a pen or pencil and a patient information questionnaire. If the new patient is illiterate or speaks English as a second language, ask the questions from the form; give the patient ample time to rspond; and then fill in the answers yourself.
2. Give new patients a pamphlet describing the office's billing practice, payment policy, business hours, telephone policies, and after-hours emergency procedures. Explain the policies if a pamphlet is not available.
3. Provide the names of all doctors sharing the practice and the names of the hospitals where the primary care physician is affiliated.
4. Ask the patient if he or she has questions, and answer them completely.
5. Show the patient where to sit when registration is complete. Point out the magazines and the water fountain and say that the physician will see the patient shortly.
6. Give the room number and ask the patient to follow you or the nurse to the treatment area.

A student at the local high school, a recent immigrant who lives with his single mother and brothers and sisters, has been referred to the medical office by the physical education teacher who senses that the teenager's recent absences may be due to an untreated physical problem. The medical assistant recognizes that the student has trouble with English.

"I need to ask you some questions for the doctor's records, so he can treat you. I will ask each question slowly. You tell me the answer, and I will write it on this form for the doctor to study." (After completing the form.) "Come with me, and I will show you where the doctor's office is located. He will want to talk with you before he examines you."

Important Points: *(1) The medical assistant explains why the questions are being asked. (2) The medical assistant walks with the patient to the doctor's office.*

Discussing Finances and Billing

Discussing finances with patients may feel awkward at first, particularly with patients who have difficulty paying their bills. Yet the ability of the practice to pay employees, suppliers, the landlord, and others depends on steady income from patients. You should maintain a relationship with patients that encourages open discussion about finances and billing. After all, it is the best interest of the patient and the doctor that you clarify with patients how their bill will be handled.

IMPORTANCE OF THE FIRST VISIT

The best opportunity to discuss finances and billing is at the patient's first visit. You should provide the patient with a written copy of the practice's payment policy and then orally review the policy, explaining any unfamiliar terms. If the patient has questions, answer them fully. A patient's frown or an uncertain or skeptical look are examples of body language that should alert you to review and clarify the payment policy.

"Ms. Klavens, Dr. Becca requires payment at the completion of medical services. In the case of your surgery, the total fee will be $1260." *(The patient states that her insurance company will be responsible for paying the fee. The medical assistant acknowledges the patient's insurance and explains that the patient must pay the physician first and then collect from the insurance company.)*

"Our policy is to ask the patient to pay the doctor's fee at the time of service; then you can file a claim with your insurance company for reimbursement. I will show you how to complete the insurance form if you like." *(The medical assistant notices that the patient is moving nervously in her chair as if she wants to speak but is uncertain.)*

"If you prefer, we can create a financial contract that allows you to pay a portion of the fee each month. A small finance charge will be added as a part of the contract."

INSURANCE COMPANY PAYMENTS

Although most patients are covered by health insurance, the patient or the patient's guardian is responsible for payment of the account when the insurance doesn't. Patients may think the insurance company will pay the entire physician's fee, but this is not always true. Private insurance and government-funded programs, such as Medicare, do not pay the total cost for many medical procedures. Therefore, you must explain to patients their responsibility to pay the balance of the bill. In the initial conversation to explain billing, you should be sure the patient understands the payment procedure in order to avoid future misunderstandings.

Medical Assistant:	Mr. Carberry, many insurance companies pay only a portion of your claim. Usually, you are responsible for paying a deductible amount of approximately 20 percent. That is why you were not reimbursed in full for Dr. Giuiella's fees.
Patient:	These darned insurance companies, you think you're covered and then you're not. How would you like to explain that, young lady? How am I supposed to make heads or tails of this insurance lingo? Doctors, insurance companies, they're all in it together.
Medical Assistant:	I can certainly see why you are upset. Is there someone at your company who can explain these forms to you? Or would you like me to make an appointment for you with our financial aid person?

Handling Emergencies

Emergencies will severely test your interpersonal skills. You may feel upset personally, while feeling responsible for keeping a calm atmosphere for the other patients, in addition to interrupting the daily schedule, walk-in emergency patients raise the anxiety level of people waiting in the reception area when the emergency patient's suffering is visible. Call-in emergency patients force the staff to change its daily schedule, and sometimes the physician may have to leave the office to attend the emergency.

RECOGNIZING AN EMERGENCY

An emergency is clearly apparent when a patient bleeds profusely, appears catatonic, shakes violently, is short of breath, complains of chest pains, or demonstrates any other symptoms that indicate severe illness. However, emergencies that are not as easy to identify, such as internal bleeding, blood clots, or allergic reactions, are potentially more harmful because if left untreated, they become life threatening. In addition, some acute illnesses, such as strep throat accompanied by a high fever, are considered emergencies by the patient, but they do not actually represent an illness for which the physician should be interrupted. The difficult responsibility of screening emergency calls goes to the medical assistant who greets patients and answers the telephone. If you have a question about whether an apparent emergency is real, you should alert the physician immediately. You do not have the medical background or the authority to determine what is an emergency and what is not. To attempt to make this decision is practicing medicine without a license and can be the basis for a malpractice lawsuit (see Chapter 4).

Whether an emergency patient arrives at the medical office or the emergency is telephoned, certain problems represent serious, potentially life-threatening situations and must receive priority status. Figure 5-9 lists examples of life-threatening emergencies.

OBTAINING SPECIFIC INFORMATION ABOUT CALL-IN EMERGENCY PATIENTS

Emergencies reported by telephone are difficult to identify because you cannot see the patient, yet you must obtain enough information to determine whether the physician should be interrupted. If a telephone caller is hysterical, crying, or too excited to provide precise information, ask the caller to put another person on the line if possible.

Medical Emergencies

Heart attack

Drug overdose

Profuse bleeding from a head or chest wound

Damage to eye

Allergic reactions (such as to a bee sting or to food)

Poisoning

Burns

Suicidal behavior

Premature labor

Foreign objects in windpipe

Extreme fever in adults

Gunshot wound

Car accident

FIGURE 5-9 Emergency medical situations

You can increase the efficient handling of an emergency by remaining calm and composed. Before emergencies arise, ask the physician to help you prepare a list of questions to ask in specific situations, such as a heart attack or premature labor. Then ask these questions each time you receive an emergency call. Several general questions are provided in the following list. Discuss these with your employer and add others appropriate for the medical specialty.

1. The name of the patient and the relationship of the caller? (Wife, mother, brother, friend, passerby?)
2. The nature of the emergency? (What happened?)
3. When the emergency occurred? (What time? Today?)
4. The extent of the emergency? (How bad?)
5. The patient's symptoms? (Is the patient bleeding? Profusely?)
6. Treatment provided? (What has been done for the patient?)
7. Has an ambulance been called? (Will the patient receive treatment from a rescue team?)
8. The name of the patient's physician? (Is your employer the patient's primary care physician?)

The situations described here demonstrate the proper method for screening emergency calls. If a caller indicates that an emergency is taking place, alert the physician immediately.

Caller:	I need to talk to the doctor right away. I'm five months pregnant, and I think I'm in labor.
Medical Assistant:	What is your name, please?
Caller:	Amelia Greene, but I need to talk to Dr. Moskowitz.
Medical Assistant:	I will get Dr. Moskowitz, but I need to be able to tell her your symptoms. Are you in pain?
Caller:	I have awful stomach cramps.
Medical Assistant:	Do you have back pain?
Caller:	No, not really, but the stomach pains make me hurt all over.
Medical Assistant:	Are you spotting blood?
Caller:	No.
Medical Assistant:	Have you lost any clear fluid from your vagina?
Caller:	No.
Medical Assistant:	Do you have a fever?
Caller:	I didn't take my temperature, but I don't feel hot.
Medical Assistant:	Is this your first pregnancy?
Caller:	Yes.
Medical Assistant:	When did you eat last?
Caller:	I had lunch with a friend about three hours ago.
Medical Assistant:	Did your pains start before or after lunch?
Caller:	After lunch.
Medical Assistant:	What telephone number are you calling from?
Caller:	555-4580. Are you getting Dr. Moskowitz?
Medical Assistant:	Dr. Moskowitz is treating another patient, but she should be finished in about five minutes. I will tell her about your symptoms immediately, and she will call you back.

The medical assistant in this situation used a list of questions prepared in advance by the physician. The medical assistant may suspect that the patient is suffering stomach cramps from lunch, but he does not have the medical background or the authority to make such a decision. The physician is notified immediately since this problem represents a potential emergency.

Caller:	My baby isn't breathing! Give me the doctor!
Medical Assistant:	I'm sorry; I can't understand you. Say that again.
Caller:	I want to talk to Dr. Petty! Right now!
Medical Assistant:	Is someone with you? I can't understand you. Please put another person on the phone.
Neighbor:	This is Myra Broadhurst.
Medical Assistant:	What is the patient's name and the problem?
Neighbor:	It's Matthew Johnson; he's eight months old, and he's having a convulsion.
Medical Assistant:	What are Matthew's symptoms?
Neighbor:	He's been sick for about four days, and today he's been listless. About ten minutes ago he cried out; then he went stiff, and now he's motionless. I think he's still breathing.
Medical Assistant:	What is the baby's temperature?
Neighbor:	He's had a high fever for two days; just about an hour ago it was 105 degrees.
Medical Assistant:	Do you have a car to take the baby to the hospital emergency room?
Neighbor:	Yes.
Medical Assistant:	Hold on just a minute while I get Dr. Petty.

This is an obvious emergency that the medical assistant recognizes should be referred to the physician. However, the medical assistant obtains specific information for the physician before interrupting another patient's treatment.

ARRANGING FOR EMERGENCY MEDICAL CARE

Immediate treatment should be provided for life-threatening emergencies. Follow these procedures for maximum efficiency in dealing with emergency patients:

1. As soon as an emergency patient appears, alert the physician and take the person to an examining room.
2. For emergencies reported by telephone, ask the physician whether the emergency patient should be brought to the office or taken directly to the hospital.

3. If the physician is out of the office briefly, ask the nurse what to do.
4. If both the physician and nurse are unavailable, tell the patient to go directly to a hospital emergency room.
5. After patients are referred to the hospital emergency room, call the emergency room to alert the staff that the patient is on the way. Give a description of the medical problem so the staff can prepare for the patient's examination. Locate the physician and provide full details about the emergency.
6. If the patient is an accident victim, call the police and provide the address of the accident. The dispatcher will send a rescue unit to the scene and alert the nearest emergency room that a patient is on the way. Once the patient has stabilized, a private ambulance can transport the person to any hospital the primary care physician designates.

REASSURING FAMILY AND WAITING PATIENTS

The medical assistant's responsibility does not end when the emergency patient receives treatment. You must reassure family members, who will be frightened, and other patients who witnessed the arrival of the emergency patient. To reduce confusion, take family members to a private room where they will not interfere with the physician's examination or further upset patients in the reception area. Check back often to answer the family's questions.

Advise patients waiting in the reception area that the emergency patient is being treated. Tell them you will let them know as soon as possible the length of delay in the physician's schedule. Some patients will ask questions about the emergency that are too private to share. Tactfully field these questions.

Curious Patient:	What happened to that man who was bleeding?
Medical Assistant:	He was in an accident.
Curious Patient:	What kind of accident? That looked like a gunshot wound.
Medical Assistant:	I don't know the details.

IN YOUR OPINION

1. How can the medical assistant assure a welcoming, uncluttered atmosphere in the waiting area, especially during busy times like flu season?
2. What are the most important things for the medical assistant to determine when answering an emergency call?
3. What would you do with a first-time patient who does not speak English very well, or read it at all, and who does not understand the payment terms?

REFERENCES

Humphrey, Doris, and Kathie Sigler. *The Modern Medical Office: A Reference Manual.* Cincinnati, Ohio: South-Western Publishing Co., 1990.*

Hyden, Janet, Ann Jordan, Mary Helen Steinauer, and Marjorie Jones. *Communicating for Success: An Applied Approach.* Cincinnati, Ohio: South-Western Publishing Co., 1994.

Smith, Leila R., and Yolanda V. Grisolia. *Communication and English for Careers.* Englewood Cliffs, New Jersey: Prentice-Hall, 1994.

*Currently published by Delmar Publishers

Chapter Activities

PERFORMANCE BASED ACTIVITIES

1. Create a plan for a welcoming reception area which would seem comforting. Two considerations are listed to help you with your planning. Add others that should be a part of your planning. List conditions or situations that should be eliminated or reduced.

Plan for a Reception Area

Furniture features to be considered	Lighting features to be considered	Other considerations
1.		
2.		
3.		
4.		
5.		
6.		

(DACUM 1.1, 1.3, 1.8, 6.1)

2. Compare behaviors that would be acceptable when you are among your family or friends but would not be appropriate in your position as medical assistant.

Work Situations	Personal Situations
1.	
2.	
3.	
4.	
5.	
6.	

(DACUM 1.6, 1.7, 2.1, 2.6)

3. Discuss your personal nonverbal behaviors with a classmate. Analyze how well you listen. (DACUM 2.1, 2.9)

4. An emergency situation affects each of the following: other medical assistants, nurses, doctors, waiting patients. Write a short paper describing how you can assist each. (DACUM 4.3, 6.6)

5. Establish guidelines for communication, including words and actions, when dealing with a bewildered, elderly, or foreign-born patient. (DACUM 1.6, 2.1, 2.2, 2.3)

6. Develop and print the dialogue you would have with a patient angry over confusing claim forms. Role play the dialogue with a classmate. (DACUM 2.3, 2.5, 3.3)

EXPANDING YOUR THINKING

1. Which situation would you give priority?

   a. A ringing phone or an arriving patient?

   b. A patient with a question or a patient ready to pay a bill?

   c. Retrieving a file for a doctor or updating a computer record?

   d. A messy waiting area or a late report?

   e. An arriving elderly patient or an arriving mother with infant?

   f. An angry patient or a weeping patient?

2. What could you say or do in each of the following situations to exemplify professional behavior?

   a. A patient is flirting with you.

   b. A child is throwing toys, and the child's mother does not seem to notice.

   c. A patient refuses to pay a bill.

   d. A patient wants to talk about a sick family member, and you have other pressing duties.

   e. A patient claims that he or she has been charged for services not provided.

3. What questions would you ask if you received each of the following emergency phone calls?

   a. "There's been a fire…"

   b. "My child fell off her bike."

   c. "There's been a diving accident at the quarry."

   d. "My mother has been asleep all day, and I can't wake her."

   e. "My husband was shoveling snow, and he collapsed."

Chapter 6

Telecommunications

ROCKFORD, ILLINOIS

I have to laugh when I talk to my mother about her days as a medical secretary. All of her reports were handwritten or typed with carbon paper for the copies. Can you imagine? We both shake our heads at the complexity of modern telecommunications. My office teammates and I are all thoroughly computer competent, but we also use the FAX machine, beepers, and pagers; arrange conference calls; call internationally; and often contact our physicians via cellular or car phones. Telecommunication manners are constantly evolving. In my office, we talk about the confidentiality aspects of using a speaker, portable, or car phone, and the proper procedure for putting and keeping patients on hold. I can't imagine how we could run our office without modern communication systems, but sometimes it seems that managing telecommunications is a full-time job in itself.

Linda Ruggerio
Medical Secretary

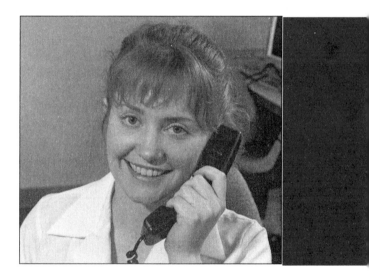

PERFORMANCE BASED COMPETENCIES

After completing this chapter, you should be able to:

1. Originate and respond to business telephone calls. (DACUM 2.8)

2. Formulate appropriate telephone greetings for a medical office. (DACUM 3.1)

3. Compare the advantages and disadvantages of station-to-station, person-to-person, direct-dialed and operator-assisted calls. (DACUM 2.8)

4. Discriminate between instances in which putting a caller on "hold" is acceptable and those in which it is unacceptable. (DACUM 2.6, 4.3)

5. Outline eight pieces of information needed for a callback message. (DACUM 2.5, 2.9)

6. Prepare a FAX message. (DACUM 3.1)

world to talk to another in a matter of minutes. The computer in your office may well have a modem, allowing you and other members of your office team to send and receive records, to access databases, and to tap medical resources worldwide.

Communicating by telephone will consume a major portion of your day as a medical assistant. Effective, courteous telephone communication will make you a valued asset in any medical environment. Whether a telephone conversation is about a patient's health, an appointment, a billing problem, or some other matter, each conversation is unique and must be handled in a professional manner. You will learn to handle multiple calls, some of which will be urgent. Your interviewing and analytical skills will help you determine rapidly (1) the nature of the call, (2) the urgency of the call, and (3) how to direct or respond to the call. Time is a scarce resource in the medical office, and your thoughtful, intelligent handling of telephone communications will improve efficient time management in your office.

Most physicians are rarely out of reach by phone. During your first days as a medical assistant, you may well be introduced to telecommunication technologies you have never seen before, including modems, cellular phones, beepers, and car phones. Knowing the scope and limitations of each type of technology will rapidly become part of your competence as a medical assistant.

The telephone links patients with the physician at all times by (1) ringing the medical office when a patient dials the correct number, (2) switching calls automatically to an answering service or answering machine when the office is closed, and (3) forwarding calls to a consulting physician when the primary care physician is unavailable. Telephone communication allows local and long-distance business transactions to be conducted quickly and efficiently. Long-distance service expands the local calling area to 500 billion telephones connected nationally and internationally. The convenience and communication capability of such a vast network is immense, allowing a person in one part of the

Answering the Telephone

The first contact most people have with the medical office is by telephone with the medical assistant. Your telephone manner and tone of voice will create the first impression. You must speak clearly and slowly, give your full attention to the caller, and use good human relations skills (Figure 6-1).

TELEPHONE TURNOFFS—I

Do not use slang in your conversations at the medical office. Although casual language may be acceptable in personal conversations, you are labeled as unprofessional when you use slang in business conversations. Words such as "hi" instead of "hello" or "yeah" instead of "yes" are typical examples of slang. You should also avoid technical language, because patients feel uncomfortable if they do not understand the terminology used.

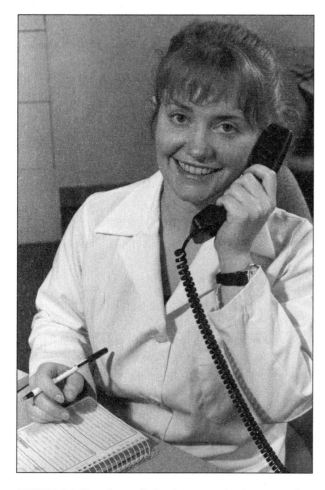

FIGURE 6-1 Since the medical assistant spends a large part of the day on the telephone, the skillful use of the telephone is an important requirement.

TELEPHONE TURNOFFS—II

Have you ever placed a call that was answered by someone who spoke so quickly you were not sure whether you had called the right number? Or perhaps the person answered with a false cheeriness that you found annoying? Because patients react negatively to annoying greetings, you should analyze your telephone answering manner and eliminate any behaviors that could be considered irritating or unprofessional.

Answer the telephone as soon as possible but no later than the second ring with a sincere, warm greeting that communicates good will. Several greetings are permissible when answering the telephone for a medical practice. Your office should have a standard greeting, used by everyone who routinely answers the phone.

This helps patients recognize that they have reached the right number. In a small practice of one or two physicians, you may use the individual names, a cordial greeting of "Good morning" or "Good afternoon," followed by "May I help you?" Identifying yourself is unnecessary.

Group practices may be large. Using all the names is time-consuming as well as confusing to the patient, a shortened greeting giving the corporate name or identifying the medical practice is acceptable. Use greetings such as these:

"Good morning, Dr. Nimet's office. May I help you?"

"Drs. Gladding and Squires. How may I help you?"

"Doctor's office. How may I direct your call?"

"Allied Medical Services. How may I help you?"

THE "HOLD" FUNCTION

Holding refers to the telephone's capability to keep a call waiting on one line while a second call is on another line. The two callers do not hear one another's conversations. When a call is placed on hold, it blocks the telephone line, making the line unavailable to incoming and outgoing calls. Asking a person to hold is often necessary, as you will usually need to retrieve a schedule or record or locate a person to answer the call. You should use the "hold" function when the person being called cannot come to the telephone immediately or when the person answering the telephone is busy with another call. Do not abuse "hold" by using this function too frequently or by keeping callers waiting for long periods.

Recipient of the Call Is Not Immediately Available

When the recipient of a call will be available within several minutes, you may ask the caller to hold. Before placing a caller on hold, ask the person's permission and give the reason for the delay. Then check back at thirty-second intervals. If the recipient of the call cannot answer within one minute, take a callback message and telephone number so the line can be freed for another call. The policy in some medical offices is to ask for a callback message first and to place the caller on hold only if the person requests, as this example shows:

Medical Assistant:	Family Medical Associates. How may I help you?
Caller:	This is Ken Oja. Dr. Ozick told me to call this morning about my son's fever.
Medical Assistant:	Dr. Ozick is on another line, Mr. Oja. May I take your number and have her return your call?
Caller:	I'd rather hold, if you don't mind.
Medical Assistant:	That's fine. I'll check back with you shortly.
	(A half minute passes.)
Medical Assistant:	Mr. Oja, Dr. Ozick is still on another line. Do you want to continue holding or would you prefer she call you back?
Caller:	I still want to hold.
Medical Assistant:	Fine. I'll put you on hold again.
	(Another half minute passes.)
Medical Assistant:	Mr. Oja, Dr. Ozick is taking much longer than I expected. I'm not sure when she will be finished. If you will give me your number, I'll give her the message and she will call you as soon as she is available.
Caller:	All right. My number is 555-2129.
Medical Assistant:	Thank you. Good-bye.
Caller:	Good-bye.

The Person Answering the Telephone Is Talking on Another Line

On busy days, you will juggle telephone calls constantly, and some calls must be placed on hold. When holding is necessary, ask the caller's permission before pressing the hold button. Take a callback message if you cannot return to the line in one minute, and remember that time will seem much shorter to you, fielding calls, than it does to the person waiting on the other end of the line. Never answer a ringing phone with the words "Hold" or "Hold, please" before giving the caller an opportunity to speak. This practice is rude and some people will hang up rather than wait.

Medical Assistant:	Good morning, Pediatric Specialties. May I help you?
Caller:	This is Gina Flynt. I'd like to make an appointment.
Medical Assistant:	Ms. Flynt, I'm on another line. May I call you back shortly?
Caller:	May I hold?
Medical Assistant:	My other call may take several minutes. I would rather call you back.
Caller:	Okay, I'm at 555-1314.
Medical Assistant:	Thank you. I'll speak with you shortly.

Abuses of the Hold Function

When the hold function is abused, it creates a negative impression for the office and for the person who answers the telephone. Basic good manners and business sense dictate when hold should be used. A list of Dos and Don'ts for holding is given in Figure 6-2. You may be able to add to the list from your personal calling experience.

Screening Calls

Most of the calls to a medical office are from people who wish to make appointments. Other calls are from patients seeking information, sales representatives, or insurance claim handlers. As a medical assistant you will screen all incoming calls and handle most of them yourself.

The physician personally takes very few telephone calls. Calls you should direct to the physician fall into five major categories: (1) emergencies, (2) calls from other physicians, (3) patients who wish to talk to the physician personally, (4) the physician's family, and (5) business calls you think should be referred to your employer (Figure 6-3).

The only people who should be routed to the physician immediately are emergency callers, other physicians, and family members if the physician requests it. Since family callers are a matter of personal preference, you should ask the physician to explain the policy on family calls. Patients who do not have a medical emergency and important business callers should be

Hold Function Etiquette

Do	Don't
Ask the caller's permission before putting a line on hold.	Put a line on hold until the caller states a reason for the call.
Check back with the caller frequently.	Leave a caller suspended on the line for several minutes.
Ask for a callback message and number.	Put several lines on hold at the same time.
Remember for whom the caller is holding.	Ask, "Who are you calling?"
Push the correct button for the line to be held.	Cut a caller off because of carelessness.
Return the call and apologize if you cut someone off by mistake.	Be rude or flippant about cutting a caller off.

FIGURE 6-2 Hold function etiquette

asked to leave a telephone number. The doctor will return the call at a convenient time later in the day. The patient who is concerned about a reaction to a medication and the physician's attorney are other examples of people who should be allowed to speak to the physician personally, depending on office policy.

Some telephone calls are difficult to screen because the caller says that the physician asked to be telephoned or that the matter is "personal business." If callers refuse to leave their name or

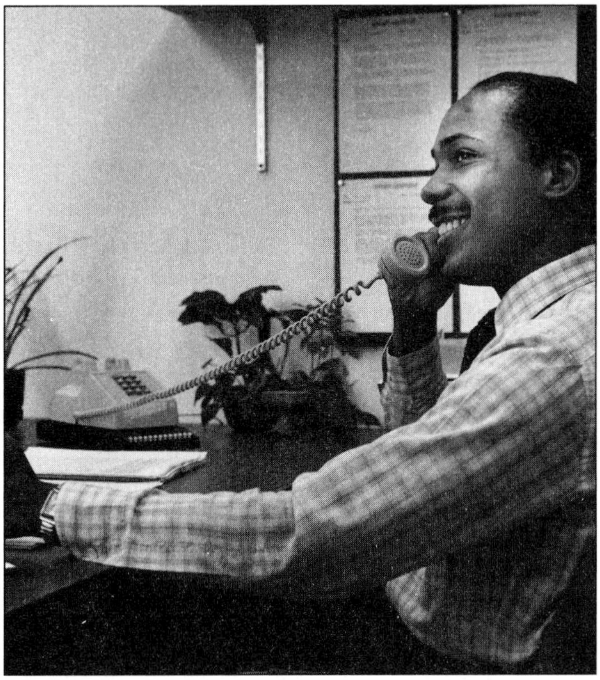

FIGURE 6-3 The medical assistant should reach an understanding with the physician concerning the screening of calls.

telephone number, suggest they write to the medical office. Remember, callers with legitimate business do not mind leaving their names.

Unless an emergency is involved, physicians rarely take telephone calls when they occur. You should take a message and a callback number for calls that the physician is to return and suggest an approximate time of day when the call will be returned. Physicians generally set aside special times of the day, such as after lunch or in the late afternoon, for making callbacks.

Procedures for Screening Calls

1. Ask the person's name and the reason for the call.
2. Ask questions that clarify the reason for the call.
3. Handle the call personally if you can.
4. Transfer the call to another staff member when appropriate.
5. Get the details for a callback message if the physician should return the call.

TYPICAL SCREENING SITUATIONS

Incoming Call—To Make an Appointment

Medical Assistant: Dr. Washington's office. Good morning.

Caller: I need to speak with Dr. Washington.

Medical Assistant: Dr. Washington is with a patient right now. May I ask who is calling?

Caller:	This is Samuel Chapman.
Medical Assistant:	Are you a patient of Dr. Washington's?
Caller:	Yes.
Medical Assistant:	Would you like to make an appointment, Mr. Chapman?
Caller:	Yes, I would.

(Continue with conversation by scheduling an appointment.)

Incoming Call—To Discuss a Medical Condition

Medical Assistant:	Dr. Mooring's office. May I help you?
Caller:	I'd like to talk to Dr. Mooring.
Medical Assistant:	Dr. Mooring is not available at the moment. May I ask who is calling, please?
Caller:	This is Clayton Ashlock.
Medical Assistant:	Are you a patient of Dr. Mooring's?
Caller:	Yes.
Medical Assistant:	Would you like to make an appointment, Mr. Ashlock?
Caller:	No, I need to speak with the doctor.
Medical Assistant:	Is your question about a medical problem?
Caller:	Yes.
Medical Assistant:	If you will tell me your symptoms, I will check with the nurse who is available.
Caller:	Well, it's my son, Clinton. Last night, he vomited several times. This morning, he has diarrhea, a sore throat, and a fever. He's diabetic, and I wondered if I should bring him in.
Medical Assistant:	Mr. Ashlock, I'm sure Dr. Mooring will want to check Clinton. Can you come in this afternoon at either 3:30 or 4:30?
Caller:	I can come at 3:30.

(Continue by making appointment.)

Incoming Call—Referral to a Consulting Physician

Medical Assistant:	Dr. Avellino's office. May I help you?
Caller:	I'd like to talk to Dr. Avellino.

Medical Assistant:	Dr. Avellino is in surgery. May I ask who is calling?
Caller:	This is Tanya Tyrell.
Medical Assistant:	Are you a patient of Dr. Avellino's?
Caller:	Yes.
Medical Assistant:	Do you need an appointment, Ms. Tyrell?
Caller:	No, I'd like to talk to Dr. Avellino.
Medical Assistant:	Is your call about a medical problem?
Caller:	Yes.
Medical Assistant:	If you will tell me your symptoms, I will check with the nurse who is available.
Caller:	Well, I think I might have broken my foot at hockey practice yesterday, and I wanted Dr. Avellino to check it.
Medical Assistant:	Ms. Tyrell, Dr. Avellino will want you to see an orthopedist. He refers all our patients to Dr. Amy Cornell who is in our same building. Dr. Cornell's telephone number is 555-8923. After checking your foot, Dr. Cornell will send a report to Dr. Avellino.
Caller:	Thank you. I wasn't sure who I should see.

Incoming Call—For Billing Charges and Insurance Information

Medical Assistant:	Dr. Wilton's office. May I help you?
Caller:	This is Elvia Alvarez with United Mutual Insurance Company. I need information about the charges for one of your patients.
Medical Assistant:	Ms. Alvarez, I will transfer your call to Joycelyn Chambers, who is in charge of insurance payments for our office.

Incoming Call—"Personal" Business

Medical Assistant:	Good morning, Dr. Darryl's office. May I help you?
Caller:	Dr. Darryl, please.
Medical Assistant:	I'm sorry, Dr. Darryl is unavailable. May I ask who is calling?

Caller:	This is a personal call. I'm a friend of his.
Medical Assistant:	Dr. Darryl usually returns calls at the end of the day. If you will leave your name and number, I will ask him to return your call.
Caller:	It's Rolfe Dijon at 555-7892.

Incoming Call—About a New Doctors' Building

Medical Assistant:	Dr. Duprey's office. May I help you?
Caller:	I'd like to talk to Dr. Duprey.
Medical Assistant:	I'm sorry, Dr. Duprey is with a patient at the moment. May I ask who is calling?
Caller:	This is Alice Russell.
Medical Assistant:	Are you a patient, Ms. Russell?
Caller:	No.
Medical Assistant:	May I ask why you are calling?
Caller:	I'd like to speak to Dr. Duprey about a new professional building we have almost completed. Many physicians in the city are relocating because of the choice location.
Medical Assistant:	Ms. Russell, I'll transfer you to our office manager, who will take the details and give the information to Dr. Duprey.
Caller:	I'd rather talk to Dr. Duprey.
Medical Assistant:	I regret that will not be possible.

Incoming Call—Refusal to Speak to Anyone but Physician

Medical Assistant:	Rosemont Medical. May I help you?
Caller:	I'd like to talk to Dr. Lesnick.
Medical Assistant:	Dr. Lesnick is not available right now. May I ask who is calling?
Caller:	This is Lance Clark.
Medical Assistant:	Are you a patient of Dr. Lesnick's?
Caller:	Yes.
Medical Assistant:	Would you like to make an appointment, Mr. Clark?
Caller:	No, I'd like to talk to Dr. Lesnick.
Medical Assistant:	Is your call about a medical problem?
Caller:	Yes.

Medical Assistant:	If you will tell me your symptoms, I will check with the nurse who is available.
Caller:	No, I just want to talk to the doctor.
Medical Assistant:	May I ask if your problem is an emergency?
Caller:	It's not an emergency.
Medical Assistant:	Dr. Lesnick usually returns her calls after seeing her last patient before lunch. That will be between 12:30 and 1:00 p.m. If you will give me your number, I'll ask her to call.

(Continue by taking the telephone number. Put the message on the physician's desk immediately with a note that the patient wanted to speak only to the doctor.)

TAKING MESSAGES

Physicians and nurses do not routinely answer telephone calls; therefore, you will take callback messages frequently.

Procedures for Taking Callback Messages

1. Write the date and time of the call.
2. Write the name of the person called.
3. Ask the caller's name and telephone number.
4. Ask whether the caller will telephone again.
5. Write down the complete message (Figure 6-4).

Be sure to ask for specifics if the message is unclear. Add your initials as the person who took the call. Figure 6-5 illustrates a telephone message pad. Some medical offices use carbon-coated telephone message pages, so a record of all incoming calls is available.

Special Screening Procedures

Patients often call physicians for advice about medication, dosage, prescriptions, side effects, symptoms, or recovery. In screening calls pertaining to a medical condition, ask questions that will help the patient give a complete explanation. Two typical situations that require in-depth screening are calls about prescriptions and calls about an illness. You must follow special procedures for screening these calls. Review

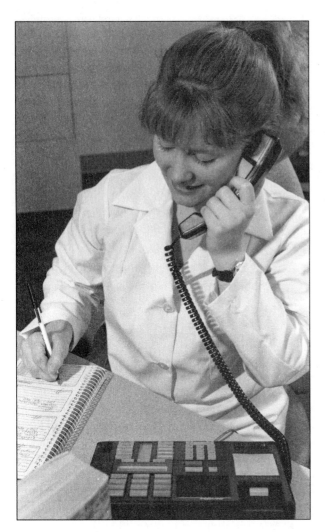

FIGURE 6-4 It is essential to keep a pencil or pen and message pad or paper by the telephone to write down the complete message.

the procedures and the screening situation. Then compare the callback form left for the physician in Figure 6-6.

Procedures for Prescription Refill Requests

Ask:

1. Name of the patient
2. Name of the medication
3. Length of time the patient has taken the medication
4. Patient's symptoms
5. Patient's age and weight, if a child
6. Name and telephone number of the patient's pharmacy
7. Patient's telephone number

Procedures for Taking Messages Regarding an Illness

Ask:

1. Name of the patient
2. Name and relationship of the caller, if different from the patient
3. When the patient's symptoms first appeared
4. Whether the patient has had similar symptoms in the past
5. Whether the patient has a fever and, if so, the temperature

Many medical offices use a specially designed message form that provides space for both medical and general information and that can be used for all types of calls. Some medical offices use a computer program that allows the medical assistant to key information on a message form shown on the computer screen as illustrated in Figure 6-7. If you listen carefully when you make business calls, you may be able to hear the sound of computer keys being struck as your message is taken. The message is

---

IMPORTANT MESSAGE

TO _Dr. Ravel_

DATE _5/2/9–_   TIME _11:15_ (A.M.) P.M.

WHILE YOU WERE OUT

M _Matthew Lee, President_

OF _Rotary_

Area Code & Exchange _000-555-7164_

TELEPHONED		PLEASE CALL	✕
CALLED TO SEE YOU		WILL CALL AGAIN	
WANTS TO SEE YOU		URGENT	
	RETURNED YOUR CALL		

Message _Would like to know if you will speak about proposed reforms in health care at 6/11 breakfast meeting_

Operator _Dawn Townsend_

FIGURE 6-5 Telephone message pad

NAME Cathi Fordham	(PHONE)	DX High blood pressure	
DATE 6/10 TIME 9:00 DR	EXAM		
FROM TO Dr. Nicole Page	RETURN PHONE # WILL CALL BACK 461-0101 RETURN TIME 4:00	TELEPHONE CONVERSATION RECORD	

MESSAGE CC/HC

Patient has taken Lopressor for 1 month and needs a refill.
She's taking bp with company nurse 2x each week at work.
Dr. Page told her to call for a refill in one month if bp had
dropped to at least 140/86

PHARMACY Eller's
PHONE ☐ 461-9423   AGE 40   WT 130

R̸ Lopressor tablets   AMT 25 mg

SIG 1/2 tablet each morning

FOR blood pressure

☑ SIDE EFFECTS   No REFILL
Drowsiness

FOLLOW UP

FIGURE 6-6 Medical callback message form

then printed and delivered by hand, or it may be sent to the recipient by electronic mail (see Chapter 8).

HANDLING EMERGENCY CALLS

Emergency calls represent potentially life-threatening situations and should be handled efficiently and quickly. The caller may be frightened and excited, and obtaining the required information may be difficult. Review the following sample conversation between a medical assistant and an emergency patient. Also refer to the section called "Handling Emergencies" in Chapter 5 for a thorough review of emergency procedures.

Incoming Call—Emergency:

Medical Assistant: Dr. Romaine's office. May I help you?

Caller: I need to talk to Dr. Romaine.

Medical Assistant: Dr. Romaine is not available at the moment. May I ask who is calling?

Caller: This is Larry Hamm.

Medical Assistant: Are you a patient of Dr. Romaine's?

Caller: Yes.

Medical Assistant: Would you like to make an appointment, Mr. Hamm?

Caller: No, I'd like to talk to Dr. Romaine.

Medical Assistant: Is your call about a medical problem?

Caller: Yes.

Medical Assistant: If you will tell me your symptoms, I will check with the nurse who is available.

Caller: I'm not feeling well. My left arm tingles, I'm sweating, and I'm having trouble breathing.

Medical Assistant: When did this start?

Caller: About an hour ago.

Medical Assistant: Does your chest hurt?

Caller: Not right this minute, but I had some really bad pains a few minutes ago. That's why I called.

Medical Assistant: Is anyone with you, Mr. Hamm?

Caller: No.

Medical Assistant: I'll get Dr. Romaine. Stay on the line; she'll be right with you.

(Get the physician immediately. This patient may be experiencing a heart attack.)

```
Call to: Dr. Ravel                          Time: 11:15 a.m.

Call from: Matthew Lee                       Date: May 2, 19—
           President of Rotary Club


Number: (000) 555-7164

Would like to know if you will speak about proposed
reforms in health care at 6/11 breakfast meeting.



Taken by: Dawn Townsend
```

FIGURE 6-7 Computer message screen

Study the techniques listed in Figure 6-8 for more suggestions on using the telephone.

IN YOUR OPINION

1. How can effective telephone techniques contribute to the efficiency of a well-functioning medical office?
2. What are the advantages and disadvantages of the "hold" function for the person calling? For the person answering the phone?
3. Why might a caller be reluctant to answer a medical assistant's screening questions?

Placing Local and Long-Distance Calls

As a medical assistant, you will place many different types of local and long-distance calls. These calls may be to patients, consulting physicians, other medical facilities, and business associates. You may also make travel arrangements for the physician(s) in your office, order

Telephone Techniques

1. **Put Yourself in the Caller's Place.** People who call a medical office are often either sick or worried about a family member. When a caller sounds unfriendly, mentally put yourself in the person's place and threat the caller as you would like to be treated in a similar situation.
2. **Give Your Full Attention to the Caller.** When you are talking on the telephone, answer questions fully, even though you may be busy. Allow the caller to explain the reason for the call, and do not interrupt unless it is necessary to encourage information.
3. **Speak Clearly and Distinctly.** As you converse, speak directly into the mouthpiece. Talk clearly and distinctly. Never chew gum or eat while you talk because the noise is offensive and distracting to the listener.
4. **Use a Courteous Tone.** Say "Please" and "Thank you" as you would in a face-to-face conversation. Close the conversation on a pleasant note.

FIGURE 6-8

supplies of drugs and equipment, or request service providers. Wait until all patients have been greeted and registered before placing outgoing calls. Then make your business calls brief and to the point. Delay personal calls until lunch or a break. If your voice carries, do not place calls within earshot of people in the reception area.

LOCAL CALLS

To place a local call:

1. Dial the seven-digit telephone number. If your call must first go through a switchboard, dial 9 for an outside line. Then dial the seven-digit number at the sound of the tone.
2. Identify yourself and the medical office when the call is answered. If you are making the call for the physician, identify the physician.
3. Leave a message or explain that you will call again, if the person you are calling is unavailable.

LONG DISTANCE CALLS—AT&T AND ALTERNATIVE SERVICES

The American Telephone and Telegraph Company, originally made up of several operating companies known as the Bell System, had very little competition for almost seventy years. However, in the late 1970s, the Federal Communications Commission opened the door for greater competition by breaking up the AT&T system and by allowing other companies to provide telephone service. Today MCI, Sprint, and many other alternative companies compete for long-distance service, resulting in reduced rates for consumers.

Long-distance users pay according to the type of call made and the amount of time spent on the line. As a medical assistant, you will be expected to know the differences among the varying services and their relative costs. Since service and rates differ among telephone companies and geographic locations, accurate national comparisons cannot be made. Contact the companies providing telephone service in your community for a complete listing of ser-

vices and fees. By spending an hour comparison shopping, you may save your practice several hundred dollars each year in telephone charges.

Direct Distance Dialing

Direct Distance Dialing (DDD) refers to calls placed directly, without benefit of an operator. They offer a low-cost alternative to calls placed through an operator. Since telephone company personnel are not needed for DDD calls, the savings is passed along to the consumer in lower long-distance rates. Area codes for direct distance dialing to all parts of the country are located at the front of the white pages. If you are uncertain of an area code, look in the listing.

To place a DDD call within the same area code:

Dial 1 plus the number.

1-555-3875

(Note: In some parts of the country, dialing 1 is not necessary. Check your local directory.)

To place a DDD call to a different area code:

Dial 1 plus the area code plus the number.

1-614-555-7927

Operator-Assisted Calls

Operator assistance is provided for person-to-person calls, collect calls, calls charged to another number, some credit cards calls, and station-to-station calls when requested by the caller.

To place an operated-assisted call within the same area code:

Dial 0 plus the number.

0-555-7927

To place an operated-assisted call to a different area code:

Dial 0 plus the area code plus the number.

0-614-555-7927

Advise the operator of the type of call you are making. If you reach an incorrect long-distance number, dial 0 and explain the problem to the operator. You will receive credit for the call.

Station-to-Station and Person-to-Person Calls

A station-to-station call means that the caller will talk to anyone who answers the telephone. A person-to-person call is made when the caller wishes to speak only to a specific person. Station-to-station charges begin as soon as the receiver is lifted, but person-to-person charges start only when the designated person answers the telephone. Station-to-station service calls cost less per minute than person-to-person service, but they may be more expensive if the recipient must be located or takes several minutes to answer the phone. Most people prefer to dial person-to-person calls directly without help from the operator, as this illustration shows. The operator will ask who is being called after you direct dial.

(Dial 0 + Area Code + Number)

Medical Assistant: Operator, I'd like to talk with Mr. Dave Ciccone at Thresh and Company. This is Erika Silk calling from Dr. Bill Burroughs' office in Philadelphia.

Operator: Thank you.

(Telephone rings and receptionist answers.)

Receptionist: Good morning, Thresh and Company.

Operator: I have a person-to-person call for Mr. Dave Ciccone.

Receptionist: May I ask who is calling?

Operator: Erika Silk with Dr. Bill Burroughs' office in Philadelphia.

Receptionist: One moment, please. I'll ring Mr. Ciccone.

Collect Calls

Collect calls are sometimes known as "reversed calls" because the charge is reversed to the answering telephone. The person who answers must agree to pay for the call before the operator will make a connection. A collect call can be station-to-station or person-to-person.

You should not accept a collect call unless the caller's identity is clear and office policy permits acceptance. Some medical offices will accept collect calls from patients with an understanding that the cost will later be billed to the patient. Acceptable collect charges might include the following: (1) a call from your employer who is attending an out-of-state medical convention; (2) a call from the physician's spouse or children; and (3) a call from a patient undergoing continuing treatment for a medical condition. (Charges for this last call would be billed to the patient later.) Examples of unacceptable collect charges include calls from a medical supply company representative or a person whose name is unfamiliar. A typical collect telephone call is shown in the following dialogue:

Collect Station-to-Station Call

(Medical assistant answers)

Operator: I have a collect call for anyone from Mr. Lawrence Babbio. Will you accept?

Medical Assistant: Operator, I can't accept this call without additional information to identify Mr. Babbio.

Operator: Mr. Babbio, will you identify yourself further?

Caller: Yes, operator. I'm the brother of Dr. Kincaid's patient, Rebecca Watson. Rebecca is visiting me in California and has a medical problem that I need to discuss with the doctor.

Medical Assistant: Operator, I will accept the call.

(The medical assistant screens the call and refers it to the physician or takes a callback message.)

Conference Calls

Long-distance calls can be arranged to include several people in different locations speaking in conference at one time. Although conference calls are more expensive than single-line calls, a net savings may occur when conversations do not have to be repeated with several different people.

To place a conference call:

1. Dial 0 and give the operator the name, area code, and telephone number of each person who will participate in the conversation. Specify a time when the call should take place, for example, 2 P.M. Eastern Standard Time.
2. When all parties to the call are on the line, the operator contacts the originator of the call, and the conversation begins.

Sometimes when a patient is extremely ill, family members who live in different places may wish to discuss with the physician the details of the illness, the length of hospitalization, and the patient's chances of recovery. The time of day is important to consider when arranging for this type of conference call. You will want to place the call at a time convenient for the family members, some of whom may live in different time zones.

Credit Card Calls

Credit cards are issued by the telephone company so customers can eliminate collect calls. Using a credit card is convenient and usually saves the caller time.

To make a credit card call:

1. Dial 0 plus the area code, if different from yours, plus the number.
2. Advise the operator that you are making a credit card call and give your credit card number. From many telephones, a long tone indicates to the caller to key the credit card number into the telephone keypad, eliminating the need for an operator.

TIME ZONES

As a medical assistant, you must understand time zones if you are to use long-distance service successfully. Because there is a three-hour time difference between the East and West coasts, a person who places a 9:00 A.M. call in New York City will awaken California residents at 6:00 A.M. and receive no answer in California offices. The time zone map in Figure 6-9 shows time zones in the continental United States and adjacent Canadian provinces. Use the map to determine the appropriate time to place a call.

The city of origination determines whether day, evening, or night telephone rates apply.

DIRECTORY ASSISTANCE

An operator can assist with locating unknown numbers. However, because you may be charged for directory assistance, requests should be kept to a minimum. You should first check available telephone directories. Your public library will carry telephone directories for major cities in the United States. The charge for directory assistance is explained in the front of the white pages.

To call directory assistance within the same area code:

Dial 1 + 555-1212

To call directory assistance in a different area code:

Dial 1 + area code + 555-1212

Operators are available to assist telephone customers, even when information is sketchy. If you need to locate someone, dial 0, give the operator any information you have, and ask for help. The operator will try to reach the designated person for you. For example, assume you need to reach your employer, who is attending a convention in another city. When you reach the convention area, you are told that the physicians are in one of three major meetings, all of which are accessible by telephone. The telephone operator will help with this problem by calling each room to ask for the physician.

TELEPHONE LOG

As a medical assistant, you should keep a log of all long-distance telephone calls so the charges can be passed along to patients or charged to the practice's account. A long-distance telephone log should show the name of the caller, the person called, the date and time of the call, the city called, whether the call was station-to-station or person-to-person, the approximate length of the call, the name of the account to be charged, and the purpose of the call. Star all col-

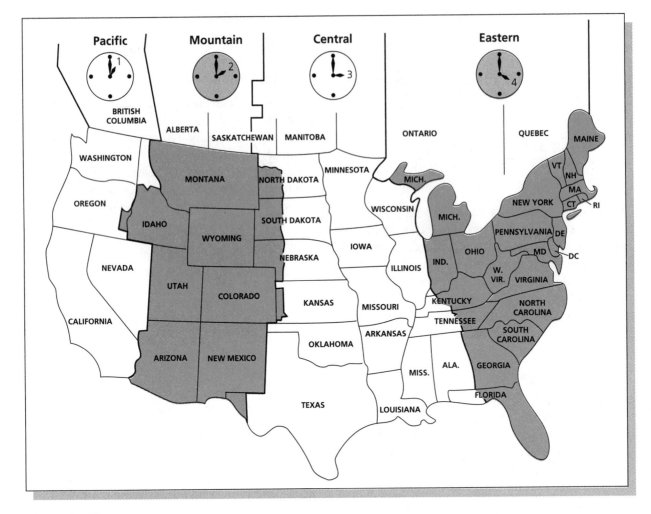

FIGURE 6-9 Time zone map

lect calls. An example of a telephone log is shown in Figure 6-10.

MONTHLY TELEPHONE CHARGES

Charges for directory assistance and long-distance calls are shown on the monthly telephone statement along with charges for local service. Each month you should check the telephone bill closely to make sure that your practice was charged properly and that directory assistance is not being abused. Too many directory assistance charges might indicate that the staff is not checking the directory before asking for assistance.

Follow these procedures for checking the monthly telephone bill:

1. Match all charged items with the telephone log.
2. Charge individual patient accounts for long-distance calls pertaining to individual patients.
3. Check all starred collect calls and charge to the appropriate account.
4. Cross through each call listing after the charge has been noted on the correct account.
5. Circle any questionable calls.
6. Calculate the total for calls to be charged to the practice and charge the proper practice account or make a note for the accountant.
7. Contact the local telephone business office about discrepancies between your records and the statement.

To	From	Date	Time	City	Type of Call	Length	Account to be Charged	Purpose
Annette Davis	Vanessa Greene	5/2	9:15	New Rochelle	P-P	8 min.	Office	Supplies shipment
Sara Dietrich	Dr. Malloy	5/2	11:45	Kansas City	S-S	20 min.	Howard Dietrich	Discuss her husband's condition
Suzanne Bourdes	Dr. Malloy	5/2	12:15	Burlington	P-P	5 min.	Office	AMA talk
Empirical Pharmacy	Vanessa Greene	5/2	12:30	Kansas City	S-S	3 min.	Howard Dietrich	Mr. Dietrich's prescription
George Motter	Sui Sing	5/2	1:00	Hesperia	P-P	7 min.	Sui Sing	Personal
*DL Dodson	Vanessa Greene	5/3	10:00	Marlington, WV	S-S	1 min.	DL Dodson	His vacation accident
DL Dodson	Dr. Malloy	5/3	11:45	Marlington, WV	P-P	8 min.	DL Dodson	His accident
Charlie Weaver	Dr. Malloy	5/3	12:00	Cape Girardeau	P-P	5 min.	Office	Review AMA talk

*Collect

FIGURE 6-10 Long-distance telephone log

IN YOUR OPINION

1. How can you save your office money if you make a great many long-distance calls to suppliers and research institutions?
2. What do you think would be a reasonable policy on making and receiving personal calls while at the office?
3. How would you find the phone number of the author of an article in a medical journal? Name several ways.

TELEPHONE NUMBER FILE

You should keep frequently used telephone numbers in a handy file at your desk. Patients' numbers are usually located in an alphabetical card file or in their medical record. In addition, you should maintain a rotary card file for business-related numbers such as the cleaning service, the electric company, and suppliers. Use a separate card for each name. Emergency numbers such as police, fire department, rescue squad, the doctor's personal physician, and local hospitals should be typed on a blank card and taped to the telephone or desk. A rotary telephone number card is shown in Figure 6-11

and an emergency telephone number list is shown in Figure 6-12.

Using the Telephone Directory

The telephone directory is a valuable but often unappreciated resource (Figure 6-13). Depending on the size of the geographic area served, one or more directories are required to contain all the information about telephone company

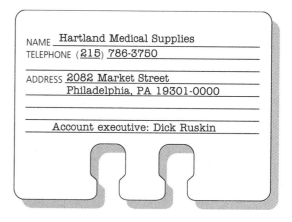

NAME Hartland Medical Supplies
TELEPHONE (215) 786-3750

ADDRESS 2082 Market Street
Philadelphia, PA 19301-0000

Account executive: Dick Ruskin

FIGURE 6-11 Rotary telephone number card

Fire department	498-1023
Police department	498-1047
Dr. Natalie Baker (Dr. Joyce's physician)	624-5542
Harris Paramedic Service	624-9443
Center City Medical Service	624-1049
Cabrini Ambulance Company	498-6169
Memorial Hospital	498-6263

FIGURE 6-12 Emergency telephone number list

customers. These are the four commonly used directories or parts of a directory:

1. The white pages list the names and telephone numbers for all telephone accounts for a specified calling area.
2. The yellow pages list business and professional accounts for the same calling area covered by the white pages.
3. The pink pages list business and professional accounts for a smaller geographic portion of the primary calling area.
4. The blue pages list special telephone numbers, including numbers for social service agencies; local, state, and federal government offices; and schools. The directories for each city vary, but typical telephone directories include some of the resource material discussed here.

LOCATING A NUMBER

Since the names listed in a telephone directory are in alphabetical order, most numbers are easy to locate. However, certain names are confusing and more difficult to find. Although the guidelines for locating names in a telephone directory are similar to basic filing guidelines, they are not identical because most telephone directories are organized in the following ways:

1. Abbreviations are spelled out. To find "St. Joseph's Center," look for "Saint Joseph's Center."
2. Names with initials are listed before full first names. "Lawson, M." comes before "Lawson, Michael."
3. Names with prefixes are listed as one word. "duPont" follows "Duke"; "McDonald" follows "MacDonald."

4. Sometimes letters are used as names. When a name, usually a business name, is comprised of all capital letters, look in the beginning of the particular letter section. For example, "CC Medical Supplies" appears at the beginning of the "C" section, and "WBL TV" appears at the beginning of the "W" section.
5. Numbers are spelled out. Numbers used as names are spelled out and listed in alphabetical order. "19th Street Cafe" appears as "Nineteenth Street Cafe."
6. "The" follows the company name. "The Emerson Drug Store" appears as "Emerson Drug Store The."
7. Company names made up of two words are listed in alphabetical order by the first name. Hyphens (-), ampersands (&), and apostrophes (') are ignored. "Hewitt-Baker Medical Supplies" comes before "Hewitt & Banks Medical Laboratory." "Medical Professional Center" comes before "Medical-Prosthetic Devices." "Jacob's Pharmacy" appears as "Jacobs Pharmacy."
8. Some names can be spelled different ways. "Smith" may be spelled "Smyth" or "Smythe";

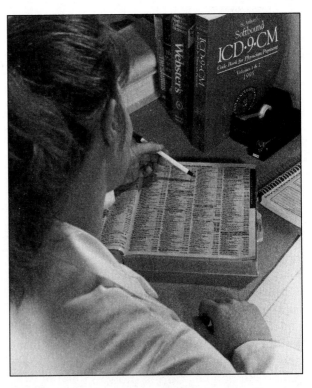

FIGURE 6-13 Telephone directories contain useful and important information.

"Cohen" might be spelled "Coan," "Kohen," "Coahen," "Cohan," "Kohan," "Cohn," "Kohn," or "Kone." Suggestions for different spellings appear at the beginning of the most common last name listings.

9. Look for alternative listings. "Marshall Warner Associates" might appear under "Warner Marshall Associates."

10. Government listings are found in the blue pages in many places. If your directory does not have a blue pages section, look for federal government agencies under "United States Government." Look for state agencies under the name of the state, city agencies under the name of the city, and municipal agencies under the name of the town.

Using Answering Services And Telephone Answering Devices

Two methods are generally used to assure that calls to physicians or their associates are answered after hours and on weekends. As a medical assistant, you will be responsible for maintaining an answering system that meets the needs of the practice and the patients. Refer to the yellow pages in your community for the names of answering services and the names of companies that sell telephone answering devices (TADs).

ANSWERING SERVICES

Answering services are twenty-four-hour services that, for a monthly fee, answer the medical office telephone number from a remote location. If a switching device is installed, the service can automatically answer the medical office telephone when it is unanswered. The service then locates the physician at an alternate number or on a paging device. If the answering service does not have the capability to switch on and off automatically, the medical assistant calls the service and advises the time to begin answering, the physician's location, and the time to stop answering. After returning to the office, the medical assistant checks with the service for messages. Because many answering services charge by the number of calls answered and the time spent tracking the physician, the service should be used only when necessary.

ANSWERING MACHINES

Answering machines give a recorded message and a number where the physician can be reached. Because answering devices appear impersonal, some physicians do not use them. Patients prefer to hear a human voice to reassure them that the physician will call back.

FAX

FAX, or facsimile transmission, allows you to send a "picture" of a document over telephone lines to anyone who has a FAX machine. Data, charts, even sketches and drawings can be sent in this way in a matter of seconds or minutes. FAX is especially useful when sending documents needed urgently some distance away.

Confidentiality issues are important to consider when using FAX. Most FAX machines are not in secure locations, and incoming FAX messages may be read by anyone passing by, so take care in using FAX for transmitting confidential data.

Newer FAX machines receive and print onto ordinary copy paper. Older FAX machines use a thermal paper which usually comes in a roll. The paper is thin and shiny and images on this paper last only about a year. If a permanent record of incoming FAX data is needed for legal purposes, the thermal message should be photocopied and the photocopy filed promptly. A FAX message is illustrated in Figure 6-14.

REFERENCES

"Jobs and Infotech: Work in the Information Society," *The Futurist*, January/February 1994.

"Managing by Wire," *Harvard Business Review*, September/October 1993.

Oliverio, John, William Pasewark, and Bonnie White. *The Office: Procedures and Technology.* Cincinnati, Ohio: South-Western Publishing Co., 1993.

Wirth, Arthur G. *Education and Work in the Year 2000.* San Francisco: Jossey-Bass Publishers, 1992.

FAX

Seriph Medical Associates

To: Petra Desmond

From: Dolores Rio

Date: October 27, 19—

Pages: 2, including cover sheet

Fax No.:   (513) 555-6956

Attached please find our purchase order #3278 for medical and surgical supplies. All items are subject to cancellation if delivered after the requested delivery dates.

Please let me know by Friday if any of the items listed require longer lead times.

Please call (513) 555-0933 if all pages are not received.

FIGURE 6-14 FAX message

Chapter Activities

PERFORMANCE BASED ACTIVITIES

1. You are taking calls at the offices of Dr. Cynthia Swinehart and Dr. Raul Lopez. They are incorporated as Heart Smart Cardiology, Inc. On the following lines, record three appropriate telephone greetings. Describe proper tone of voice.

Telephone Greetings

1. _____

2. _____

3. _____

(DACUM 1.6, 2.5, 2.8)

2. Analyze the advantages of (a) station-to-station and person-to-person calls and (b) DDD versus operator-assisted calls. Infer an appropriate occasion for using each.

Station-to-station		*Person-to-person*	
Advantages	*Disadvantages*	*Advantages*	*Disadvantages*
1. _____	1. _____	1. _____	1. _____
2. _____	2. _____	2. _____	2. _____
3. _____	3. _____	3. _____	3. _____

Appropriate Occasions for Use

1. _____	1. _____
2. _____	2. _____
3. _____	3. _____

Direct Distance Dialing		*Operator-Assisted*	
Advantages	*Disadvantages*	*Advantages*	*Disadvantages*
1. _____	1. _____	1. _____	1. _____
2. _____	2. _____	2. _____	2. _____
3. _____	3. _____	3. _____	3. _____

Appropriate Occasions for Use

1. _____	1. _____
2. _____	2. _____
3. _____	3. _____

(DACUM 2.6, 2.7)

3. Prepare a FAX message on the form below stating that Dr. Dave Marcum will arrive in Dr. Anna Ravinsky's office at 10:00 a.m. on March 9. Ask for confirmation by FAX that Dr. Ravinsky will be available.

Doctor's Office
FAX Note

To: _____

From: _____

Date: _____

Fax #: _____

No. of pages: _____

(DACUM 2.5, 2.7)

4. Compile a packet of materials on cellular communication from your local telephone office. Develop a summary of service offered by the company. (DACUM 1.7, 2.6, 3.6)

EXPANDING YOUR THINKING

1. Role play screening the following callers to determine their business.

   a. Sales person from a pharmaceutical firm

   b. Golf partner of the physician

   c. Fund raiser from the physician's alma mater

   d. Patient with excessive pain the day after outpatient surgery

   e. Mother with a child with a fever of 104.5 degrees F

   f. Patient who does not understand instructions on medication

   g. Insurance company seeking records

2. Locate the following, and compile name, address, and phone number for each:

   a. A medical supply house in your state

   b. A medical school in your state, or in an adjoining state

   c. A service that searches medical databases and can provide articles on requested topics

   d. A local uniform supply business

   e. A British dermatologist

   f. A manufacturer of medical instruments

   g. Three associations that serve the medical field

3. Assemble a list of emergency phone numbers that you think should be posted in the average home. Compile a similar list of emergency numbers for a medical practice.

   Home

   1. _____
   2. _____
   3. _____
   4. _____
   5. _____
   6. _____

   Medical Practice

   1. _____
   2. _____
   3. _____
   4. _____
   5. _____
   6. _____

Scheduling Appointments

HESPERIA, CALIFORNIA

I'm amazed by how much difference good scheduling makes to the quality of our workday. When I first began working here at Sonrisa Medical Center, our office manager, Kate, trained me in scheduling so that I could take over while she went on maternity leave. My first week alone was very challenging. Patients were waiting; doctors were waiting; the day just didn't seem to flow.

There's a lot more to good scheduling than you think. Each doctor has his or her own pace. Some patients and conditions take longer than others. No one wants to wait, and no one wants to be rushed.

I learned from this experience that well-managed scheduling is an important factor in delivering quality care to patients. Yes, there will always be emergencies and interruptions, but learning how to react to them is part of managing the schedule.

Rosemarie Kao
Medical Assistant

PERFORMANCE BASED COMPETENCIES

After completing this chapter, you should be able to:

1. Evaluate different means of scheduling. (DACUM 3.1)

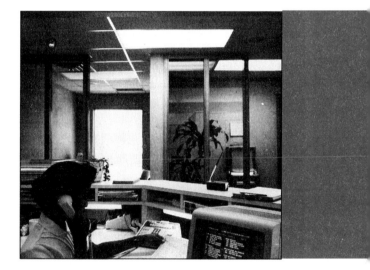

2. Schedule patient and nonpatient appointments. (DACUM 3.2)
3. Analyze the time required by different patients and procedures. (DACUM 3.2)
4. Choose among options for handling delays to the schedule. (DACUM 6.6)
5. Screen nonpatient appointments. (DACUM 2.5)
6. Prepare the daily master schedule. (DACUM 3.2)
7. Coordinate scheduling of patients at other medical facilities. (DACUM 3.2)
8. Measure the performance of the actual to planned schedule. (DACUM 3.2)

Management of the schedule is vital to the delivery of quality medical services to patients and quality of work life to the medical staff. Time is a scarce resource, like money, and scheduling is the tool for managing that resource. Whether appointments are scheduled by hand in a day book or with a computer using scheduling software, the entire staff depends on a smooth flow of patient traffic in order to maintain a workable schedule. Appointments must be made so they allow sufficient time for each patient's medical problem to be treated thoroughly, yet without long waits, which waste the time of the medical staff.

As a medical assistant, you will schedule appointments based on several factors such as the availability of time, the type of patient being treated, the type of specific medical problem, and the personal preferences of the medical staff at your office. Trade-offs will always occur because days are not long enough during cold season, emergencies and sudden schedule interruptions, and assorted other reasons. Learning to manage these interruptions is part of learning how to manage the schedule.

To make rational decisions about the allocation of time, you will screen and evaluate callers. If the call is truly urgent, you will have to find time for the patient to see the physician. For other problems, you will work with the patient to schedule a convenient appointment.

You will find human relations and organizational skill to be important qualities in balancing your schedule (Figure 7-1). As you monitor

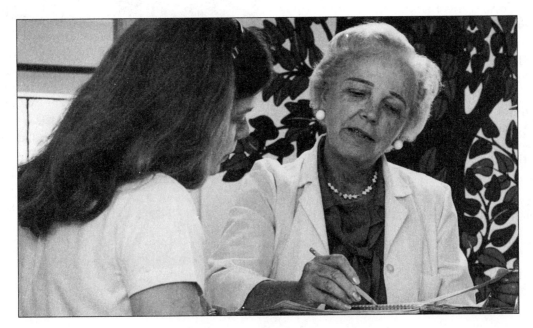

FIGURE 7-1 Scheduling appointments requires good judgment and organizational skill on the part of the medical assistant.

patient flow, you must strive to maintain both a calm and unhurried environment and an efficient system. Although these two characteristics may appear to be opposites, they actually complement one another.

Maintaining the Appointment Schedule

 Appointments for patients and other visitors are recorded in the appointment book or in a computer software system such as *The Medical Manager,* published by Delmar Publishers. With either arrangement, the appointment schedule serves as the daily planning guide by showing (1) the names of all patients to be seen each day, (2) the time of each patient's appointment, (3) the patient's telephone number, and (4) a brief reason for the visit. From this information, the doctors and other office personnel determine approximately how much time is needed for their portion of the patient's treatment, and which medical instruments and supplies will be required for the examination.

PATIENT APPOINTMENTS

Patient appointments are usually requested by the patient or a relative, by notes or messages from the physician or nurse, or by a referring physician. Appointments are scheduled for varying amounts of time, based on the patient's symptoms and on the particular medical specialty, but most practices develop a formula for scheduling that will help you decide the amount of time needed for each patient. Figure 7-2 shows a typical formula for an internal medicine practice.

When a patient requests an appointment, ask for a specific description of the symptoms. If, in your judgment, the complaint is serious enough to justify an immediate examination, look through the day's schedule for the first vacant time period. If no openings exist, find a time when the patient can be "worked in." For example, an elderly patient suffering from chest pain might be in the preliminary stages of a heart attack and should be seen as soon as possible. In this case, you must make room in the schedule for an immediate appointment, even though other patients will be delayed. If the patient's request is not urgent, such as for a routine physical exam, a recheck, or a minor ache or pain, search the appointment schedule for the first vacant time period. Give the patient one or two alternative times and then schedule the appointment according to the patient's wishes.

Ask established patients if their addresses or telephone numbers have changed recently. If so, note any changes in their medical record. To increase efficiency, ask new patients to arrive at the office about fifteen minutes early so that they can complete forms needed to open accounts.

In some medical offices, specific appointment times are set aside during the day or week for certain types of patients. For example, all patients requiring physical examinations might be scheduled for early morning or late afternoon, and all consultations might be scheduled during a designated time. In an obstetrics and gynecology practice, all new mothers might be seen on a specified day of the week and all expectant mothers at another specific time. Pregnant patients might be scheduled after lunch when their "morning sickness" has disappeared. When patients can be scheduled according to a specific category, the physician and staff increase their efficiency.

Many reasons exist for not scheduling a day completely full. Last-minute adjustments will almost certainly occur, and you will be able to react to them more easily if you have built some flexibility into your plan. Cancelled patient appointments and other time vacancies allow other patients to come in for earlier appointments. When a cancellation occurs, review the

---

Scheduling Formula for Internal Medicine Practice

New patients	30 minutes
Patients for consultation	45 minutes
Patients requiring complete physical examinations	45 minutes
All other patients (minor illnesses, routine checkups, etc.)	15 minutes

FIGURE 7-2 Scheduling formula for internal medicine practice

schedule to determine which patients can be moved to the opening caused by the cancellation. Then call the patients until you locate person who wishes to make a change. Always try to fill openings made available through cancellations so all patients can be served and the physician and staff can practice at top efficiency.

Acquiring Information

Some patients prefer to provide information about their symptoms to the doctor only, but part of your job will be to screen requests for appointments and make rational determination of their relative urgency. This will be an opportunity to use your human relations skills to acquire the necessary information. Patients frequently decide to talk after a little encouragement. Determining a patient's condition involves asking several questions, such as the following:

Procedures to Help Identify a Patient's Complaint

Ask these questions:

1. Are your symptoms related to a previous illness?
2. Has the doctor treated you for this condition before?
3. How long have you been ill?
4. Is your problem urgent or routine?
5. Would you like a consultation with the doctor (if the patient refuses to talk about the illness or the reason for the visit)?

Most appointments are made by telephone, and you will not always recognize the name or the voice. When you don't recognize the patient's name, ask, "Are you a new or an established patient of our office?" You may also ask, "Have you seen Dr. Cooper previously?" or "When were you last seen by anyone in this office?"

RECORDING THE APPOINTMENT

 You will record appointments either manually in a daily appointment book or electronically using computer software such as *The Medical Manager*. With an appointment book, you will search for "holes"

in the schedule by flipping through each page until you find an opening appropriate for the patient's symptoms. With a computerized system, you will enter information about the appointment, and the system will provide information that allows you to maintain an optimal plan.

The Appointment Book

A typical appointment book is divided by days of the week, with each day broken into fifteen-minute segments. You will block out as many fifteen-minute segments as necessary to provide time for each examination. For example, a new patient visit, which in most offices requires thirty minutes, would use two fifteen-minute segments as shown in Figure 7-3. To record an appointment, follow these procedures:

Procedures to Record an Appointment in the Appointment Book

1. List the patient's first and last names in ink.
2. Draw a slash after the name; then list the patient's complaint or reason for the visit.
3. Draw another slash; then write the patient's telephone number.
4. Write "New" if the patient is visiting the physician for the first time.
5. Mark out additional time periods with an arrow if more than fifteen minutes are needed for the examination. By doing so, you will not schedule two patients for the same time.
6. Make sure your handwriting is legible.
7. Review the appointment book at the end of each day to be sure it is accurate for all patients seen that day. This step is important because the appointment book might be used as evidence in a court case.
8. Make a note of changes and interruptions to the schedule, and measure how well the staff was able to perform against the schedule. This will allow you to improve the effectiveness of future schedules.

Physicians must often be away from the office to make hospital rounds, perform surgery, or handle personal business, and these absences are also recorded in the appointment book. When the physician will be out of the office, draw an "X" in pencil through the appropriate

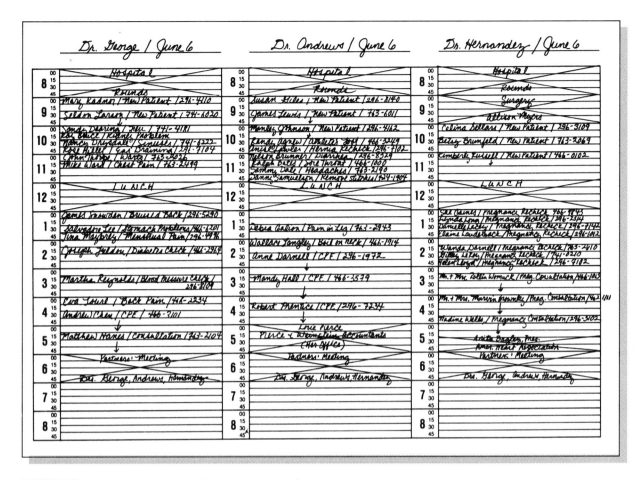

FIGURE 7-3 Appointment book page from a group practice

time period and date; then write a brief explanation. This information is for staff knowledge only and should not be given to patients. The appointment book in Figure 7-3 shows Dr. Andrews' planned absence at 5:00 P.M. on June 6.

Computer Scheduling

 Appointment scheduling can be done by computer using a variety of scheduling software, including The *Medical Manager.* When you want to allocate time for an appointment, the computer system searches through the database of current appointments for an open slot and then schedules the appointment according to your instructions. In some systems, you must enter a code for the type of appointment required. For example, after entering the code "CPE" to request an appointment for a complete physical examination, the computer searches for the first opening with the appropriate time length. If the patient agrees

to the time, you enter the person's name and the computer automatically schedules the appointment. With other systems, you can request a specific date and time, and the computer will search for time availability. If the time is unavailable, the program will request an alternate time. You can continue your search until the computer locates a time slot the patient prefers. Figure 7-4 shows a medical assistant using computerized scheduling software to arrange patient appointments.

Wave Scheduling

One method for managing the schedule is called wave scheduling. Groups of patients are scheduled to arrive all at the same time. For example, a "wave" of several patients may be scheduled to arrive at Oakdale Family Practice at 9 A.M. The office staff routes each patient differently, according to the patient's needs and the availability of practice facilities. While one

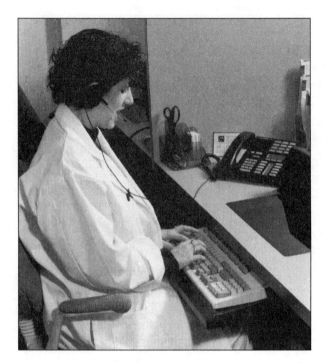

FIGURE 7-4 Appointment scheduling on computer can save time.

patient is having vital signs measured, others complete paperwork, undergo laboratory testing, consult with the physician, or meet with the office manager. Wave scheduling allows full use of the practice staff and facilities while minimizing patient delay.

OVERBOOKING PATIENTS

Overbooking or **double tracking** refers to scheduling more patients than the physician can see during a reasonable period of time. Overbooking is not recommended because it often delays the schedule and frustrates the patients, physician, and staff. You should avoid overbooking unless an emergency patient or a very sick patient must see the doctor immediately. Many physicians like to schedule a thirty-minute break once or twice a day to ease scheduling pressures. In Figure 7-3, on page 129, Drs. George and Hernandez have set aside thirty unscheduled minutes at 11:30 A.M. to compensate for any delays in the morning. Dr. Andrews has thirty minutes unscheduled at 1:00 P.M., allowing the lunch hour to be pushed back if necessary to accommodate patients. However, if physician assistants perform preliminary examinations, patients can be scheduled more closely.

RESCHEDULING AND CANCELING APPOINTMENTS

A patient may sometimes need to reschedule an appointment for a later date, or may decide to cancel the appointment altogether. Since rescheduling and canceling appointments disrupt the schedule, patients should be encouraged to give early notice when they will not be able to keep an appointment. Follow these procedures to reschedule or cancel an appointment:

Procedures to Reschedule an Appointment in the Appointment Book

1. Erase the patient's name at the original appointment time to indicate that the slot is once again available for scheduling.
2. Give the patient one or two alternative dates and times; then ask which time is more convenient.
3. Transfer the patient's name and the reason for the visit to the new date and time.

Procedures to Cancel an Appointment in the Appointment Book

1. Erase the patient's name.
2. Record the cancellation in the patient's medical record. (If the same patient cancels several appointments, tactfully suggest that no further cancellations should be made. You may say, "Mr. Reynolds, will you check your calendar, please, before we schedule this appointment? You had to cancel your three previous appointments.")

Procedures to Reschedule or Cancel an Appointment by Computer

In most computer systems, rescheduling and cancellations are accomplished by deleting the patient's name from the appointed time slot and adding it at another time. The first slot then becomes available for other appointments. Because it is important to maintain a list of cancellations for legal purposes, refer to your software manual to determine whether your system provides a method of record keeping for canceled appointments. If not, maintain a separate list of all cancellations. Also, record the cancellation in the patient's medical record. Refer to the software manual that accompanies your system for specific instructions about rescheduling and canceling appointments.

HANDLING EMERGENCY APPOINTMENTS

An emergency patient should receive top priority and be allowed to see the physician immediately, even though the emergency delays other patients. When emergencies occur, you should call all patients who are affected by the delay and reschedule their appointments for another time. Advise patients already in the office of the emergency and give them the option of waiting for the physician or rescheduling their appointments. When a patient's complaint is serious, work the waiting patient into the schedule as soon as possible the same day. To avoid overcrowding the schedule, delay the other appointments until a later date. Most people are understanding of the need for rescheduling because of an emergency. They will appreciate it if you can give them a choice about waiting, returning, and rescheduling.

COORDINATING DELAYS AND UNEXPECTED APPOINTMENTS

The appointment schedule cannot be followed at all times even in the most efficient and organized medical office. Delays are caused by (1) examinations that take longer than expected, (2) patients who arrive late for their appointments, (3) tests that the doctor orders for patients, (4) important telephone calls that the physician must take between appointments, (5) patients who wish to talk to the physician following their examinations, and (6) other unforeseen reasons. When delays interrupt the appointment schedule, you must adjust the daily routine so the medical staff can return to the schedule. This can be done using these procedures:

Procedures to Adjust the Daily Schedule

1. Alert the physician and medical staff that appointments are behind schedule.
2. Volunteer for some tasks that other office personnel ordinarily handle; for example, clearing examination rooms and preparing them for patients.

3. Determine whether later appointments can be rescheduled for another time. Check with the physician before taking this step.

When the physician will be delayed more than thirty minutes, inform patients waiting in the reception area. They can select magazines, engage in conversation with other patients, or run errands. You will avoid complaints by advising patients of the approximate length of the delay.

RESCHEDULING MISSED APPOINTMENTS

Some patients miss appointments without calling to cancel. When a patient misses an appointment, draw a line through the name in the appointment book and write "Missed" or "No show" beside the name. Refer to your computer software manual for instructions for noting a missed appointment in the computer system. Record the missed appointment in the patient's medical record and mail a card to the person as a reminder. Figure 7-5 illustrates an appointment book page showing a missed appointment. Figure 7-6 shows the reminder that is mailed to the patient.

Some medical offices charge for missed appointments because the doctor wastes valuable time and they cost the medical practice income. You should review office policy carefully regarding this issue since the ill will generated by a missed appointment charge may be too big a risk. When missed appointments are charged, print the notice on the bottom of monthly statements and in any other materials given to patients.

NONPATIENT APPOINTMENTS

People besides patients frequently request appointments with physicians. These may be sales representatives for pharmaceutical companies, medical equipment manufacturers, medical supply companies, or office supply companies; the doctor's accountant or attorney; representatives from civic or charitable organizations; or other doctors. You should ask your employer which visitors should be scheduled routinely. Do not schedule others unless you believe their business can be handled only by

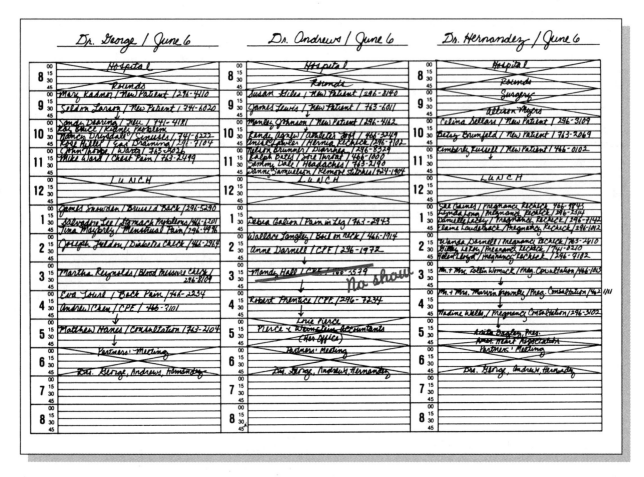

FIGURE 7-5 Appointment book page showing a missed appointment

the physician. When you think the physician would like to see a person who is not a patient, schedule the appointment at a time that will not interrupt the daily routine, such as in the late afternoon.

You can handle many of the nonpatient appointments personally, or if not, you may decide to refer them to other staff members. Since nonpatient callers can take up a great deal of time, only those who have important business or who can be helpful in some way to the practice should be scheduled. Figure 7-5 on this page shows a nonpatient appointment for Dr. Hernandez at 5:30 P.M. on June 6.

Sales Representatives

Most physicians are interested in new pharmaceutical products and innovative or improved medical equipment and supplies. Your responsibility is to distinguish between the sales representatives whose products should be seen per-

sonally by the physician and the representatives whose products can be evaluated by you or someone else. An appointment with a sales representative should be scheduled for approximately fifteen minutes, unless the physician agrees to a longer appointment. Because most sales representatives believe their product is

---

DID YOU FORGET...

your appointment on _____ June 16 _____ at
_____ 9:45 am _____?

Please let us know when you would like to reschedule your appointment.

Molly Bertrand, M.D.
89 Lancaster Highway
Philadelphia, PA 19301
(215) 555-0293

FIGURE 7-6 Missed appointment card

valuable, some may be intimidating in their efforts to convince you to schedule an appointment. Therefore, you must be firm in denying the appointment if you think it is unnecessary.

Most sales representatives are open and straightforward about their business; however, some may attempt to see the physician without disclosing the purpose of the call. For this reason, you must screen all visitors carefully. Ask questions that will extract the information you need. Then if a caller does not provide an adequate explanation, consider the business unimportant and do not schedule an appointment.

SITUATION ONE

Medical Assistant: May I help you?

Visitor: Dr. Benjamin is expecting me.

Medical Assistant: Do you have an appointment?

Visitor: No, but she wants to see the results of the first clinical testing of our new product.

Medical Assistant: Our the staff members review new products first and then make recommendations. Would you like to make an appointment with the office manager?

Visitor: No, I'd prefer to see Dr. Benjamin. If she's too busy today, I'll come back another day.

Medical Assistant: Dr. Benjamin will not see you until your product is reviewed by other staff members.

Visitor: This will only take a minute. I'll just wait and you can work me in between patients.

Medical Assistant: I regret that I can't do that.

Visitor: I know you're trying to do your job. But I think Dr. Benjamin will be very upset if she learns that you wouldn't allow me to see her.

Medical Assistant: As I mentioned, you may make an appointment with the office manager if you like. I'll advise her that you'd like to see her.

Visitor: All right, I'll wait.

SITUATION TWO

Medical Assistant: May I help you?

Visitor: I'd like to see Dr. Hawthorne.

Medical Assistant: Are you a patient?

Visitor: No.

Medical Assistant: Does this concern one of our patients?

Visitor: No.

Medical Assistant: May I ask the purpose of the appointment then?

Visitor: It's personal.

Medical Assistant: Are you a friend of Dr. Hawthorne?

Visitor: No, I just need to see him.

Medical Assistant: You need to give me additional information before I can schedule an appointment. Would you give me your name and the name of your company, please?

Visitor: Elinor Post, from Eastern Office Technology.

Medical Assistant: Is this a sales call regarding one of your products?

Visitor: Well, I want to show him the new computer software we've developed especially for medical offices.

Medical Assistant: Perhaps I could review your software. If you will leave me a brochure and any special information you think I should have, I'll be glad to study it.

Visitor: Do you make the purchasing decisions?

Medical Assistant: I review all office products and make recommendations to Dr. Hawthorne.

Visitor: Since this represents a major purchase, I think I should talk to the doctor.

Medical Assistant: He is not available without an appointment.

Visitor: I'll come back next week.

(Note: If this visitor returns, she should not be given an appointment with the physician.)

Representatives from Charitable Organizations

Physicians often are asked to contribute their time or money to charities. Although most physicians are supportive of charitable organizations and participate in their activities when possible, they do not have time to speak to each representative. Therefore, you should ask the representative for complete details about the organization, the nature of the request, and the date and time of any events in which the doctor might participate. Leave a note for the doctor to review and ask the representative to call you back for the doctor's decision regarding participation or a donation. If the physician wants to participate and wishes to talk to the representative, you can arrange an appointment later. If the physician makes a donation, you can forward a check to the organization.

The Physician's Business Associates

The physician's accountant, stockbroker, or other business associates may occasionally ask for an appointment. Check with the physician in advance to determine which of these people should routinely be given an appointment. If you have a question about a person requesting an appointment, do not schedule it until after you have talked to the physician.

Occasionally other physicians may wish to meet with your employer. As a professional courtesy, escort them to a private office immediately and advise your employer of their presence. Do not ask a visiting physician to wait with patients in the reception area.

IN YOUR OPINION

1. What are the characteristics of good and poor scheduling?
2. How do you know a schedule is a good schedule?
3. What are the different factors you must balance in maintaining a schedule?

Preparing a Daily List of Appointments

The daily list of appointments is prepared at the end of each business day for the next day or in the morning before patients begin arriving. The list shows the names of all patients who will be seen, the time of their appointments, and the reason for the visit. The list is typed neatly on plain paper with the doctor's name and the date centered near the top of the page. A copy is made for each person who works with patients, including the physician, nurses, medical assistants, and others.

 Each staff member places a check mark (✓) beside the patient's name after seeing or treating the person. The medical assistant checks off the name after preparing the patient's medical record for the nurse, the nurse or medical assistant checks off the name after routine tests have been administered, and the physician checks off the name following examination and treatment. Figure 7-7 shows a computerized daily list that was automatically prepared by *The Medical Manager*.

Scheduling Patients for Other Medical Units

Physicians refer their patients to hospitals for out-patient care, in-patient care, and surgery; to laboratories for tests; to other physicians for consultations; to nursing homes and rehabilitation centers for long-term care; and to other medical facilities that treat special problems. You, as a medical assistant, will be responsible for coordinating the patient's arrangements, whether this means simply providing the patient with the name, telephone number, and address of another physician or making complete arrangements, including calling for the appointment and scheduling the tests (Figure 7-8).

SCHEDULING PATIENTS FOR THE HOSPITAL

One of your duties will be to make arrangements for patients who must be admitted to the hospital. Based on the physician's instructions, you will call the hospital admitting clerk and provide the following information:

- Patient's name, address, and telephone number
- Admitting physician's name

```
Slot  Time     Patient                 Len    Reason                    Rm

..............................................................................

02/16/—  Thursday

..............................................................................

1     8:30
2     8:45
3     9:00
4     9:15
5     9:30
6     9:45
7    10:00
8    10:15
9    10:30     30.0 League,Claire       1     1 -General Check-up        0
10   10:45
11   11:00
12   11:15
13   11:30     21.0 Edwards,Portia       2     5 -General Examination     0
14   11:45     21.0 Edwards,Portia       -     5 -General Examination     0
14.1 11:45     14.0 Evans,Deborah        2     5 -General Examination     0
15   12:00     14.0 Evans,Deborah        -     5 -General Examination     0
16   12:15
17   12:30
18   12:45
19    1:00     10.1 Carlson,Sharon       1     1 -General Check-up        0
20    1:15
21    1:30
22    1:45
23    2:00     14.1 Evans,Gene           1     1 -General Check-up        0
24    2:15
25    2:30
26    2:45
27    3:00
28    3:15
29    3:30
30    3:45
31    4:00
32    4:15
33    4:30
34    4:45
35    5:00
```

FIGURE 7-7   Computerized daily list of appointments. (Courtesy of Gartee and Humphrey, *The Medical Manager, Student Edition, Version 5.3,* copyright 1995, Delmar Publishers)

- Date of admission
- Admitting diagnosis
- Consulting physicians' names

After making hospital arrangements, you must call the patient to give him or her the admission date and check-in time. Any special instructions, such as no food or drink after a certain hour, must also be communicated at this time. As a courtesy, you should always ask if the patient has any questions about the hospitalization.

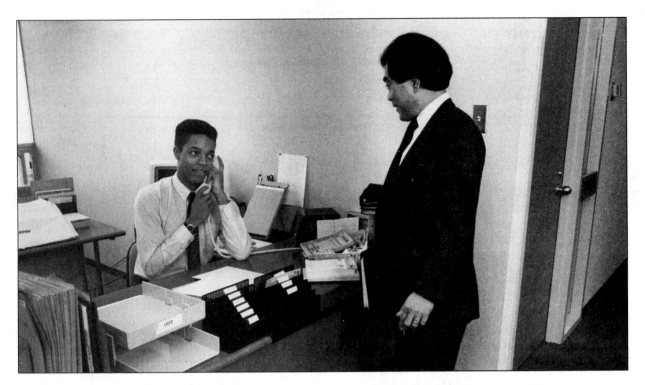

FIGURE 7-8   The medical assistant may need to schedule patients for outside facilities or for referral to other physicians.

SCHEDULING PATIENTS FOR SURGERY

When surgery is to be performed, the time for the surgery is arranged with the surgery scheduling clerk, who must be given the following information:

- Patient's name and address
- Nature of the surgery
- Surgeon's name
- Assisting surgeon's name
- Names of other assisting physicians, such as the anesthesiologist or the pediatrician, in the case of a child's surgery
- Names of other operating room personnel

After arrangements are complete, call the patient with full information about the surgery. Provide any special instructions, for example, how many hours before surgery the patient can eat. Tell the patient the name of the surgeon and all assisting physicians; then try to answer any questions. If the patient has questions you cannot answer, ask the physician to call. Schedule the surgery in the practice's appointment book or computer as shown in Figure 7-9 so that the staff will know the physician will be unavailable during this time period.

SCHEDULING PATIENTS FOR OUTSIDE FACILITIES

Patients frequently require medical service that must be performed outside the physician's office, either by another physician, a laboratory, or a specialty medical service. These patients may be asked to schedule their own appointments, or you may be asked to schedule the appointment for them. If you make the arrangements, call while the patient is in the office. Provide the scheduling clerk with the patient's name, the physician's name, the diagnosis, any necessary details regarding the service to be performed, and the previous treatment. When arrangements are complete, give the patient a card showing the date, time, and place of the appointment.

7:00 A.M.	
7:15 A.M.	Angelea Stern/D & C
7:30 A.M.	
7:45 A.M.	Antona Carpenter/Hysterectomy

FIGURE 7-9   Appointment book showing surgery schedule

```
_____Gary Lutel_____ is scheduled for an

appointment with Dr. _____Concord_____ at

____2____ a.m./p.m. on _____June 19, 19—_____ .


                            Mabel Buck, M.D.
```

FIGURE 7-10 Referral card

SCHEDULING PATIENTS FOR REFERRAL

Primary care physicians sometimes refer patients to consulting physicians for additional tests and examinations or for a second opinion. You may be asked to make the appointment or to give the name and telephone number of the consulting physician to the patient. Keep a handy list of names, addresses, and telephone numbers of all physicians to whom patients are routinely referred.

Give the following information to the medical assistant at the consulting physician's office:

- Patient's name
- Preliminary diagnosis
- Previous treatment
- Service to be provided
- Referring physician's name

Prepare an information card for the patient who is being referred. Include (1) the name of the referring physician, (2) the address and telephone number of the consulting physician, and (3) the date and time of the appointment. A preprinted form or a blank 3" × 5" card may be used for this purpose. A referral card is shown in Figure 7-10.

Follow-Up Appointments

Monitoring an existing health condition and preventive medicine are accomplished through follow-up appointments. These can be either progress appointments designed to check on and control an existing condition or periodic routine appointments that allow the physician to evaluate a patient's health. Both types of follow-up appointments are important for the overall care of patients, and you must assist patients in arranging follow-up appointments that will encourage good health practices. Follow-up appointments can be tracked easily by computer. You will enter a command to store the patient's name for a follow-up appointment in the future, usually for a specific month. Later, when you recall all follow-up appointments needed that month, you will be given the patient's name. The computer can also print a follow-up reminder card.

PROGRESS APPOINTMENTS

Many patients see their physician for follow-up appointments to monitor the progress of their treatment. When appointments are to be scheduled for the near future, ask the patient to make arrangements before leaving the office at the time of the current visit. Then prepare a card showing the date and time of the next appointment and give it to the patient. A progress follow-up card is shown in Figure 7-11.

ROUTINE PERIODIC APPOINTMENTS

Patients who see their physicians for routine appointments on a regular schedule, for example, every six months or once a year, may prefer to wait until a time close to the required date to make arrangements. You should maintain a tickler file containing the name and approximate follow-up date for each patient. A few weeks before the follow-up is due, mail a reminder notice to the patient.

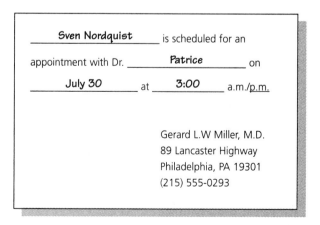

```
_____Sven Nordquist_____ is scheduled for an

appointment with Dr. _____Patrice_____ on

____July 30____ at ____3:00____ a.m./p.m.


                        Gerard L.W Miller, M.D.
                        89 Lancaster Highway
                        Philadelphia, PA 19301
                        (215) 555-0293
```

FIGURE 7-11 Progress appointment follow-up

Chapter 7 Scheduling Appointments   **135**

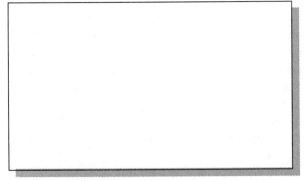

Front of card

IT'S TIME for your _____ month check up.

Please call the office for an appointment.

Jennifer Tinnari, M.D.
89 Dick Lane
Trevose, PA 19301
(215) 555-0293

Back of card

FIGURE 7-12   Reminder card

Some offices use a different system. You may ask patients to address a preprinted reminder card before leaving the office at the current visit. A few weeks before the appointment is due, stamp and mail the card, thus giving the patient adequate time to schedule a follow-up. Medical offices that are computerized may instruct the computer to print reminder notices on a regular schedule. For example, once-a-month reminders can be printed for all patients who need to schedule an appointment within the next month or two. A reminder card is shown in Figure 7-12.

IN YOUR OPINION

1. Explain this statement, "A schedule is a good servant, but a poor master."
2. What would cause the following practices to need flexibility in scheduling: (1) pediatrics, (2) orthopedic surgery, (3) obstetrics, and (4) dermatology?
3. How can good scheduling improve patient satisfaction? The financial performance of the practice?

REFERENCES

Humphrey, Doris D. *Pediatric Associates, P.C.* Cincinnati, Ohio: South-Western Publishing Co., 1988.

Humphrey, Doris D., and Kathie Sigler. *The Modern Medical Office: A Reference Manual.* Cincinnati, Ohio: South-Western Publishing Co., 1990.*

*Currently published by Delmar Publishers.

Chapter Activities

PERFORMANCE BASED ACTIVITIES

1. Debate with a classmate the advantages and disadvantages of scheduling on a computer versus in an appointment book. Key and print a summary of your point of view. (DACUM 3.2, 6.6)

2. Develop a plan for the following schedule interruption. A blizzard has caused the physician and much of the office staff to be late. Several patients negotiated roads and are waiting. (DACUM 1.8, 3.1)

3. Create practice guidelines for building flexibility into a schedule. (DACUM 2.11, 3.7)

4. Prepare a form showing information to be acquired before scheduling patients for hospital admission. Using a fictitious patient, fill in information you might already have as part of the patient's file. (DACUM 4.6, 5.2)

EXPANDING YOUR THINKING

1. You think that the current scheduling policies of the practice result in overbooking and delay. How could you measure scheduling success to support your opinion?

2. Your practice consists of three physicians. One is a single mother and the other two are a married couple with children. The practice is open six days a week. Each physician wishes to work five days a week. Construct two different schedules for a one month period, and assess the advantages of each.

3. Linda Hebert has a condition the physician is unable to diagnose and is being referred to Dr. Raisa Van Doren for consultation. Your employer asks you to make the arrangements. List the steps you will follow and include any conversations you will have.

Referral Procedure

Information Needed   *Person to Contact*

1. _____

2. _____

3. _____

4. _____

5. _____

6. _____

Portfolio Assessment

DACUM 2.8, 2.9, 3.1–3.7

1. Use Portfolio Figure PII-1 to schedule by hand the appointments shown in Portfolio Figures PII-2 through PII-8. Key and print a daily list of appointments for July 15.
2. Arrange an appointment with your mentor to observe practice scheduling methods used in your mentoring practice. Complete Portfolio Figure PII-9; then summarize in paragraph form what you learned from this experience.
3. Interview the senior medical assistant at your mentoring practice asking the questions listed below. Audiotape the interview or prepare a two-page summary of your conversation. Comment on how your thinking has changed or remained the same regarding a medical assistant's job.

   Questions

   a. How many patients are seen daily and what are the office hours?
   b. What security procedures does the office have for drugs kept in the office?
   c. What three types of incoming calls to the medical office are the most difficult to screen?
   d. What is the greatest problem the medical assistant has in maintaining medical records?
   e. What method is used for internal/external billing?
   f. Why did the medical assistant choose the medical profession as a career?
   g. Compile a list of magazines and toys kept in the waiting room.
4. Ask for permission to interview three patients. Prepare a list of five questions that focus on what they like about the practice. Compile, compare, and prioritize their answers to determine what patients at your mentoring practice consider most important about the practice.
5. Form a group with four other class members. Combine your responses for No. 4 and reach a consensus about what is important. Form a panel and present your responses to the class.

MONDAY _July 15_

9:00	Matthew Jackson / Tired, can't sleep / 555-44??	
9:30	Martha McClendon / gastric?/ 555-0010	
10:15	John Rhenholt / urinary problems / 555-1918	
10:45	Richard Duncan / Checkup / 555-341	
11:00	Paula Roses / Sore throat / 555-1261	
11:30–12:45	Lunch	
1:15	Leslie Roland / Complete physical exam / 555-1000	
1:45	Suzanne Cadle / eye tearing / 555-4391	
2:30	Barbara Boyer / old knee injury / 555-1192	
3:30	Nancy Armand / Pap / 555-6868	

TUESDAY _July 16_

9:00	Jane Morley / Diabetes / 555-4949	
9:15	Martha Drake / cough / 555-1904	
10:15	Anna Qusics / complete physical exam / 555-4111	
11:30–12:30	Lunch	
12:45	Franch Shuler / Sinuses / 555-1918	
1:30	Barbara Knoeli / Back pain / 555-4685	
2:00	Frances Dodd / Kidney infection / 555-1191	
2:30	William Morgan / remove cast / 555-1931	
3:00	Betty Eddins / Back Pain / 555-4014	
3:30	Sandy Weasley / checkup / 555-9011	

WEDNESDAY _July 17_

11:30–12:45	Lunch	

PORTFOLIO FIGURE PII-1

MEMO FROM
    DR. REBECCA CRANE

Please schedule a consultation appointment for Leslie Roland on July 17, so I can review the results of his CPE. He needs an early a.m. or late p.m. appointment.

RC

PORTFOLIO FIGURE PII-2

TO *DR. CRANE'S SECRETARY*   DATE __7/15/—__
                               TIME __9:00 a.m.__

TELEPHONE MESSAGE

M *RS. NANCY ARMAND* ___ OF _____

ADDRESS _____

CALLED	✓	WANTS TO SEE YOU		RETURNED YOUR CALL	
PLEASE CALL	✓	WILL CALL AGAIN		URGENT	

MESSAGE *Cancelled her 3:30 appt. today. Wants to reschedule for 7/17 at 3:30. Please change the appointment. Call her if change cannot be made.*

PHONE NUMBER __505-6868__   TAKEN BY *Tina*

PORTFOLIO FIGURE PII-3

TELEPHONE MESSAGE

DATE 7/15/— TIME 9:30 a.m. DR. Crane

NAME Mrs. Waasdorp PATIENT'S NAME Sandy Waasdorp

[X] TELEPHONED   RETURN PHONE NO. _____   RETURN TIME _____   [ ] WILL CALL BACK

TO Dr. Crane's secretary   FROM Victoria Ramonez

PHARMACY _____

PHONE _____

AGE _____ WT. _____

MESSAGE   Sandy Waasdorp will not be in at 3:30 p.m. tomorrow for her checkup. Ms. Waasdorp has rescheduled the appointment for July 17 at 2:00 p.m. You need to make the changes in the appointment book. I confirmed the time with Ms. Waasdorp.

Rolf

PRESCRIPTION STRENGTH _____

AMOUNT _____

LABEL _____
_____
_____

FOR _____
[ ] SIDE EFFECTS ___ REFILL

FOLLOW-UP _____
_____
_____

PORTFOLIO FIGURE PII-4

TO Dr. Crane's secretary

DATE 7/15/—
TIME 10:30 a.m.

TELEPHONE MESSAGE

Mrs Abernathy, secretary OF Dr. Linda Bronner's office

ADDRESS _____

CALLED	✓ WANTS TO SEE YOU	RETURNED YOUR CALL
PLEASE CALL	WILL CALL AGAIN	URGENT

MESSAGE Dr. Bronner is referring Mrs. Sally Fields to Dr. Crane for a consultation. Make an appointment for Mrs. Fields for 7/16 or /17; then call Mrs. Fields and tell her the date and time.

PHONE NUMBER 555-1283   TAKEN BY Jose

PORTFOLIO FIGURE PII-5

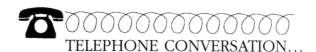

TELEPHONE CONVERSATION...

Telephone Rings:

Medical Secretary: Good morning. Dr. Crane's office. May I help you?

Patient: This is Waltyer Burgham. We are going out of town Thursday. I would like to come to the office Tuesday afternoon or Wednesday morning for a recheck of my strep throat. Is that possible?

Medical Secretary: I'll check the appointment book. One moment please. (Pause) Dr. Crane can see you at 2:45 p.m. Tuesday or between 9 and 10 a.m. Wednesday. Which time is more convenient for you?

Patient: May I come in Tuesday at 3:30 instead of 2:45?

PORTFOLIO FIGURE PII-6

MEMO FROM
DR. REBECCA CRANE

July 16, 19--

Sheila Duckworth of Medical Micrographics, Inc., would like to demonstrate micrographics equipment to us on Wednesday, July 17. I have asked my new medical assistant to arrange my calendar, so I can see the demo at 4 p.m. and I would like you to attend also. We may soon lease micrographics equipment for our inactive medical records.

PORTFOLIO FIGURE PII-7

DESK NOTES

From: **Rebecca Crane, M.D.**

7/16

Scott Lansing, my attorney, needs
to see me for about an hour
on Wednesday. If there is an hour
free immediately before or after
lunch, make the appointment then.
He will call you this morning for
a confirmation.

RC

PORTFOLIO FIGURE PII-8

Analysis of Scheduling in Mentoring Practice

Scheduling Method   *Check One*

         Manual   _____

         Computerized   _____

Factors Determining When Patients Will Be Given an Appointment

1. _____
2. _____
3. _____
4. _____
5. _____
6. _____

Amount of Time (in Minutes) Reserved for Appointments

    New Patients

         Level I   _____

         Level II   _____

         Level III   _____

         Level IV   _____

    Established Patients

         Level I   _____

         Level II   _____

         Level III   _____

         Level IV   _____

Number of Patients Seen Each Day

    Average Day   _____

    Busy Day   _____

    Slow Day   _____

Staff Members Who Will Be Involved with Patients

    Title   *Responsibility*

1. _____
2. _____
3. _____
4. _____
5. _____
6. _____

PORTFOLIO FIGURE PII-9

Method for Handling Cancellations

Procedure for Responding to Emergencies

Physicians' Preferences for Scheduling Personal Appointments

Other Special Scheduling Considerations

What I Learned About Scheduling:

PORTFOLIO FIGURE PII-9 (continued)

Computers and Information Processing in the Medical Office

Computers, originally used in the medical field by hospitals for billing and administration, have taken on an important function in private medical practices as well. Computers are now used for most administrative tasks, such as billing and collection, check writing, payroll management, accounts posting, personnel records, drug and supply inventory, recall notices, and financial and tax applications. In addition, computers give physicians access to the most current medical research and opinion from around the world through medical databases and bulletin boards.

Computerizing a medical office usually leads to increased productivity, efficiency, and organization. Computers simplify tasks that are difficult, repetitive, and time-consuming. Consequently, employee morale improves, and patients receive speedier service with fewer mistakes.

As a medical assistant, you will be expected to know about computers in general and medical computing applications in particular. Office automation is just one part of information management. You will create, maintain, store, retrieve, and route data and documents of many types. In addition to conventional U.S. mail, you will use various forms of expedited mail, such as Federal Express, UPS, Priority Mail, and even couriers. Intelligent selection among these choices will result in high quality, cost-effective service.

The following section will give you an overview of what to expect from medical computing and communication systems.

Chapter 8

Information Equipment and Processes

MADISON, WISCONSIN

My sister asked me if I thought she should take some computer courses, and I said, "Absolutely!" She's also thinking of going into the medical field, and I told her I can hardly believe all the pieces of electronic equipment I use at work. When we moved our offices recently, I even set up my own personal computer and connected it to the printer and modem.

I've taken some courses for searching online medical databases, and we may soon be purchasing a medical reference library stored on laser disk. I often dial into our university library here in Madison, but I've also networked with practices as far away as Taiwan and Scotland. We receive very few journals anymore, but keep up with the latest research in our specialty by scanning the literature every week for selected topics.

Dana Howard
Medical Librarian

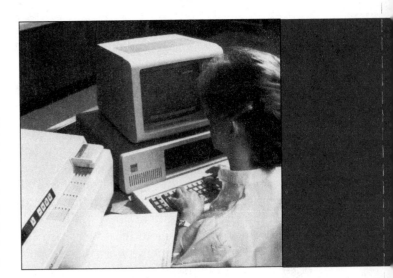

3. Analyze and choose among available special mail services. (DACUM 3.6, 6.4)
4. Compare available telecommunications services and match their capabilities to office needs. (DACUM 6.2, 6.4)

PERFORMANCE BASED COMPETENCIES

After completing this chapter, you should be able to:
1. Compare the components of the information processing system and explain how each is used during the information processing cycle. (DACUM 2.7, 3.4)
2. Categorize and prioritize incoming mail. (DACUM 2.5, 3.1)

HEALTHSPEAK

Central processing unit (CPU) Electronic circuitry that performs computer instructions.

Data Numbers and letters keyed into a computer.

Data processing Organization of data into understandable information that can be used in decision making.

Disk drive Internal or external storage device for computer documents and programs.

Function keys Extra keys that expand the computer's capacity.

Hardware Machines in a computer system.

Keyboard Input device that allows the operator to key data into the computer.

Micrographics Photographic process that miniaturizes documents and stores them on magnetic film or cards.

Modem Device that converts a sender's computer signals into telephone signals.

Monitor Television-like screen on which words, charts, letters, and other data appear.

Optical character recognition Process by which handwritten or printed characters are converted into electronic impulses that a computer or word processor can understand.

Reprographics Process of making copies.

Software Programs or instructions that operate computers.

Word processing Processing of words to form narrative documents, using a computer and software package instead of a typewriter.

Information processing is a broad term that describes the flow of information from its creation to its permanent storage. The path a letter takes from the time it is dictated until it is stored in a file cabinet is an example of the flow of information.

The term information processing also refers to the use of electronic equipment, including computers, word processors, facsimile or FAX machines, and cellular and satellite communications. Medical offices without information processing technology are the exception rather than the norm.

The Information Cycle

Information flows in a cycle of five stages: (1) input, (2) processing, (3) output, (4) storage, and (5) distribution, as shown in Figure 8-1. Whether a medical office uses traditional means or electronic equipment, each piece of information moves through each stage of the cycle. Figure 8-2 traces the information processing cycle of a dictated document for a patient record and describes each phase of the cycle.

Consider the time saved in the processing, output, and distribution stages when electronic equipment is used in the information processing cycle. In addition to saving time, electronic equipment usually results in less paper handling and improved morale because the staff does not have to perform dull, repetitive activities.

These steps show the information flow in a linear route, moving directly from one step to another. However, information does not always flow in a straight line. By adding other typical steps in the information processing cycle, increased efficiency becomes even more apparent (Figure 8-3). Study Figure 8-4 to see how the stages of the cycle overlap.

The Computer System

 A computer system consists of hardware and software. Hardware refers to the equipment; that is, the machines that are visible and tangible in a computer system. This includes the central processing unit, the keyboard, the monitor, and the disk drives.

INPUT	Data collected from a variety of sources is compiled. This includes the patient information questionnaire, laboratory reports, consulting reports, and other background information. The physician dictates a case history into a dictating machine.
PROCESSING	Some treatment is given to the information, either with pen and paper or by computer. This step involves the work of organizing facts and transforming them into something meaningful; for example, processing the physician's dictated report to develop a patient's history.
OUTPUT	The finished report is shown on paper or on a computer screen. Copies are made if needed.
STORAGE	The processed report is filed for later retrieval.
DISTRIBUTION/ COMMUNICATION	The information is delivered to the source for whom it was intended.

FIGURE 8-1 The five steps involved in information processing in a medical environment

	Traditional Office	**Electronic Office**
INPUT	This stage is the same for both types of offices unless the document has previously been keyed and stored electronically. Data is collected, compiled, and given to the physician who dictates a patient history.	
PROCESSING	Medical assistant keys the dictation on a typewriter and uses correction materials or a correcting key for mistakes. Corrections are visible on the original document, though they may be neat. If corrections are excessive or too messy, the document must be rekeyed.	Medical assistant keys the dictation using a keyboard and an electronic device, either an electronic typewriter, a word processor, or a computer with word processing software. Corrections are made on the screen and saved in the machine's memory. The central processing unit arranges, edits, tabulates, or performs some other function to organize the data.
OUTPUT	The finished document is removed from the typewriter.	An original document with no visible corrections is printed.
STORAGE	A copy of the patient's history is filed by hand in the medical record folder.	The patient's history is filed either on a floppy disk or on a hard disk. A hard copy is filed by hand in the medical record folder. (This step can be eliminated when patient records are stored electronically; however, some medical offices continue to maintain both paper and electronic files.)
DISTRIBUTION/ COMMUNICATION	An envelope is keyed; the report is enclosed and mailed to the referring physician, if appropriate for the patient's case.	An address is retrieved from electronic memory, and an envelope is printed, so the report can be mailed to the referring physician. If an electronic mail system is available between the two physicians, the document can be transmitted electronically.

FIGURE 8-2 Comparison of dictation in traditional office and electronic office

Software refers to the programs or instructions that operate the computers. *The Medical Manager,* for example, is medical billing software. Hundreds of different software programs can be used with almost any computer.

Hardware and software can be compared to a VCR machine and a videotape. The VCR machine by itself is useless unless the tape is inserted. The main menu screen from *The Medical Manager* is shown in Figure 8-5.

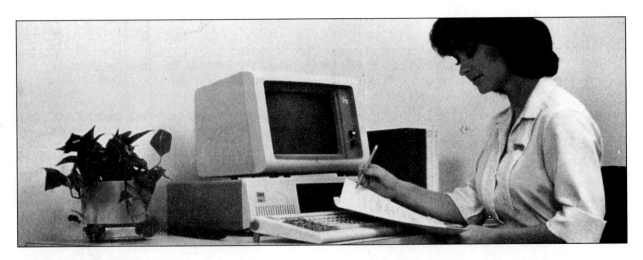

FIGURE 8-3 The introduction of electronic equipment into the information processing cycle results in considerable time saving in processing, output, and distribution.

Stage	Problem	Solution—Traditional Office	Solution—Automated Office
PROCESSING	Several mistakes are made during keying.	Correction fluid or paper, erasure, or an electronic correction key is used. If corrections are excessive, the entire report must be rekeyed.	Corrections are made on screen and are saved in the memory; a perfect copy is printed.
OUTPUT	Physician makes changes in or adds to report.	Report must be rekeyed.	Report is retrieved from electronic memory and changes are keyed. The entire document is not rekeyed.
DISTRIBUTION	Physician asks for an additional copy of the report.	Report is retrieved from the medical record, photocopied, and then returned to the medical record.	Report is retrieved from electronic memory, and an additional copy is printed. The medical record is not involved.

FIGURE 8-4 Information flowing across cycles

HARDWARE

Computer hardware and software change very rapidly. Today's computers have more processing power than those of a few years ago, yet they are smaller and less expensive. Personal computers and even laptops will run most of the medical software in use; however, personal computers do not have the memory capacity to run some of the comprehensive medical programs. Many medical offices, especially larger

```
01/10/--          Personalized Programming, Inc.            Menu 1
                         The Medical Manager

                  Sydney Carrington & Associates, PA

      1 - NEW Patient Entry         6 - BILLING Routines

      2 - PROCEDURE Entry           7 - FILE Maintenance

      3 - PAYMENT Entry             8 - OFFICE Management

      4 - DISPLAY Patient Data      9 - SYSTEM Utilities

      5 - REPORT Generation        18 - (Reserved)


                  Enter Desired Option : .....
```

FIGURE 8-5 Main menu screen (Courtesy of Gartee and Humphrey, *The Medical Manager, Student Edition, Version 5.3,* copyright 1995, Delmar Publishers)

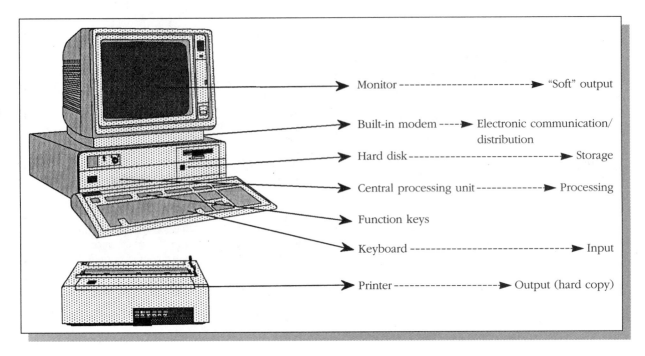

Monitor ----------------------▶ "Soft" output

Built-in modem ----▶ Electronic communication/ distribution

Hard disk -------------------------▶ Storage

Central processing unit -------------▶ Processing

Function keys

Keyboard -------------------------------▶ Input

Printer -------------------▶ Output (hard copy)

FIGURE 8-6 Computer hardware components

group practices, purchase or lease minicomputers, which are larger and more sophisticated than personal computers.

Figure 8-6 shows typical computer hardware for a medical office. The function of each hardware component is also listed. Review the functions of each piece of hardware. Compare these functions to the information cycle shown in Figure 8-1 on page 149 for additional understanding of the role of each piece of equipment.

Keyboard

The keyboard is an input device that allows the operator to key data into the computer. A computer keyboard looks like a typewriter keyboard except that it has extra keys, called function keys, that expand the computer's capacity. Function keys are shown above the keyboard in Figure 8-6. By pressing a function key designated by the software program, the user can tell the computer to perform such tasks as edit, format, delete or save text, check for spelling errors, and print. Some newer and enhanced systems replace function keys with a mouse and menu-driven software.

Monitor

The television-like screen on which words, charts, letters, and other data appear is called the monitor. Full-color monitors supported by software that displays graphics and pictures are becoming more prevalent, though older, monochrome systems may show only gray, green, or amber.

Central Processing Unit

The central processing unit (CPU) is the electronic circuitry that performs instructions stored in software programs. For example, after keying a medical report, you may use a function key to tell the CPU to format the report for printing. The CPU follows the command of the function key and arranges the words and paragraphs into an attractive medical report format ready for printing.

To store data, the CPU uses temporary memory. Computer memory works in the same way as human memory, with the computer holding the information temporarily for tallying, organizing, editing, or changing. Just as human memory is invisible, neither can one see the computer's memory. It is built in at the factory in computer chips, hidden inside the machine,

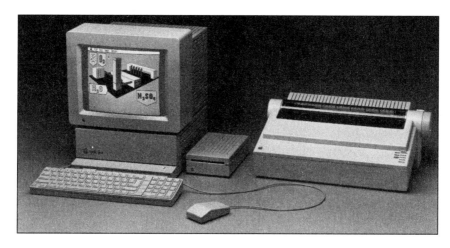

FIGURE 8-7 The Apple IIGS with AppleColor RGB monitor (Courtesy of Apple Computer, Inc.)

and available for use as needed. The cost of a computer is largely determined by the amount of Random Access Memory (RAM) it contains—the greater the amount of RAM, the more expensive the computer.

Random Access Memory, sometimes called working memory, is measured in thousands of units or bytes of information. A typical 486 computer has 4 megabytes of RAM or 4,000,000 characters. This translates into about 800,000 words or 3,200 pages. Since some temporary memory is required for the program instructions, not all of the temporary memory is available for documents.

Disk Drive

Documents and computer programs are stored on disks housed in a computer's disk drive(s). The disk drives allow data either to be read from a disk or to be written onto a disk. They may be built inside the computer, or they may be detached.

A medical assistant wishing to add information to a patient's medical history would command the computer to retrieve the history from the disk and make changes as directed by the physician. After finishing the document and saving the revisions, the medical assistant would close the file and save it either on the hard drive or on a floppy disk.

Drives are available for both hard and floppy disks, but the trend in medical offices is to use hard disk storage. With a hard disk, the operator does not physically touch the disks since they are airtight, inflexible (or hard), and permanently stored in the computer. Hard disks are faster and more efficient than floppy disks, and they are relatively trouble-free. In addition, a hard disk allows for storing a large volume of data. Since even small medical offices have several hundred or a few thousand patients, storage capacity is important. Typically, a medical computing consultant recommends a minimum of 100 megabytes of storage for a growing practice. The term *mega* means million.

You may use floppy disks in your classroom. Floppy disks are commonly used when a minimum amount of storage space is needed or when data is to be transported from one location to another. Lengthy documents and records may be sent on a disk rather than on paper.

Printer

As with most computer equipment, the choices among printers have blossomed in recent years. Laser printers, once quite expensive, are now affordable. Ink-jet printers provide near laser quality documents at a lower cost. Most printer manufacturers also offer high quality portable printers. Printers come in many types with varying characteristics. The price is determined by the quantity of advanced features.

Modem

Computers can transmit data to one another across telephone lines if they are connected by a modem. A modem is an external or internal device that converts a sender's computer signals into telephone signals so they can be sent to a computer in a different location. The receiving computer must also have a modem to convert the telephone signals into computer messages.

Information Processing Components

Although the term "word processing" has often been used incorrectly to describe a broad range of office procedures and technology, it is actually only one component of information processing that interacts with other components to move data through the cycle. Nine separate office technologies are linked together to process information as shown in Figure 8-8. The volume of data to be processed establishes which components are used. For example, a large hospital might use all the technologies, whereas a small private practice might use only a few components. This chapter explores the information cycle as it pertains to a small medical office.

A solo practice with one medical assistant will need, at least, a telephone and typewriter or word processor. As the practice grows, requiring more sophisticated methods of managing its paperwork, it may add a computer for billing, word processing, and scheduling. If the practice continues to grow, several or perhaps even all nine components may be required to process information. Each electronic component and the role it plays in a medical office are discussed in the next section.

DATA PROCESSING

Every day, billions of unrelated facts such as names, addresses, dates, ages, symptoms, illnesses, and diagnoses are used in medical offices. These unrelated facts, or data, are of no value unless they are organized or related. Data processing describes the organization of data into information that can be used in decision making. Although office personnel can process this data manually, the large volume of work, even in a small practice, makes manual processing unrealistic.

WORD PROCESSING

IBM invented the term word processing to describe the processing of words to form narra-

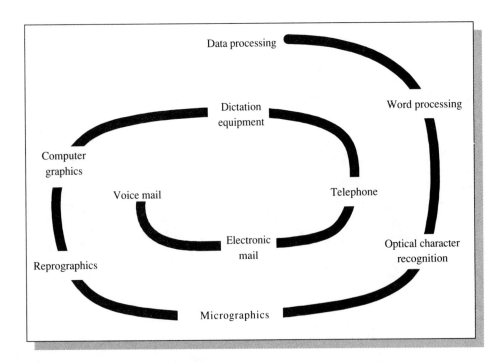

FIGURE 8-8 Information processing components

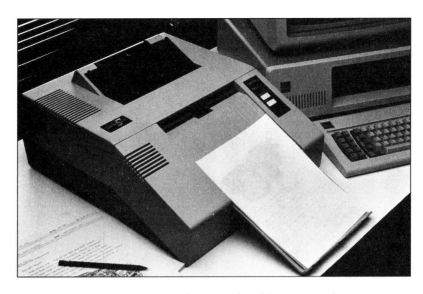

FIGURE 8-9 OCRs are used to scan documents for editing or storage by a computer.

tive documents. In medical offices, word processing is used widely to produce printed copies of medical reports, letters, research articles, business documents, and other communications. Although documents can be stored electronically on disk and retrieved as needed, a paper or "hard" copy of a document may also be printed for filing. After you begin work as a medical assistant, you may create correspondence on a word processor and print copies for manual storage.

OPTICAL CHARACTER RECOGNITION

Optical character recognition is performed by a machine called an optical character reader (OCR). It is able to scan the characters on a previously typed or handwritten document and convert them into electronic impulses that a computer or word processor can understand (Figure 8-9). OCRs are valuable because they scan documents and enter information into a computer system faster and more accurately than a person can key the same information.

Hospitals use OCR equipment to scan incoming documents for editing or storing by a computer, and insurance companies use OCR equipment in their claim departments to input information from hundreds of insurance claim forms that arrive daily. This saves time and money.

An OCR machine works very much like an electronic copier. An operator places a document on the machine's glass plate where it is scanned by an electronic eye. Instead of a copied document appearing in a copy bin, however, characters from the original document are transmitted by electronic signals to the memory of a computer or word processor. The documents are stored or they are edited and reprinted. Similar electronic scanners are used at grocery checkout counters, in department stores to read pricing information from labels, by automated bank tellers to read the magnetic strip on bank cards, and by the post office to sort mail by ZIP code.

MICROGRAPHICS

A photographic process called micrographics miniaturizes standard size documents and stores them on magnetic film or cards. Since the miniatures are about 1/100th of the original document size, the use of micrographics greatly reduces the storage space required for files. Microfilm, which resembles a roll of movie film, and microfiche, a small magnetic sheet of film, are two popular forms of micrographics used in medical facilities (Figure 8-10). Cameras reduce, photograph, and store regular size documents on microfilm or microfiche. Later, an individual can enlarge the documents for viewing and

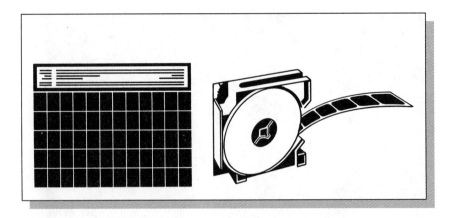

FIGURE 8-10 Microfiche and microfilm (From Humphrey and Sigler, *The Modern Medical Office: A Reference Manual,* copyright 1991, Delmar Publishers)

printing with a special microfilm or microfiche reader as shown in Figure 8-11.

Medical offices use microfiche and microfilm primarily for storing inactive medical records. Since medical practices, hospitals, and other facilities must maintain medical records for several years for legal purposes, storage space can become costly. Operating expenses are reduced when records are miniaturized before storage.

Medical records may be sent to an outside filming company for reduction, or they can be converted to microfilm or microfiche at the office. Advanced technology called Computer Output Microforms (COMs) allows computers to store information directly on microfiche or microfilm.

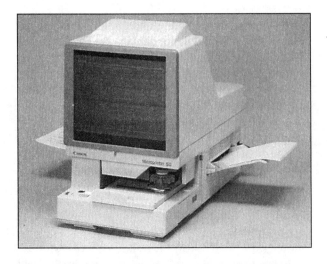

FIGURE 8-11 Microfilm reader-printer machine. (Courtesy of Canon, Inc.)

REPROGRAPHICS

Reprographics is a fancy term for making copies. The quantity of material to be duplicated determines the type of machine that should be used, although computer printers and electronic copiers are most commonly used in small medical offices. Copy work can be sent out to a company that specializes in high-volume reproduction and can produce color copies. A medical facility that produces a large volume of documents usually leases or purchases a high-speed copier.

COMPUTER GRAPHICS

Computer graphics—the pictures, diagrams, and graphs drawn with a computer—are used to clarify narrative data, illustrate a point, or interpret data visually. Pictorial illustrations can be made on the screen or printed on hard copy.

In a medical office, computer graphics are useful for representing visually a practice's financial analysis, illustrating the results of medical research, or following medical trends. For example, using the data from a daily log, a bar graph can illustrate which physicians contribute the greatest income to a practice or which procedures are performed most frequently, as shown in Figures 8-12 and 8-13.

DICTATION

Dictation is a major source of input to the information processing cycle. The physician can dictate medical reports, examination results, doc-

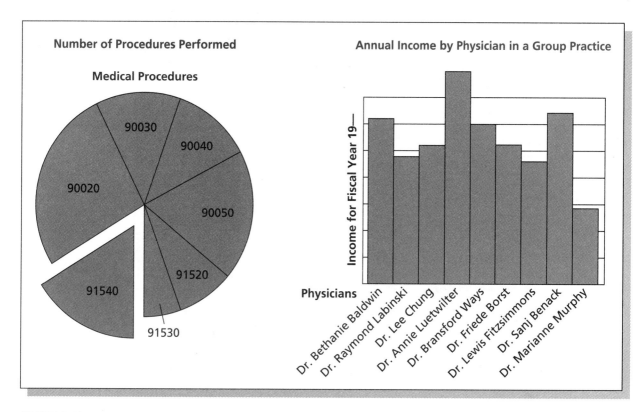

FIGURE 8-12 Example of computer graphics

tor's notes, and other information when it is convenient without disrupting the daily schedule. The medical assistant or a medical transcriptionist then transcribes the dictated material. Voice-activated computers, which will become more common in the future, transcribe the physician's oral reports. Some large hospitals have this technology now. By the time patients are returned to their rooms following procedures or examinations, the nurses can view computerized reports giving all information needed for follow-up care.

In large medical institutions, special dictating areas equipped with telephones are set up in a central location so that physicians can dictate medical notes and reports. The dictation is recorded on magnetic tapes in the dictation center and transcribed by specially trained medical transcriptionists in the medical record department.

TELEPHONE

Telephone technology combined with computer linkage has vastly expanded possible applications of the telephone. Physicians can use telephones to link patients in hospitals to machines that conduct tests and monitor the results, even though the testing facility may be hundreds of miles away. Experts predict that telephone and computer technology will soon become so intertwined that the general population will be unable to tell where one system ends and the other begins.

ELECTRONIC MAIL/ELECTRONIC COMMUNICATION

Computers and word processors can communicate, either through cables connecting the machines or through telephone lines. This process of sending messages using electronic devices is called **electronic mail** or **"e-mail."** Electronic mail allows an individual at one computer terminal to send a message to another computer terminal across the room, across the city, or across the world in much the same way that mail is delivered from one postal address to another.

With electronic mail, each user has a mail location identified by a special address code,

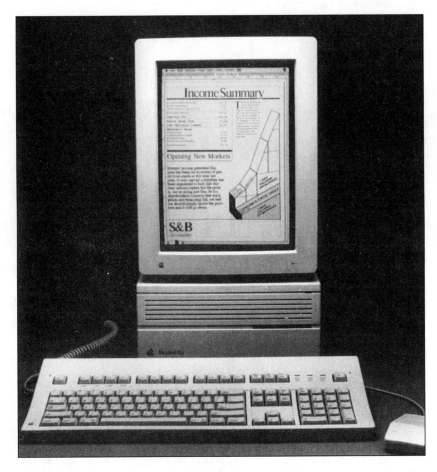

FIGURE 8-13 Computer graphics help clarify, illustrate, and interpret data. (Courtesy of Apple Computer, Inc.)

sometimes as simple as the person's name. When staff members want to send mail to one another, they simply key the mail address code, the message, and the "send" command. The receiving computer makes a beeping sound or a message blinks on the screen when an electronic mail message is received to alert the user. Mail messages can then either be read from the screen or printed.

As a medical assistant, you may arrange meetings between your employer and the hospital on an electronic calendar, a form of electronic mail. You may also send medical reports, patient information, medical instructions, and other information to the medical records department of a hospital electronically. In major hospitals, nursing stations are connected to the hospital's main computer, allowing for electronic communication among the nurses, pharmacy, and physicians.

Electronic communication, made possible by modems, is growing in popularity in medical offices. Users can access medical news and journals, computer-based education programs, consultation with specialists worldwide, and dosage and patient care instructions. Other electronic communication options are discussed later.

VOICE MAIL

Voice mail refers to a special system of communicating by telephone and computer hookup using voices instead of typed messages. A recording answers a telephone when the correct number is dialed, tapes the voice message, stores it in memory, and signals the recipient of the waiting message. Voice mail is sometimes used instead of an answering service. Messages can be retrieved even when the recipient is not at the location of the voice mail system.

Making Computerization Decisions

Leasing or purchasing hardware and software requires careful planning and extensive research. Lack of thorough planning and knowledge can result in frustrating, ineffective results at great expense. Since the investment in a medical computing system can be very large, from $20,000 for a small office to many times that amount for larger offices, a physician is unlikely to make a major change once a system has been chosen.

Consultants are available to provide guidance regarding the purchase of medical office systems. Selecting good software is a primary concern when purchasing computers. The medical staff involved in this decision should spend the largest part of its time previewing software packages and making sure they perform the functions needed by the practice. Since not all software programs run on all computers, the computer selected must be compatible with the software chosen. Some medical offices make the mistake of first purchasing the computer and then locating software that runs on that brand of computer. Because the software may be inappropriate for their needs, the result may be the loss of dollars and time. This checklist provides some guides for making important software decisions.

CHECKLIST FOR PURCHASE OF COMPUTER SOFTWARE

1. How easy is the system to use?
2. How many software programs are currently available in the field?
3. How long has each software company been in business?
4. Will the company provide names of current users? If not, forget about the company. Be sure to check out the referrals. They will be more informative than the salesperson.
5. Will the company train the office staff as much as necessary, and how much after-sale support will it guarantee?
6. How much training will be necessary before the system can be operated by the staff? Is this training included in the cost of the system?
7. Is the salesperson understandable? If no one in the office can understand the salesperson, confusion will result.
8. Will staff members be able to enter data into the system and see the reports or see only a prearranged demonstration?
9. Will the company provide on-site maintenance? What is the cost?
10. What about software updates? Will current users receive a lower price than new purchasers for updates? Is the present system new, or has it had several revisions to "get the bugs out?"
11. Does the company offer one-step service or will the practice have to deal with two, three, or more vendors to maintain the system? With more than one vendor, it is possible no one will accept responsibility if a problem arises.
12. How clear is the software manual? Is it easy to use and well organized?
13. What enhancements is the company developing?
14. What report formats does the computer supply? Can reports be customized?
15. How is the office protected in case of power failure or system malfunction?
16. Can hard copy printouts be made for all applications?
17. Who manufactures the hardware and how reliable is it? Check with current users about this.
18. How many patients can the system handle?
19. How many doctors can the system handle?
20. How many transactions can the system handle daily?

21. How many patients can be maintained with complete ledgers for one year?

22. Does the system maintain a permanent record of all patients' names, or is a patient removed every time the balance is 0?

23. How well do other hardware and software vendors support the system?

24. Can the system be easily and cost-effectively expanded and upgraded?

25. Can the present manual system perform the same task as rapidly and accurately?

IN YOUR OPINION

1. What are some good sources for information about medical billing software?

2. Will good information systems most improve administrative processes or patient processes? Defend your answer.

3. What are the most popular word processing and medical billing programs in your and your classmates' mentoring practices?

Communication and Mail Distribution

The information processing cycle is not complete until data is communicated or distributed to the final recipient. In a medical office, this may involve a combination of telecommunications, the U.S. Postal Service, and private express delivery services. As a medical assistant, you should have a good understanding of all three forms of communication and distribution.

Telecommunications

Telecommunications is the process of transmitting information over distances by telephone lines, cables, microwaves, satellites, and light beams. Telecommunication includes (1) voice or spoken communication, (2) data communication via modems, (3) message communication such as telegrams, mailgrams, and teletypewriters, and (4) image communication such as FAX or facsimile communication. A FAX machine is shown in Figure 8-14.

MEDICAL TELECOMMUNICATIONS SERVICES

Telecommunication services that expand a medical office's computer capability have proliferated in the past few years. By providing a personal computer with a telephone modem and by using the proper software and a subscription to one of the many public or private data services, a medical practice can increase the turnaround time for insurance claims, access diagnosis and treatment information, search databases for drug information, and access a wide variety of other services around the country. The following section explains several of these medical telecommunication services.

Electronic Communication

A medical office can send claims to participating insurance carriers instantly over telephone lines when the computer is installed with special software. Electronic Data Interchange (EDI) is rapidly becoming the technology of choice for this process. The trend is toward open, accessible systems with uniform standards and forms rather than proprietary systems, which make it necessary to learn a new system for each company. EDI enables a practice to deliver medical claims to participating insurance carriers within hours after the physician treats a patient. One telephone call allows the computer to send all the information needed to process a practice's claims to multiple carriers, including Medicare and commercial and private carriers.

These systems reduce the administrative costs for processing claims and the number of claims rejected because of incomplete or incorrect information, as well as speeding up the claims payment, a very attractive feature to most physicians. The future of EDI is toward "electronic commerce," including eligibility checking and patient enrollment in addition to the billing process.

Biomedical, Clinical, and Other Databases

Because technology is changing so rapidly, physicians must stay up to date on medical and health developments. A biomedical database, essentially a library of health information that can be accessed by a personal computer and modem, allows a physician to search available literature for a topic or combination of topics.

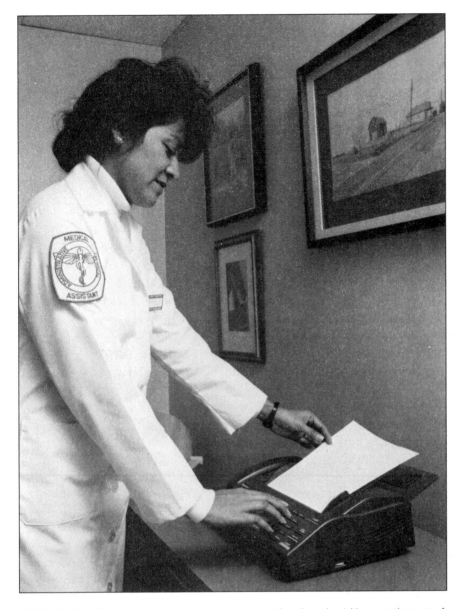

FIGURE 8-14 FAX machines are used to transmit material easily and quickly to another part of the country or world. (Courtesy of Murata Business Systems, Inc.)

As a medical assistant, you may be assigned the task of researching available databases before the physician subscribes to a particular database service. You may also be asked to search for specific pieces of information the physician requires. If so, look for a database that gives you information from around the world. A good biomedical database should index at least 4,000 journals, including foreign journals.

Clinical databases are another aid in researching questions about drugs or chemicals.

These databases index drugs and their interactions, poisons and their antidotes, emergency illnesses and their treatments, as well as scores of other clinically related topics. A practice seeking a service of this type should contact the local medical association, the American Medical Association, or a major vendor of medical software for the names and addresses of the most widely used clinical database services. Poisindex™, Drugdex™, Emergindex™, and Identidex™ are typical information services. Each is offered by Micromex, Inc., in conjunction with the Rocky Mountain Poison and Drug Center and the University of Colorado.

Hospitals, such as Massachusetts General, routinely use databases such as MedLine, Cumulative Index for Nursing and Allied Health Literature (CINAHL), GENONE (genetic information), and Micromedics. Massachusetts General users access these databases through networks such as Prodigy, CompuServe, Dialog, and Internet.

Nonmedical databases such as Nexus, which might occasionally be used in large medical offices, provide information on just about every imaginable subject, from travel schedules to financial information, art history, and physics.

Electronic databases work in the same way as magazine subscription services. A subscriber selects a particular database service, then pays a monthly fee. In addition, the subscriber pays long-distance telephone charges for the amount of time on-line each month with the database service.

Teleconferencing

Teleconferencing refers to pre-planned conferences that allow people in different locations to see and talk with one another. Unless you go to work in a hospital, a research center, or some other large medical facility you probably will not arrange teleconferences. However, you should be familiar with the concept.

Teleconferences are usually arranged for convenience when the various parties find it difficult or time consuming to travel to one location for a meeting. By arranging the conference in a central location and transmitting the proceedings by computers and telephone lines to special teleconference rooms in another part of the country, the people in all the locations can see one another and talk back and forth. A typical teleconference room is shown in Figure 8-15. For example, doctors in a San Francisco teleconference room could talk with doctors in a similar room in New York City (Figure 8-16).

Cellular Service

Today, many physicians have car or portable phones. Car phones are convenient when the physician is running late or when an emergency occurs. As cellular signals are not secure, other people may be able to listen in on the conversation. Therefore, the staff and physician may want to create a code that refers to patients without using their full names and allows discussion without revealing details. For reasons of driver safety and confidentiality, car phone discussions should be kept brief and used only when important.

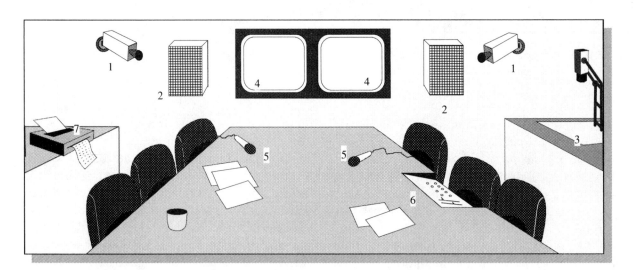

FIGURE 8-15 Teleconference room (1: Video camera; 2: Speaker; 3: Visual aid equipment; 4: TV monitor; 5: Microphone; 6: Control console; 7: FAX machine)

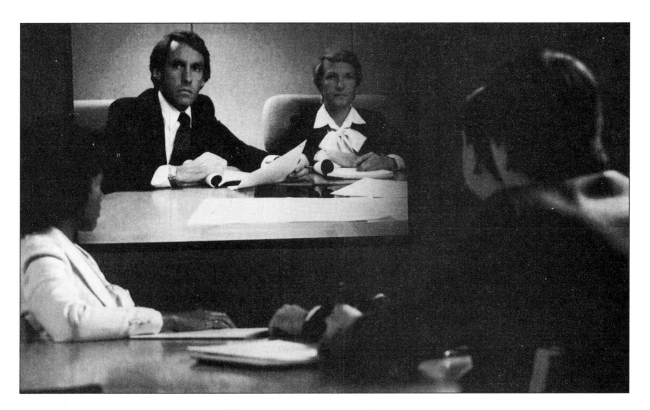

FIGURE 8-16 in a teleconference, parties in different locations can see and talk with one another.

IN YOUR OPINION

1. How can patient confidentiality be protected when using modern telecommunications systems?
2. When would teleconferencing be helpful?
3. Would employees in your mentoring medical office welcome or resist a new computer system? Why?

Postal and Delivery Services

Traditionally, the letters, x-rays, medical reports, and related materials going to and from a medical office were transmitted by first class or express mail via the U.S. Postal Service. However, private mailing and shipping services compete today with the postal service. In some cases, as with x-rays, special attention must be paid to packaging in order to protect the contents of the material. The categories of mail services are discussed below.

PRIVATE MAILING AND SHIPPING SERVICES

Several national and international delivery services, such as Federal Express, UPS, Emery Worldwide, Purolator, and others compete with the U. S. Postal Service for delivery of mail and packages. Most services will pick up parcels to be shipped from the office, and many offices use them because of convenience. Speed is also an important factor, with private services often delivering faster than the post office. Taxicabs and bus service may also be used for delivery in small towns and cities. Big cities may offer door-to-door courier services via bicycle.

DOMESTIC MAIL SERVICES

Domestic mail service can be categorized as follows:

- **Express Mail:** The fastest class of postal service. Items deposited at the post office by 5 P.M. are guaranteed for delivery by 10 A.M. the following day if the receiving post office has express service. Letters, legal documents, or other items needing fast delivery may be sent through Express Mail. Express service is more expensive than other classes of mail service. Since postal fees change from time to time, check the post office for the current rate for Express Mail.

- **Priority Mail:** Second day delivery, not guaranteed, for items weighing over 11 ounces. The maximum weight for priority mail is 70 pounds, and the maximum size is 100 inches combined length and girth. Charges are assessed according to zones, with the fee increasing as the distance increases. Priority mail is used for sending medical records when a former patient changes to a new physician in another city or when a package needs to be shipped by a fast method.
- **First Class:** The second fastest class of postal service. Service includes items weighing up to 11 ounces, such as letters, laboratory reports, and medical reports. Items weighing over 11 ounces are considered priority mail. The charge for this service is by the ounce. First class is used for most of the printed communications leaving the office.
- **Second Class:** Printed newspaper and periodicals. Contact the local post office for second-class fees. Although medical offices receive a great deal of second-class mail they rarely send items by this method.
- **Third Class:** Any material that does not fall in the categories of first-class or second-class mail and weighs less than 16 ounces, such as merchandise, printed matter, and keys. Bulk advertising material is third-class mail. Third-class mail is used for such mailings as a newsletter to patients.
- **Fourth Class:** The same as parcel post, including all mailable matter not in first, second, or third class that weighs 16 ounces or more. Rates are charged according to the weight of the parcel and the distance it will travel. Fourth-class mail is used for packages such as returned medical supplies or office supplies sent by the postal service.

SPECIAL MAIL SERVICES

Special mail services can be classified as follows:

- **Registered Mail:** First-class and priority mail of monetary value that must be guaranteed against loss or damage by the postal service. Fees are based on value of the contents.
- **Insured Mail:** Third- or fourth-class mail or priority mail with third- or fourth-class contents valued at $400 or less.
- **Return Receipt:** Evidence that mail was received by the Restricted Mail addressee. A return receipt should be requested and attached to the patient file any time a letter is mailed advising that the physician is withdrawing from a case. A return receipt is shown in Figure 8-17.
- **C.O.D:** Merchandise for which the cost is collected at delivery. Merchandise ordered from a supplier with arrangements to pay for it when it is delivered is a C.O.D. item.
- **Certified Mail:** A record of delivery of a letter by the post office, attached to letters and other items that have no insured value but for which evidence is needed that the item was actually delivered. Certified mail might be used on final collection notices before an account is turned over to a collection agency. A certified mail receipt is shown in Figure 8-18.
- **Special Delivery:** Immediate delivery by post office messenger to prescribed locations in a mailing area. X-rays might be sent by special delivery.
- **Special Handling:** Method of moving third- and fourth-class packages with first-class mail. Check the first-class rate for sending the package. It may be cheaper than special handling. Medical instruments are sometimes sent by special handling.
- **Metered Mail:** Postage that is affixed by a postage meter machine at the medical office, reducing handling time at the post office. Postage meters may be electronic; feeding, sealing, and stacking the stamped envelopes. The actual metering device maintains a record of postage expenditures and the number of pieces that have passed through the machine. Pitney Bowes is a major lessor of postage meters (see Figure 8-19).

UNITED STATES POSTAL SERVICE

Official Business

PENALTY FOR PRIVATE
USE TO AVOID PAYMENT
OF POSTAGE, $300

U.S.MAIL

Print your name, address and ZIP Code here

Mr. B. J. Bunyon
618 Harris Drive
New Orleans, LA   70126-4178

SENDER:
- Complete items 1 and/or 2 for additional services.
- Complete items 3, and 4a & b.
- Print your name and address on the reverse of this form so that we can return this card to you.
- Attach this form to the front of the mailpiece, or on the back if space does not permit.
- Write "Return Receipt Requested" on the mailpiece below the article number.
- The Return Receipt will show to whom the article was delivered and the date delivered.

I also wish to receive the following services (for an extra fee):

1. ☐ Addressee's Address

2. ☒ Restricted Delivery

Consult postmaster for fee.

3. Article Addressed to:

Rene Hebert
7 Pease Hall
New Orleans, LA   70122-0161

4a. Article Number

4575231

4b. Service Type
☐ Registered   ☐ Insured
☒ Certified   ☐ COD
☐ Express Mail   ☐ Return Receipt for Merchandise

7. Date of Delivery

3/11 /9- -

5. Signature (Addressee)

Rene Hebert

6. Signature (Agent)

8. Addressee's Address (Only if requested and fee is paid)

Is your RETURN ADDRESS completed on the reverse side?

Thank you for using Return Receipt Service.

PS Form **3811**, December 1991   ✩U.S. GPO: 1993—352-714   **DOMESTIC RETURN RECEIPT**

FIGURE 8-17 Return receipt

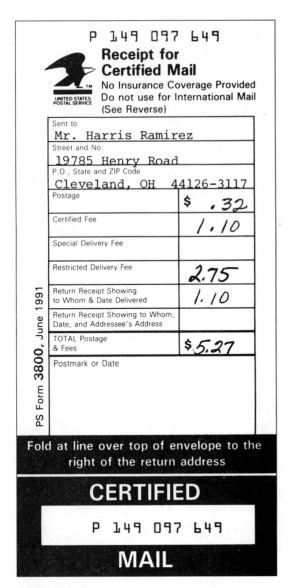

P 149 097 649

Receipt for Certified Mail

No Insurance Coverage Provided
Do not use for International Mail
(See Reverse)

UNITED STATES POSTAL SERVICE

Sent to	
Mr. Harris Ramirez	
Street and No.	
19785 Henry Road	
P.O., State and ZIP Code	
Cleveland, OH 44126-3117	
Postage	$ .32
Certified Fee	1.10
Special Delivery Fee	
Restricted Delivery Fee	2.75
Return Receipt Showing to Whom & Date Delivered	1.10
Return Receipt Showing to Whom, Date, and Addressee's Address	
TOTAL Postage & Fees	$5.27
Postmark or Date	

PS Form 3800, June 1991

Fold at line over top of envelope to the right of the return address

CERTIFIED

P 149 097 649

MAIL

FIGURE 8-18 Receipt for certified mail

PACKAGING AND SORTING MAIL

Some mail sent from medical offices requires special attention and packaging. For example, x-rays should be backed with cardboard and placed in a sufficiently large envelope so that they will not be damaged, folded, or bent. An envelope containing x-rays should never be run through a postage meter. Instead, it can be hand stamped or postage meter tape can be attached to the envelope. When shipping medical records, the contents should be secured with rubber bands and cardboard backing and then placed in an envelope strong enough to contain the material.

Letters and packages should be clearly identified with the type of mail service desired. For example, "Registered" or "Special Handling" should be written with a felt tip pen in block letters under the stamp area on items sent in these manners.

Metered mail should be bundled and identified with the coding labels provided by the postal service. All mail for one state is identified by an orange label marked by an "S," and all mail from the same medical office is identified with a blue label marked "F," for "Firm." Delivery of an office's mail can further be expedited by separating the mail according to major ZIP code categories, such as local and out of town.

RECALLING THE MAIL

Occasionally, a piece of mail may be sent in error. Mail that has been metered or stamped and mailed can be recalled if the sender acts quickly. First, an envelope identical to the one posted must be produced. The envelope must be taken to the local post office if the letter was mailed to the same ZIP code. The sender would have to call the local post office to determine where to take the envelope if the original was mailed out of town.

The sender would then complete a Sender's Application for Recall of Mail and give it and the duplicate envelope to a postal clerk. The original would be returned immediately if it were still at the local post office. If it had already been shipped to another ZIP code area, the postal clerk would contact the post office serving the area and attempt to have the letter returned. Letters that have already been delivered obviously cannot be recalled.

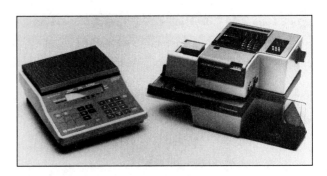

FIGURE 8-19 Postage meter machine. (Courtesy Pitney Bowes)

PROCESSING INCOMING MAIL

The size of a medical practice determines the steps followed in processing incoming mail. Large physician groups usually have a mail room where one person receives and sorts all incoming mail and delivers it to the appropriate medical assistant. In smaller offices, the mail is typically delivered by a postal employee to the medical assistant who sorts it and delivers it to the appropriate people (Figure 8-20). The following section discusses how a medical assistant should process mail once it is delivered.

Follow five basic steps to process incoming mail—sorting, opening, reading and annotating, expediting, and distributing. Use these procedures for each step.

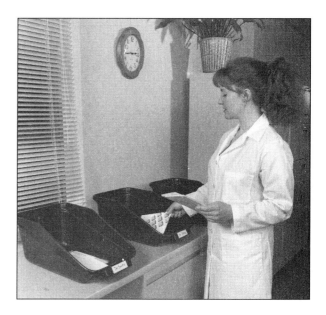

FIGURE 8-20 The first step in processing incoming mail is sorting.

Procedures for Processing Incoming Mail

Sorting Mail

1. Separate the mail according to class. Put special delivery, express, registered, certified, and first-class mail into one stack. Put second- and third-class newspapers and magazines in another stack. Place fourth-class parcels and packages in still another stack.
2. Organize the special classes and first-class mail according to what appears to be most important. Place letters together in one group, medical reports in another, and other related items in their own groups according to their content. Sometimes several items for one patient will arrive from different sources, such as laboratories. Organize all materials concerning one patient in a group and paper clip together.

Opening Mail

1. Leave any envelopes or packages marked "Personal" or "Confidential" for opening by the person to whom they are addressed. *Do not* open these letters or envelopes unless you have been specifically requested to do so by the addressee. If you open a personal letter by mistake, reinsert the letter in the envelope, tape the opened edges of the envelope, and write "Sorry, Opened by Mistake" on the front.

Be alert for any letters that look personal or confidential even if they are not identified as such. In a medical office, this is a challenge, as patients often handwrite the envelopes in which they send payment for their accounts. Enclosing a pre-addressed envelope with the bills helps with this problem.
2. Collect these supplies for opening the mail: a letter opener, stapler, paper clips, tape, and a date and time stamp.
3. Open the most important-looking material first and scan the contents to see if you need to keep the mailing envelopes. If so, paper clip the envelope to the contents. Repair any damaged items. Envelopes should be kept in the following situations:
   a. Look in the envelope for enclosures. If the letter refers to enclosures and none are found, underline the enclosure notation and write "No" beside the notation. Attach the envelope missing the enclosure to the letter.
   b. Paper-clip all checks to the envelopes in which they were received.
   c. Determine if the date on the letterhead matches the date on the envelope. If a major discrepancy exists, attach the envelope to the document and write a note about the date difference.

Courtney Wavens
2203 Merck Road
Malvern, PA 19355

Dr. Edna Mornick
33-B Foster Court
Wayne, PA 19087

Postmarked
6/8/94

Dear Edna:

It was good to see you and Raul at the jamboree. How our kids can eat! I don't care if I don't see a hot dog or hamburger for a while.

Curt Wetland date of birth

As a I mentioned to you at the jamboree, Curt, our oldest, is off to Penn State in a few weeks. He hasn't had any allergy problems lately, but I want to make sure that he takes a copy of his medical records to college, as well as a list of his allergies and the names of the medications you have prescribed for asthma and his related conditions. Curt certainly doesn't look asthmatic. We call him the Hulk! He has grand ideas about playing football, but we're warning him not to be too optimistic. He may transfer to a smaller school if his gridiron dreams don't materialize.

records
attached

Also, could you send a refill for his inhaler prescription. He and I will both feel better knowing he has it with him.

See you soon.

Courtney

FIGURE 8-21 Annotated letter

d. Attach all envelopes that hold legal documents to the document. The envelope may be needed for evidence in the future.

4. Discard remaining envelopes unless office policy dictates otherwise.

5. Date and time-stamp all mail, either with a commercial date/time stamp or by hand. This is very important in a medical office when a question arises regarding an insurance payment, a legal paper, the date a document was mailed, or any other controversial matter. Some offices maintain a log of all incoming mail as documentation in the event of legal problems.

6. Open packages after first-class mail has been processed.

Reading, Underlining, and Annotating Mail

1. Read all the first-class mail unless the employer requests otherwise. Most physicians expect medical assistants to read their mail. It is not necessary to read the medical reports pertaining to individual patients.

2. Make calendar notations and notes based on the contents of the letters.

3. Highlight or underline words and phrases that will speed the physician's understanding of the message and add notes where helpful. Use a highlighter or pen in a color that contrasts with the paper and print of the letter. Check before annotating letters, since some physicians prefer to read a "fresh" letter. See the annotated letter in Figure 8-21.

4. Make filing notations or follow-up comments if the letter may be returned for additional filing or processing.

Expediting Mail

1. Determine whether background information, previous correspondence, a medical record, or other information is needed for understanding a specific piece of mail. If so, attach the necessary information.

   For example, a consulting physician may ask the primary care physician to answer a question about the patient's previous history. In this case, retrieve the medical record and paper-clip the consulting physician's letter to the folder or file before giving the letter to the physician.

2. Prepare an action slip for materials that are routinely handled in a particular way. For example, laboratory reports often need to be filed in the medical record without further action from the physician. An action slip can be attached to the lab report before giving it to the physician; the physician can then simply pass the report back to the medical assistant when it is ready for filing. An action slip is shown in Figure 8-22.

3. Fill out a routing slip and attach it to materials that the physician may send to others. For example, magazines often are routed among the staff or used in the lobby after the physician has read them. Time can be saved by attaching a routing slip to the magazine before giving it to the physician. See Figure 8-23.

Distributing Mail

1. Distribute mail to the individual to whom it is addressed after sorting materials that need only to be filed, "junk" mail, and magazines to be placed in the waiting room. Stack all the mail for each individual into categories according to importance:
   a. To be answered immediately
   b. To be answered routinely
   c. To be answered by someone else
   d. To be read for information
   e. To be filed
   f. To be forwarded
   g. To be discarded

Action Slip

_____ File in the medical record.

_____ Send to bookkeeping.

_____ Please make _____ copies.

_____ Please follow up.

_____ Please record in tickler.

FIGURE 8-22

Please pass the attached periodical to the next name on the list after you finish reading it.

_____ Dr. Mallaney

_____ Dr. Ricardo

_____ Ellyn Kincaid

_____ Henry Plunkett

FIGURE 8-23 Routing slip

2. Distribute mail addressed to the practice to its proper destination. For example, all checks should be sent to the bookkeeper even though they are addressed in care of the practice name.

3. Return all mail that was delivered incorrectly. Write an appropriate comment, "Not at this address," or "Delivered to the wrong address."

IN YOUR OPINION

1. Under what circumstances might a letter need to be recalled?
2. If you are in charge of sorting the mail, how can you save time for recipients of the mail?
3. In what ways might procedures for processing mail in a medical office be different from the procedures used in a business office?

REFERENCES

Feldstein, Paul J. *Health Care Economics,* 4th ed. Albany, New York: Delmar Publishers, 1993.

Johnson, Joan, Marie Whitaker, and Marcus Wayne Johnson. *Computerized Medical Office Management.* Albany, New York, Delmar Publishers, 1994.

Oliverio, John, William Pasewark, and Bonnie White. *The Office: Procedures and Technology.* Cincinnati, Ohio: South-Western Publishing Co., 1993.

Van Huss, Susan, and Daggett, William. *Electronic Office Systems.* Cincinnati, Ohio: South-Western Publishing Co., 1992.

Waggoner, Gloria A., and Jonathan Price. *Computer Concepts.* Cincinnati, Ohio: South-Western Publishing Co., 1991.

Chapter Activities

PERFORMANCE BASED ACTIVITIES

1. In the chart below, list the benefits in cost and service a medical practice can expect when billing, payroll, scheduling, and patient records are computerized instead of being handled manually.

	How Costs Can Be Saved	*Service Benefits*
Billing		
Payroll		
Scheduling		
Patient records		

(DACUM 2.6, 2.7, 5.1)

2. In what ways could each of the following types of practices use medical databases—rural medical practice, teaching hospital, family practice, sports medicine clinic?

Type of Practice	*Database Use*
Rural	
Teaching hospital	
Family	
Sports medicine	

(DACUM 3.4, 3.6, 5.3)

3. What type of postal or communication service do you recommend in each of the following situations, and why?

Situation	*Service Recommended*
a. *Letter advising that the physician will no longer treat a patient*	
b. *Letter from you renewing a magazine subscription*	
c. *X-rays needed across the country tomorrow*	
d. *Final collection letter to a patient*	
e. *Letter to a consulting physician*	
f. *Letter announcing a new partner*	
g. *Newsletter to all patients*	

(DACUM 1.8, 2.7, 3.1)

EXPANDING YOUR THINKING

1. Assume that you are a medical assistant who has been with a small group practice for several years. You are quite familiar with the doctors' preferences and needs regarding mail. Tell what you might do with each of the following pieces of mail as you sort it, and why.

   Smithsonian Magazine

   JAMA

   Telephone bill

   Patient x-rays

   Halloween card from patient

   Medical supply catalog

   Supermarket flyer

   L.L. Bean catalogue

   New England Journal of Medicine

   Professional Medical Assistant

   Invitation for a physician to speak

   New patient admission guidelines from a local hospital

2. Visit the library in your school and view a microfilm and a microfiche on any subject of your choosing. Then write a paragraph in which you answer the following questions:

   a. How many pages were contained on each microform you viewed?

   _____

   b. What was the subject?

   _____

   c. What type of material was included? Was it all narrative? Were there charts?

   _____

   d. What did you like and not like about the miniaturized format?

   _____

3. Prepare a short scenario in which you recommend teleconferencing as the answer to a meeting problem. Describe the subject to be discussed, explain why teleconferencing would be helpful, and tell why you think other forms of communication are not advantageous. Include information about the costs.

   _____

   _____

   _____

   _____

   _____

   _____

4. Underline and annotate the following letter for the physician.

April 10, 19—
Seiji Ohira, M.D.
230 Water Tower Road
Paoli, PA 19301

Dear Dr. Ohira:

Your patient, William A. Clyde, came in as you requested for a cardiology consultation. In reviewing his file that you mailed earlier, I note that Mr. Clyde had an EKG on March 15 of last year and another on December 15; however, I am unable to find a report of either test. Will you please see if you can locate the results so that I may review them?

I also would appreciate your calling me so we can discuss other phases of Mr. Clyde's health which seem to affect his cardiac condition.

I will be out of the office until April 14.

Sincerely,

Anton Van de Ven, M.D.

Chapter 9

Computerizing the Medical Office

TUCSON, ARIZONA

I find our office computer system so fascinating. Each month, I put together for our staff a package of reports which includes not only financial results, but a variety of other reports. We measure, for example, the average length of appointment by doctor and by medical complaint to aid in better scheduling. I run an inventory report, which shows the number and type of medical and office supplies we use and compares usage to last year. This way, we don't run out of things, but we also don't keep a lot of extra stock.

Once a year, I create a "State of the Practice" report, which summarizes the types of patients and ailments we have treated during the past year and how this has changed over the years. For example, with all the retirees moving into our area, we've seen an increase in the average age of our patients. Looking back ten years, our patients in this age group are healthier than they used to be.

This type of analysis helps us run the practice intelligently and plan better for the future.

Bonnie Malloy
Medical Assistant

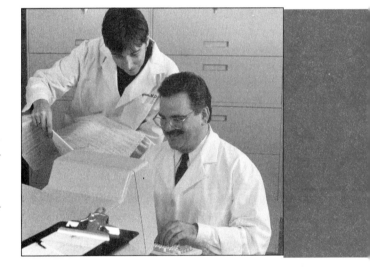

PERFORMANCE BASED COMPETENCIES

After completing this chapter, you should be able to:

1. Plan the computerization of medical office functions. (DACUM 3.4, 5.1, 5.2)
2. Analyze critical components of computer maintenance agreements. (DACUM 5.2, 6.4)
3. Manage inventories of equipment and supplies. (DACUM 3.1, 6.3)
4. Choose the appropriate computer application for medical office tasks. (DACUM 3.4, 8.6)

Computers have brought revolutionary change to medical offices in the last few years, primarily because of two factors: (1) spectacular advances in computer clinical applications, and (2) a drop in the price of computer processing power. The introduction into the practice of the whole-body scanner, computerized analysis of test results, and computerized laboratory equipment allows physicians to perform procedures in the office that previously were performed only at hospitals.

Today's personal computers, which are small enough to sit on a desk top and cost less than $5,000, have the processing power of the room-size computers of the 1960s. Lower prices for high-powered systems make computing affordable for even the smallest practice, and many solo practitioners are adding personal computers to handle office applications that previously were performed manually or by a contracted computer service. When you consider that the first microcomputer, an Apple I, was introduced in 1975 and that today almost all medical offices either use computers or are considering computers for the future, the significance of this office tool becomes clear.

Any person who works in a medical office should be knowledgeable about computers and proficient with applications software. As a medical assistant, you may be the most knowledgeable person about computers in the office, since your training will be recent. This chapter will help define overall responsibilities for computing and the broad issues involved in computerizing a medical office.

Planning for Computerization

Computerizing a medical office requires careful planning and extensive research. Lack of thorough planning and knowledge can result in ineffective results at great expense. When computerization is approached in a systematic, well-planned manner, it streamlines office activities and becomes an invaluable asset (Figure 9-1). Computerization can lead to increased productivity, efficiency, and organization and can simplify once difficult and time-consuming tasks. As more and more medical offices computerize, the physician's practice will benefit from availability of increased information and more efficient office procedures.

 A summary of what computers can and cannot do for a practice will be helpful. A computer cannot solve an unspecified problem. The specific task to be accomplished, for example, calculating fees or posting debits and credits, must be communicated. Secondly, only a properly designed computer system, such as *The Medical Manager,* discussed previously in Chapter 8, will result in increased efficiency. A poorly designed system may lack vital functions or may not be integrated among tasks, requiring the medical assistant to enter data twice. The system may be inflexible, forcing the staff to "work around" it.

Although automation eliminates repetitive manual work, it also requires accuracy and precision. The computer can change the type of work to be done but cannot replace needed skills. By giving up repetitive, often boring, tasks to the computer, the medical staff has more time for management tasks, including

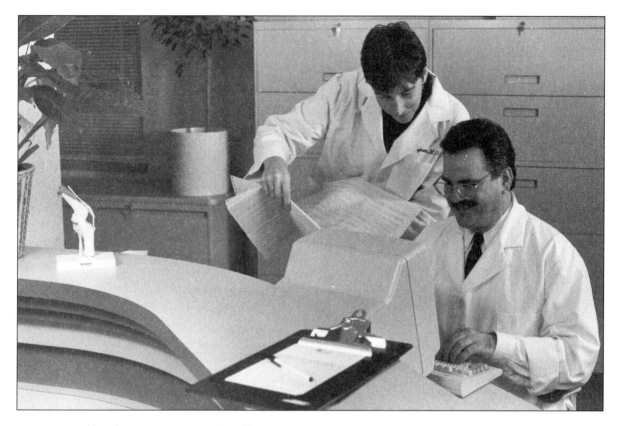

FIGURE 9-1 Although computerizing a medical office requires careful planning and research, the result can be increased productivity.

thinking creatively about reports that can be generated, other office tasks that can be computerized, and the way the practice can further serve patients through computerization. The chart shown in Figure 9-2 gives a brief review of computer software applications discussed throughout this text.

CHOOSING AND USING A MICROCOMPUTER

Computerizing a medical office requires careful planning and extensive research. An employer may hire a practice management consultant to help with selecting and converting to a computer system, and almost certainly you as a medical assistant will take some training courses in the software packages selected. Because the medical assistant is the person whose daily activities will be most directly affected by the computer, you will work very closely with the consultant, the equipment, and the software supplier. As a medical assistant, you should take full advantage of this opportunity to learn everything you

can about the system. After the consultant leaves, you will be on your own, although most consulting services offer a telephone hotline for questions or problems.

Hardware and software are always accompanied by extensive documentation. In addition, most computer manufacturers, software developers, computer retailers and consulting services offer telephone hotlines for questions or problems after initial training.

The following section outlines the guidelines a medical assistant should follow to make the transition from a manual system to a computer system as painless as possible. The key point to remember is: Ask lots of questions. The best time to get the necessary information is during the initial phases of implementation.

GUIDELINES FOR CONVERTING A MANUAL SYSTEM TO A COMPUTER SYSTEM

1. Visit similar practices that have installed computer systems and ask the medical assis-

Scheduling
Appointment scheduling
Follow-up scheduling
Patient recall lists
Patient reminders

Word processing
Articles
Consultation reports
Correspondence
Labels and addressing
Memos
Thank you letters
Welcome-to-practice letters

Clinical
Access to national data banks
CME (continuing medical education) programs
Drug interaction and allergy checks
Medical records
Patient education
Prescription writing
Protocols, diagnosis, and treatment
Research
Retrieving medical research

Accounting
Accounts payable
Annual statements to patients
Cash report
Cash register
Check writing
Cross-posting in multiphysician practices
Daily log
Deposit slip
General ledger
Income and expense statement
Payroll
Profit and loss statements
Retirement plan accounting
W-2 forms

Billing, collecting, and insurance
Accounts receivable
Aging accounts receivable
Billing forms
Collection letters
Insurance claim processing
Patient billing

Practice management
Employee vacation and sick-time records
Hospital lists and charges
Inventories and drug supplies
Ordering drugs and supplies
Patient profiles by age, diagnosis, etc.
Practice profiles by diagnosis, procedure, service
Production reports by physicians
Referrals

FIGURE 9-2 What computers can do

tant responsible for computing to share problems or questions that arose when the practice became computerized. Make a list of issues and concerns.

2. Prepare a detailed list of the tasks the computer is to perform. Be as specific as possible. If it is not clear whether a task can be computerized, ask the salesperson or consultant. Do not be afraid to show inexperience with computer systems.

3. Study the vendor's written guidelines for conversion to the computer. If something does not seem right, say so. Any problem clarified now will save headaches later.

4. Visit at least one practice that uses the software package you are interested in and watch how the staff performs the functions. Make sure the software will perform the majority of tasks you need without modification; or ascertain that you can easily modify your office procedures to conform to the software function.

5. Plan enough time to enter data from existing records into the new system. If possible, delegate your other responsibilities to someone else during this period, or hire a temporary worker to work under your supervision. All of the data that is re-keyed must be thoroughly audited and proofread for errors.

6. Suggest to the physician that data entry can best be accomplished when the office is closed for vacation. If this is impractical, perhaps your employer will agree to see a limited number of patients during conversion. After hardware and software are installed, data can be entered in the late evenings and on weekends.

7. During a pilot period, enter only a few data records and test all the functions to make sure they work as specified, and that you understand them.

8. If possible, run both the manual and automated systems for several weeks or months until the staff is convinced that the new system works properly. This is double work but may be worthwhile if other staff members need to be convinced about the new system. If you run both systems simultaneously, you will not only be doing twice the

work for a while, but you will also have to spend time comparing the output of the two systems. Otherwise, the overlap will be a waste of time.

CONTRACTS

One of your responsibilities as a medical assistant will be to review equipment and software contracts. Use the guidelines given in Figure 9-3 to review contracts of all types.

COMPUTER SERVICES

A computer service is commonly used by small practices that do not find purchasing or leasing a system to be cost-effective. When a service is used, the practice pays a monthly fee for processing statements and financial records. The service prepares statements and reports and delivers them to the practice, or mails them directly to patients.

When a practice uses a computer service, coordination with the service vendor is important. Initially, each statement should be audited to make sure accounts are being charged and billed correctly. When the vendor has established a track record for accuracy, a random sample of statements should be checked each month. The same number of statements should be pulled each month, regardless of the total number of statements sent. When the vendor makes an error, the cause of the error should be determined to prevent its recurrence.

Medical Software Applications

Medical offices can purchase or lease medical software packages, both ready-made or customized, for a specialty or an individual office. In addition, a wide variety of general-use computer software programs, such as Lotus 1-2-3, a spreadsheet program; dBase IV, a database management program; WordPerfect, a word processing program; and hundreds of others are available. However, general programs do not offer the special features of programs developed

1. Specify all terms and conditions of the contract. Write as part of the contract any verbal agreements between the physician and the vendor or between you and the vendor related to the system's performance.
2. Is the price standard or is it a negotiable item? Does it include the printer, hard disk, monitor, modem, mouse, central processing unit, and keyboard?
3. Make sure the maintenance support agreements and guarantees are detailed to identify how the equipment and software will perform.
4. Have the physician's accountant or attorney review the contract. Will the vendor assume liability when the computer is down?
5. Does the practice's current insurance coverage include financial losses when extended maintenance for the system is required?

FIGURE 9-3 Guidelines for reviewing contracts

specifically for medical computing, and their use is diminishing while the use of specialized medical software is increasing. A practice will likely choose a system with such features as scheduling and billing capabilities developed especially for medical offices.

No one piece of software can handle all computing functions, and the specific needs and priorities of each medical office must be analyzed to determine how software can be most useful. Ready-made software packages, customized software packages, or a combination of the two may provide an electronic alternative to traditional paper methods of running a medical office. Word processing, database management, spreadsheets, graphics, communication, and practice management software are used extensively to improve efficiency in medical offices.

Medical offices use software programs to process data. For example, when a patient visits the physician, a data processing program calculates the charges keyed by a medical assistant, subtracts payments and adjustments, adds the previous balance, and produces a current balance. As a medical assistant, if you key a number incorrectly, the computer will produce an incorrect result. The term "GIGO," or "Garbage In, Garbage Out," is applied to the computer mistakes that occur because of human error. Perhaps you have received an incorrect bill for your doctor's services. When you questioned the mistake, you may have been told "the computer made a mistake." Most of the time, the computer only processed a mistake made by a human.

Most common software packages are based on four types of applications; word processing (covered extensively in Chapter 10), spreadsheet, database, and graphics. Many software packages are integrated, which means that all four of these applications "talk to" one another, allowing you to use spreadsheet data, for example, to create charts and graphs, and to "paste" them into documents.

WORD PROCESSING

The major advantages of word processing over typing are ease of making changes, and the ability to cut and paste from various documents already in your system to create a new document. Many packages also provide the ability to integrate graphics and data into your text. Word processing is one of the most frequently used medical software applications.

SPREADSHEET

Applications that involve rows and columns of numbers requiring calculation usually use spreadsheets. Financial reporting, tax, and money management packages are spreadsheets that have been customized. General spreadsheet packages such as Lotus 1-2-3, Excel, and Quattro allow users to enter their own formulas. For example, instructions in the expense sheet in Figure 9-4 tell the computer to add both down and across, so that day and expense category totals can be seen. The medical billing packages used for patients are based on spreadsheet software.

DATABASE

Computers are excellent at sorting and arranging data. Applications that involve many records, such as patient files and inventory records, are good candidates for database applications. Each piece of data in the record, such as the patient's name, address, age, and sex, is stored separately. The value of databases is that they can sort by any of these characteristics. For example, how many patients are six years old and under? How many are female? How many are more than six feet tall? Lists can be produced and printed in alphabetic or numeric order using any characteristic in the database, including number of visits, number of prescriptions issued, or average length of appointment. Only data put in can be extracted, so database applications require good planning. Medical scheduling software is developed around database guidelines.

The medical assistant should meet with the medical staff to draft the types of reports need-

	Ground Trans	Meals	Lodging	Mileage	Parking/Tips	Other	Totals
Monday		23.41		10.08		25.6	$59.09
Tuesday	65.14	26.24	52.19				$143.57
Wednesday	43.80	20.44	87.75				$151.99
Thursday	43.96	16.40	80.64	10.08	26.00	1.40	$178.48
Friday							$0.00
Totals	$152.90	$86.49	$220.58	$20.16	$26.00	$27.00	$533.13

FIGURE 9-4 Expense sheet

ed before entering data. Collecting and storing data costs money, so storing data that is "nice to know" rather than "needed to know" should be avoided. The medical assistant should review the reports periodically, and make sure they are really being used by the staff. A good way to audit this is to continue to run a report without distributing it and see if anyone complains. High volume, repetitive transactions are the most cost-effective to complete by computer.

GRAPHICS

Graphs and charts are excellent for presenting information that can be interpreted at a glance. Integrated software converts spreadsheet or database data into charts and graphs such as those shown in Figures 9-5a, b, and c.

Choose the type of chart that pictures the information most effectively. For example, data tracked across time, such as monthly financial data, can be graphed to show how the dollars change over time. When data is divided into groups, such as patient types, bar graphs and pie charts show the division clearly. Intelligent use of graphics can save the medical staff valuable time when they read reports.

Developing Practice Lists and Reports

One of your responsibilities as a medical assistant will be to develop weekly or monthly lists and reports. The software manuals accompanying your system will illustrate many types of reports pre-programmed into the software. You can use these to create similar reports or you may wish to customize report formats specific to your practice. Figure 9-6 shows a database of drugs and codes used in one practice. The following guide suggests several lists and reports that are generally helpful in a medical practice. Most of these are easily created by using information stored in the computer's database. This list is not intended to be comprehensive, but it should serve as a guide to the types of reports that are available.

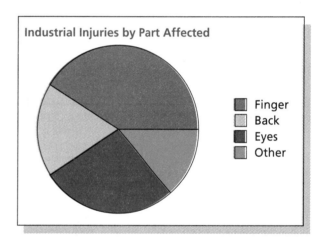

FIGURE 9-5b Medical pie chart

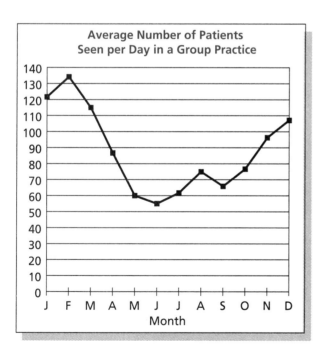

FIGURE 9-5a Medical line graph

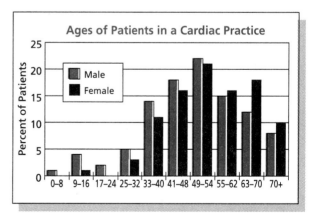

FIGURE 9-5c Medical bar chart

```
                    DRUG CODE LIST                    03/17/—
                                                     Page 1
==============================================================
   Index        Drug Code        Name
==============================================================
    54)          ADRIA           ADRIAMYCIN
    15)          ALBUT           ALBUTEROL
    24)          ALDOMET         ALPHA METHYL DGPA
    35)          ELAVIL          AMITRIPTYLINE
    18)          AMP             AMPICILLIN
    12)          ASA             ASPIRIN
     6)          ATEN            ATEOLOL (TENORMIN)
    61)          BRONK           BROKOSOL
    66)          CAPTO           CAPTOPRIL
    55)          CARD            CARDIAZEM
    63)          LIBRIUM         CHLORDIAZEPOXIDE
    25)          CATPRES         CLONIDINE (CATAPRES)
    17)          TRANX           CLORAZEPATE
    62)          LOTRIM          CLOTRIMAZOLE
    51)          PREMAR          CONUGATED ESTROGENS
    31)          CORG            CORGARD
    50)          COUM            COUMADIN
    26)          B12             CYANOCOBALAMIN
     9)          DEPOSE          DEPO-ESTRADIOL
    69)          DESIMPR         DESIMPRAMINE
    68)          DESIP           DESIPRAMINE
    46)          DIAB            DIABINESE (CHLORPRO)
    11)          DIG             DIGOXIN
    47)          PERSANT         DIAPYRIDAMOLE
    21)          DYAZ            DYAZIDE
    53)          ESDERM          ESTRADERM
    36)          LIDEX           FLUOCINONIDE
    49)          LASIX           FUROSEMIDE
     4)          FASIX           FUROSEMIDE
    64)          GLUC            FLUCOTROL
    43)          HYDER           HYDERGINE
     7)          HCTZ            HYDROCHLOROTHIAZIDE
    27)          NUPRIN          IBUPROFEN
    37)          IMIP            IMIPRAMINE
    22)          ISORDL          ISOSORBIDE DI (NO3)
    59)          ALUPENT         METAPROTERENOL
    28)          MINI            MINI-PRESS
    52)          NAP             NAPROSYN
    10)          NAPROS          NAPROXEN
     1)          NTG             NITROGLYCERIN SL
     3)          NPH             NPH INSULIN U-100
    20)          TALWIN          PENTAZOCINE
    41)          PERIAC          PERIACTIN
    45)          PERS            PERSANTIN
     8)          KCL             POTASSIUM CHLORIDE
    33)          MINPRES         PRAZOSIN
    60)          PRED            PREDNISONE
    30)          PREM            PREMARIN
    23)          PROCAN          PROCAINAMIDE
    56)          INDERAL         PROPRANOL
```

FIGURE 9-6 Drugs and codes used in one practice

USEFUL COMPUTERIZED LISTS AND REPORTS

Patient-Related Information

- Patient names, addresses, telephone numbers, and patient numbers, if used
- Frequently used insurance company names and addresses
- Frequently used provider names, addresses, and telephone numbers, including hospitals, laboratories, and consulting physicians
- Emergency medical services in the area
- ICD codes and descriptions not listed on the superbill but frequently used
- CPT codes and descriptions not listed on the superbill but frequently used
- Codes for drugs commonly used by the practice (see Figure 9-6)
- ZIP codes of nearby towns and cities

Practice Management Information

- Staff names, addresses, telephone numbers, and social security numbers
- Vacation and holiday schedules
- Payroll information, including FICA and other taxes paid by each employee and the practice
- Transaction report for each physician by day, week, month, or year. A daily transaction report created by *The Medical Manager* is shown in Figure 9-7.

```
02/02/—                        DAILY REPORT FOR 02/02/—                          Page 4
                            Sydney Carrington & Associates, PA

                                    Totals for 02/02/—


...............................................................................................
Doctor                 Charges   Receipts  Adjustments  Net A/R   Total A/R  # Proc.  Serv Chg  Tax Chg
...............................................................................................
1. James Monroe, M.D.    70.00     0.00       0.00        70.00     202.00      2       0.00      0.00
2. Sydney Carrington, M.D. 533.00  0.00       0.00       533.00   1,240.00     10       0.00      0.00
...............................................................................................
TOTAL                   603.00     0.00       0.00       603.00   1,442.00     12       0.00      0.00


                        PERIOD-TO-DATE TOTALS FOR 01/01/— - 02/02/—


...............................................................................................
Doctor                 Charges   Receipts  Adjustments  Net A/R   Total A/R  # Proc.  Serv Chg  Tax Chg
...............................................................................................
1. James Monroe, M.D.   202.00     0.00       0.00       202.00     202.00      7       ....      ....
2. Frances Simpson, M.D. 128.00    0.00       0.00       128.00     128.00      3       ....      ....
3. Sydney Carrington, M.D. 1,240.00 0.00      0.00     1,240.00   1,240.00     23       ....      ....
...............................................................................................
TOTAL                 1,570.00     0.00       0.00     1,570.00   1,570.00     33       ....      ....


                        YEAR-TO-DATE TOTALS FOR 01/01/— - 02/02/—


...............................................................................................
Doctor                 Charges   Receipts  Adjustments  Net A/R   Total A/R  # Proc.  Serv Chg  Tax Chg
...............................................................................................
1. James Monroe, M.D.   202.00     0.00       0.00       202.00     202.00      7       ....      ....
2. Frances Simpson, M.D. 128.00    0.00       0.00       128.00     128.00      3       ....      ....
3. Sydney Carrington, M.D. 1,240.00 0.00      0.00     1,240.00   1,240.00     23       ....      ....
...............................................................................................
TOTAL                 1,570.00     0.00       0.00     1,570.00   1,570.00     33       ....      ....
```

FIGURE 9-7 Daily transaction report (Adapted from Gartee and Humphrey, *The Medical Manager, Student Edition, Version 5.3,* copyright 1995, Delmar Publishers.)

- Productivity report by procedure; for example, the number of EKGs performed in one week
- List of all clinical and office equipment and dates of purchase or contract renewal, if leased
- Calendar of warranty requirements and maintenance dates of all equipment

IN YOUR OPINION

1. What are some of the ways you could assist the medical staff in making the transition to a new computer system?
2. What are some of the barriers that might prevent a medical office system from being used to its fullest extent?
3. What are the most important criteria in selecting a vendor for hardware and software?

Inventories

A well-managed supply of office and clinical equipment and supplies enables a medical practice to deliver good service efficiently. The objective of an inventory system is to have the needed item available on time without excess stock. Items must be of the quality needed at the best price available.

EQUIPMENT INVENTORIES

Once a year the medical assistant should review the inventory list of all equipment to make sure it is current. Clinical and office equipment may be listed together or separately. If all items are included in one list, the inventory may be easier to maintain; however, some medical assistants prefer to separate the inventory according to clinical or office functions or disposable or nondisposable. Some offices also include paintings, rugs, and other office furnishings. This decision should be made in coordination with the practice's financial advisors, as they may wish to categorize equipment for tax purposes.

After the first equipment inventory is created and keyed into the database, it is a simple matter to add or delete items. For example, when any item is purchased, sold, traded, or replaced, the appropriate information should be immediately keyed into the inventory database. In the partial inventory list shown in Figure 9-8, notice that a typewriter at the reception desk was replaced with a computer terminal on December 15, 1994. The disposition of the typewriter is shown, as well as information about the new terminal.

The computer can be instructed to print a current inventory at any time. Using the example in Figure 9-9, the medical assistant could instruct the computer to print a list of all items available as of today. The typewriter and the old copier would not be included on the list.

CLINICAL SUPPLIES

Keeping a separate list of clinical and office supplies is a good idea. Depending on the type of practice, the clinical supplies will vary from a

---

OFFICE EQUIPMENT INVENTORY

Item	Serial Number	Purchase Date	Location	Disposition Date
Pitney Bowes Postage Meter	XL 10243	6/24/80	Billing	
IBM Selectric II Typewriter	196-40268789	6/24/80	Reception	12/15/94 Trade In
IBM System 2 PS 50	2-244581190	12/15/94	Reception	
Xerox Copier	AB-L0142	9/18/84	Billing	2/10/90 Trade In
Xerox Copier	AB-LA961	2/10/90		

FIGURE 9-8 Complete inventory of current and noncurrent equipment

OFFICE EQUIPMENT INVENTORY				
Item	**Serial Number**	**Purchase Date**	**Location**	**Disposition Date**
Pitney Bowes Postage Meter	XL 10243	6/24/80	Billing	
IBM System 2 PS 50	2-244581190	12/15/94	Reception	
Xerox Copier	AB-LA961	2/10/90		

FIGURE 9-9 Current inventory of equipment

very few to a large quantity. For example, in a psychiatric practice, the number of supplies is usually small, consisting primarily of medications. However, a pediatric practice requires bandages, tapes, medications, adhesive bandages, suture supplies, scissors, needles, and a wide variety of other items. A complete inventory must include a count of each of these (Figure 9-10).

OFFICE SUPPLIES

Paper, pens, scratch pads, superbills, ledger cards, daily logs, staples, paper clips, printer or typewriter ribbons, and other office supplies are listed by number of boxes, reams, or packages in the inventory. An up-to-date stock of both clinical and office supplies is basic to a successful practice, and it will be your responsibility as

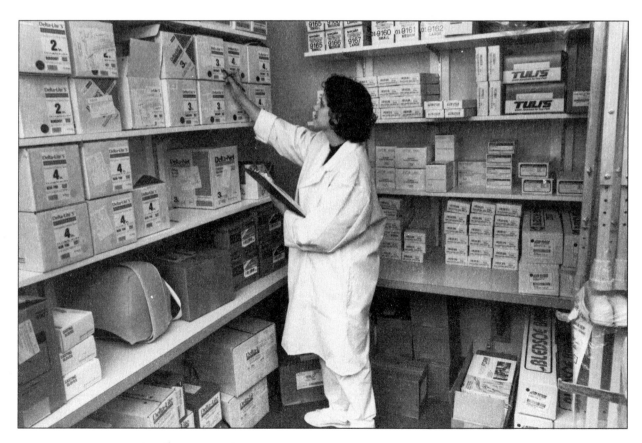

FIGURE 9-10 A complete list of supplies must be kept accurate and up to date to assure the required item is available when needed without keeping excess stock.

a medical assistant to have supplies available when needed. There are two goals that may seem contradictory in managing an inventory: "do not run out and do not have excess." Some tips for managing inventories are listed below:

1. Know what you have. If you do not know what you have, you will not know what to buy and may maintain expensive duplication. Think of supplies as money sitting on the shelf.
2. Keep track of how fast you use supplies. When you run out of something, check to see the last time you purchased it. Buy in quantities appropriate to your rate of usage. Do not tie up extra money in inventories.
3. Categorize your inventory.

Type of item	Inventory objective
Inexpensive, often used, like tongue depressors	Buy in bulk, never run out
Dated supplies	Review for expiration date, discard properly, do not store excess
Items similar to one another, such as gauze pads of different sizes	Eliminate duplication where possible and buy only needed sizes
Expensive, often used	Monitor often and buy carefully
Expensive, rarely used	Locate a source that can rapidly supply this item
Items that have not been used for six months or more	Review for possible disposal; storage costs money and prevents you from keeping a tidy supply area
Items that have a long "lead time"	Order far enough ahead of time to avoid last-minute crises and expensive delivery charges
Items that can be substituted for out-of-stock items, for example, a larger gauze pad could be used if the smaller size is out of stock	Develop a list of substitutes

4. Some office and medical suppliers may be willing to hold inventories in order to get your business. They will bill you only when you "call out" or order supplies. This can save your employer thousands of dollars in supplies and office space. The supplier may even agree to come in weekly to review supplies and replenish them to your desired level. This saves the practice administrative costs.
5. Label shelves where supplies are kept, and group supplies of a similar type. On a monthly basis, review the most frequently used supplies to make sure the actual supply matches your computer record. If it does not match, review your procedure for updating receipts and issues of supplies at the time when they occur.

PURCHASING

Purchasing is an important function that can save your practice a lot of money. The objective of the purchasing function is to buy the right quality of supplies for the right price. The right price is not always the cheapest initial cost but should take into consideration the total cost of using the item over its period of use. A piece of equipment that rarely breaks down, for example, may easily justify a higher initial cost than a cheaper alternative.

Purchasing software is available. This type of software shows inventory balances, prints orders, tracks items on order, shows inventory transactions such as issues and receipts, and tracks prices paid. An office that uses a modem may be able to order supplies directly if the supply house provides this service.

Miscellaneous Computer Tips

The following suggestions will help with office computerization.

MECHANICAL FAILURES

Do not be concerned about whether a computer will ever malfunction. Sooner or later it will. The essential question is how rapidly can you get it repaired. All hardware should be covered by a maintenance agreement that guarantees service within a few hours. It is important for the medical assistant to make sure that the turnaround time is short. This is a matter on which you should insist.

When a medical office is fully automated, the computer's down time can destroy the practice's schedule and organization. Consider, for example, the office that stores all patient accounts and medical records in a computer. If the computer is down, no financial transactions can be completed, and medical histories cannot be reviewed unless a paper file exists.

Maintenance agreements are invaluable. Computer equipment should be covered by a contract, preferably by the same vendor who sold it. Otherwise, each vendor may say someone else is responsible for maintenance and repair.

BYPASSING FRUSTRATION

Computers do not always do what the user wants. Software generally causes more problems than hardware because each program has its own quirks. The best way to bypass frustration is to refer to the software manual. For example, when unable to print, find the section on printing in the manual and read the troubleshooting tips. To eliminate the frustration of lost data, back up your files on a daily or weekly basis.

DON'T PANIC: CALL THE 800 NUMBER

Many software vendors provide a toll-free 800 number for the moments when all best efforts fail, even though all the manual's instructions have been conscientiously followed. The 800 number should be used any time assistance is needed because a technical support representa-tive who will understand your problem is sitting by a telephone waiting for such calls. As a caller, you must, however, be able to specify exactly what happened before, during, and after a procedure. Generalities are not good enough. For example, someone who cannot print from a particular program might say, "When I de-pressed CODE and PRINT, the screen locked. Just before that I had saved my document to a new disk." The representative will offer suggestions until the trouble has been cleared up. It is also a good idea to be sitting at the computer terminal and to have the machine on during the call.

IN YOUR OPINION

1. What transactions in a medical office might not justify the time and money to computerize?
2. Name medical supplies for which quality is more important than initial cost.
3. The computer says you have sutures, but there are none on the shelf. What could have caused the discrepancy?

REFERENCES

Clark, James F., and Beverly Oswalt. *Computer Confidence.* Cincinnati, Ohio: South-Western Publishing Co., 1991.

Gartee, Richard, and Doris D. Humphrey. *The Medical Manager.* Cincinnati, Ohio: South-Western Publishing Co., 1995.*

Oliverio, John, William Pasewark, and Bonnie White. *The Office: Procedures and Technology.* Cincinnati, Ohio: South-Western Publishing Co., 1993.

*Currently published by Delmar Publishers.

Chapter Activities

PERFORMANCE BASED ACTIVITIES

1. Interview a knowledgeable person at your mentoring practice about the practice's implementation of a word processing, billing or scheduling software package. Determine the stages of implementation and the time required. Ask what should have been done differently. Complete the chart below and make recommendations that would have improved the process.

Implementation of Software at Mentoring Practice

Type of Application: _____ *Name of Software:* _____

Steps Followed	Time Required	Recommendations
1. _____		
2. _____		
3. _____		
4. _____		
5. _____		
6. _____		

(DACUM 2.6, 2.7, 3.4, 5.1, 5.2)

2. Compare two maintenance agreements from your mentoring practice for office or lab equipment. Using the format below, analyze the features of each to determine which is a better contract. Summarize the pros and cons of each contract.

Type of equipment _____ *Purpose* _____

Contract Features

Contract 1	Contract 2
1. _____	
2. _____	
3. _____	
4. _____	
5. _____	

Summary of advantages

1. _____
2. _____
3. _____

Summary of disadvantages

1. _____
2. _____
3. _____

(DACUM 5.2, 6.4)

3. Develop a list of guidelines that will help you maintain an accurate inventory count. (DACUM 3.1, 6.3)

4. Decide whether word processing, spreadsheet, graphics, or database software is the best application to accomplish each task named below. Justify your answer.

Task	Software Applications	Reason for Application
Indexing medical journals	Database	Alphabetizes sorts a lengthy list
Determining rate of usage of disposable supplies	Spreadsheet keeps up with quantity used and time frame	
Creating holiday card list		
Calculating mortgage payments		
Maintaining patient records		
Logging vehicle mileage		
Writing memos		
Preparing income statements		
Presenting a research paper		
Compiling credit card expenditures		
Creating correspondence		
Maintaining payroll records		

(DACUM 3.4)

EXPANDING YOUR THINKING

1. List several ways computers can help each of the following:
   a. The physician
   b. The medical assistant
   c. The nurse
   d. The laboratory assistant
2. Develop a list of questions to ask a prospective maintenance company that wishes to service your computer system.
3. Assume that you are speaking with a new medical assistant who has reservations about assuming a job in a computerized office because his computer skills are weak. Prepare a role-playing situation with a friend and present it to the class.

Chapter 10

Medical Documents and Word Processing

HARTLAND, MAINE

Our practice has very high standards for the documents and correspondence we send out. A perfect, well-laid-out letter gives a good impression of our professionalism and attention to detail, qualities that people want in their medical care. I know that when I open a letter and notice a misspelling or awkward construction it makes me wonder about the standards of the office that mailed it.

We use customized formats for all of our documents. Our custom-designed forms are stored in the computer for FAX, memos, letters, research papers, and other documents. We spell check each document before printing and have someone other than the person who keyed the document do the proofreading. These quality control procedures help us maintain our standards. The best part of this is that our physicians provide a lot of freedom in creating documents because they trust us to adhere to high standards.

Angela Sebastini
Medical Secretary

PERFORMANCE BASED COMPETENCIES

After completing this chapter, you should be able to:

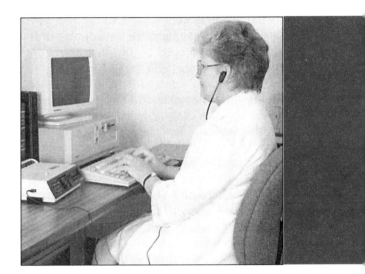

1. Create written communication appropriate to the reader's ability to understand. (DACUM 2.3)
2. Demonstrate comprehension of guidelines for medical correspondence by developing form letters and medical documents. (DACUM 3.1, 3.3, 3.4)
3. Adapt available word processing technology to medical applications. (DACUM 2.6, 3.4)
4. Apply proofreading techniques to rough draft and finished copy. (DACUM 3.1)
5. Use proper methods in transcribing by machine. (DACUM 3.5)

HEALTHSPEAK

Block Letter format in which all lines begin at the left margin.

Formatting Placement of the parts of a letter or medical document.

Gender bias Subtle form of verbal sex discrimination.

Gender neutral Language that is not biased toward either sex.

Modified block Format in which the date and closing lines begin at center.

Proofread To examine a document for errors.

Redundancy Unnecessary repetition of words.

Stored letter parts Standard paragraphs that are stored in the computer's memory.

Thesaurus Reference book or word processing feature containing synonyms and antonyms.

Tone Sound of letters; what is said and how the writer chooses to say it.

Transcription To write from one source to another.

As a medical assistant, you may compose some of the general correspondence and reports for your practice. Letters concerning business matters, such as leases or equipment repair, and reports about office management, such as a comparative study of computer systems, are items that physicians usually do not have time to write themselves. They will leave these and similar writing responsibilities to the medical assistant. As a result, the medical assistant must be prepared to create documents that represent the practice. This involves an understanding of writing principles and objectives as well as writing practice.

For some people, writing well is an ability developed during their formative years. Everyone else can learn and improve their ability to produce clean, clear documents and letters. The ability to write well increases your value as a medical assistant. If you have the skills to develop a topic and write an interesting, well-organized letter, you will have more opportunity to advance in your career.

Your professional writing will probably include: (1) correspondence for your personal signature, (2) correspondence for the physician's signature, (3) informal notes to other staff members, (4) standard fill-in forms or cards to

be mailed, and (5) occasional practice or research reports. If you are also the office manager, your writing responsibilities will be even greater.

Letter Writing

The Dartnell Institute, a research organization, produces an annual study of the cost of producing letters. Their current estimate ranges from $12.28 for a letter produced using machine dictation and word processing software on a computer, to an astonishing $18.54 for a letter produced using face-to-face dictation and an electric typewriter. A practice that creates fifty letters per week spends $31,928 to $48,204 annually on correspondence. A medical staff that can rapidly create accurate, effective correspondence will have a dramatic effect on the practice's productivity. Success at letter writing depends on skill in these two areas: (1) creating the proper tone and (2) using the correct words.

DEVELOPING TONE

Musicians tune their instruments before every concert so that the sound will be pleasing to listeners. Good orchestra leaders know that an out-of-tune instrument can spoil the effect of a lovely composition. In the same way, the tone or sound of letters should be pleasing to the readers. What is said and how the writer chooses to say it determines a letter's tone. Appropriate tone in a letter is conversational, informal, and businesslike. It is not too familiar, chatty, or pretentious.

"You" Viewpoint

A letter is written for the benefit of the reader. Therefore, the reader's wants, needs, feelings, and emotions come before the writer's wants, needs, feelings, and emotions. For example, a letter requesting a patient to pay an overdue account should focus on the reader's desire to maintain a good credit rating, not on the practice's desire to collect money. Commonly called the "you" viewpoint or the "you" attitude, this concept of letter writing might be described as "putting yourself in the reader's place." The "you" viewpoint is accomplished through a positive, pleasant tone that focuses on the reader. It does not mean that the word "you" is overused.

The opposite of the "you" viewpoint is the "I" (or "we") viewpoint; a letter based on the writer's needs. "I" letters sound selfish and turn the reader off from the message. Read the following examples of the two viewpoints.

"YOU" VIEWPOINT

Dear Mr. Wisczniewski:

Good health is the key to a good life, and you obviously had that thought in mind when you asked us to remind you of your annual physical examination. It is once again time for your annual checkup.

If you will call the office at your convenience, we will schedule an appointment for a day that won't interfere with your work. The telephone number is 555-3867.

"I" VIEWPOINT

Dear Mr. Wisczniewski:

Our calendar shows that it is time for your annual physical examination, and I would like to schedule an appointment that fits Dr. Carerra's schedule within the next month. Please call me so I can determine what time is available for an appointment.

Use Positive Words Instead of Negative

Positive words add pleasure to letter reading and should be used abundantly. Negative words are worthwhile only if they add meaning or make an important point. By reconstructing sentences, positive words can usually be substituted for most negative words. In addition to "no," "not," "never," and other generally recognized negatives, the connotations of some words also set a negative tone. Figure 10-1 lists some negative words and phrases.

Saying "No" in a "Yes" Way

Letters should speak of what can be done instead of what cannot be done. Letters whose purpose is essentially negative, even credit rejection letters, can be written to say "no" in a "yes" way. The following two letters were written by a medical assistant for the physician's sig-

---

Negative Words and Phrases

dumb	inconsistent
unsuccessful	reject
useless	in vain
impossible	mistake
failed	oversight
inadvertent	mess
fiasco	limit
sorry	withdraw
stupid	beg your pardon
correct me if I'm wrong	disagree

FIGURE 10-1

---

nature. Compare the ways in which the negative letter was rewritten to say "no" in a positive way.

NEGATIVE TREATMENT

Dear Ms. Tariela:

I am sorry to say that your failure to keep your last two appointments forces me to withdraw from treating your medical condition. It is useless for me to continue to make recommendations, since my efforts are in vain.

POSITIVE TREATMENT

Dear Ms. Tariela:

Your good health is important to me, so I was naturally concerned when you missed your last two appointments. Routine appointments to evaluate your condition are important for your continuing successful recovery.

Unless we can arrange a suitable schedule of checkups, I will be unable to continue as your physician. Will you please call me so we can discuss the future direction of your treatment?

CORRECT WORD CHOICE

Using the right word at the right time is a gift for some letter writers. However, even the person who is not naturally gifted in writing can develop skill in choosing the right words. A few liberally applied guidelines, as well as a thesaurus for strengthening vocabulary and a dictionary

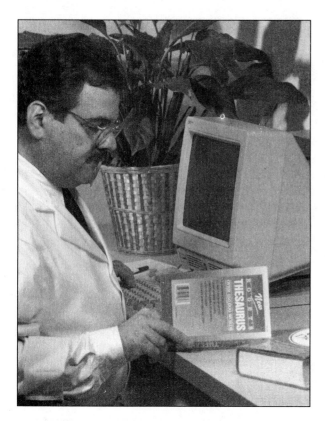

FIGURE 10-2 A thesaurus and dictionary are invaluable resources for choosing appropriate words and strengthening a medical assistant's vocabulary and spelling skills.

for correct spelling, will ensure correct word choice (Fingure 10-2).

Communicating at the Reader's Level

To understand the importance of writing to a specific audience, consider these questions:

- Should a teacher write a first grader a note using twelfth-grade words?
- Should an engineer use engineering terms in a memorandum to a botanist?
- Should a medical assistant write to a patient using technical medical terminology?

The answer to all of these questions is "no." Unfortunately, some writers fail to consider the reader's background. Because of this, they write letters that fail to deliver their messages because the language is too technical or too sophisticated for the reader to understand. Direct the message to the educational level, maturity, and experience of the reader. For example, a letter to a consulting physician to arrange an appointment may use medical terminology, which should be understood. Patients, however, may not understand medical terminology, and letters sprinkled with medical terms may confuse and frustrate them. A comparison of technical terminology and ordinary words is shown in Figure 10-3. A letter to a medically trained person may use the terminology on the left. A letter to a nonmedical person should use the common language substitutes.

Gender Bias

Occupations that once were male-dominated or female-dominated are now gender-neutral because of federal legislation to eliminate bias in employment. It is difficult to change habits of thought and speech, so gender-restrictive terms continue to be a part of language. Although the number of female physicians has grown in

Technical Terminology	Common Language Substitute
myocardial infarction	heart attack
hypertension	high blood pressure
diabetes mellitus	diabetes
carcinoma	cancer
arteriosclertic heart disease	hardening of the arteries
deglutition	swallowing
erythrocyte	red blood cell
h.s.	at bedtime
hyperglycemia	excessive sugar in the blood
inspiration	breathing
trauma	injury

FIGURE 10-3 Comparison of medical and nonmedical terminology

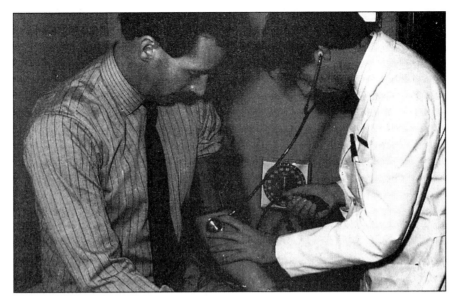

FIGURE 10-4 Be aware of gender biases you may have. Occupations that were once dominated by one sex, such as nursing, are now considered gender-neutral.

recent years and male nurses are becoming more common, some people still visualize "doctors" as male and "nurses" as female (Figure 10-4). Always strive to eliminate gender bias in writing. Sometimes this is as simple as being aware of the subtle biases that exist in the subconscious. Thinking in nongender terms will make writing gender-neutral prose much easier. By substituting a word, reworking the structure of a sentence, or changing the pronoun from singular to plural, gender bias can usually be eliminated from writing. Review the lists in Figure 10-5 to learn some acceptable substitutes for sexist words or phrases.

Use Active Instead of Passive Voice

Active verbs make writing more direct and easier to read. The difference between an enticing and a boring piece of communication may rest in the choice of verbs. Review the examples of sentences with active verbs or passive verbs in Figure 10-6.

Use Short Sentences and Paragraphs

Short sentences and paragraphs are more readable than long sentences and paragraphs. A sentence should state the point directly and concisely. Usually, twenty words is considered the maximum limit for a good sentence. Eliminate

Gender-Biased Language	Substitute for Gender Bias
female nurse	nurse
male orderly	medical attendant
stewardess	flight attendant
foreman	supervisor
cleaning ladies	cleaning crew, janitorial staff
physician wore his lab coat	physician wore a lab coat
nurse called her husband	nurse called a spouse
medical assistant spoke her mind	medical assistant commented
her mind reviewed his paperwork	reviewed the paperwork

FIGURE 10-5 Substitutes for gender-biased language

Comparison of Active and Passive Verbs	
Active Voice	**Passive Voice**
The medical assistant filed the patient's records.	The patient's records were filed by the medical assistant.
An emergency physician saves lives daily.	Lives are saved daily by an emergency physician.
The mother brought her baby in for a checkup.	The baby was brought in by the mother for a checkup.
The young children disrupted the entire staff.	The entire staff was disrupted by the young children.

FIGURE 10-6 Active and passive voice

unnecessary words and phrases that do not contribute to the sentence and combine short sentences that sound choppy and monotonous. Constructing sentences that are clear, yet not wordy or choppy is a challenge to writing skills. Study the sample sentences in Figure 10-7.

Finally, a paragraph should cover only one point and contain from two to five sentences. Readers lose interest when a paragraph is too long.

Eliminate Redundant Words

The remark "I didn't have time to write a short letter, so I wrote a long one" means that a writer finds it easier to be wordy than concise. Paraphrased, this comment means "Never use two words when one word will do." Excessive use of words makes a piece of communication tedious to read and undermines its effectiveness, causing the reader to yawn figuratively and lose interest.

Redundancy means the unnecessary repetition of words. Redundant use of language shows up too often in business correspondence. Does that mean the writer is lazy? Or does the writer not understand how redundancy affects the communication process? After each letter, memo, or report, analyze the paragraphs to check for redundancy. Eliminate or rephrase any part that bogs down the message. Figure 10-8 lists some common redundant expressions. In each case, the phrase can be replaced with one word.

Developing Your Communications

Consider a request to compose letters, reports, memorandums, and other materials as a compliment. Only the person with advanced grammar, punctuation, spelling, human relations, and organizational skills is given this assignment. A medical assistant asked to compose a communication should start by developing a plan. One system that works well is the simplified five-step

Short, Choppy Sentences:
Dr. Ashley examined the patient. The patient complained of headaches to the doctor. The doctor prescribed medication. The patient took the medication and felt better.

Long Sentence:
The patient complained to Dr. Ashley about headaches; then Dr. Ashley examined the patient and prescribed medication which the patient took before feeling better.

Well-Constructed Sentence:
Dr. Ashley examined the patient who complained of headaches. The patient felt better after taking the medication the doctor prescribed.

FIGURE 10-7 Comparison of sentence structure

Redundant Expression	Replacement
repeat again	repeat
forever after	forever
reverse order	reverse
close up	close
very latest	latest
now and forever	always
first and foremost	first
each and every	each
absolutely free	free
invisible to the eye	invisible
physician's patient	patient
patient's illness	illness

FIGURE 10-8 Redundant expressions and substitutions

plan developed by Frank Andera of Montana State University, which significantly reduces the time required for composing. The plan is given below in Figure 10-9.

Writing for the Physician's Signature

Composing a letter to be signed by another person poses a challenge because the writer must duplicate the other's writing style and philosophy. As a medical assistant, you will routinely key the physician's dictated communications and thus gain a feel for the person's style of writing. You can also review other documents written by the physician at an earlier time to see the particular style he or she employs. When you are asked to write a letter, search the files for a letter on the same subject that the physician previously dictated or wrote. Substitute current details in the appropriate spots and update the letter with names, times, and specific details. The first two or three times you compose a document for the physician, submit a rough draft for approval or revision. After keying the changes, print the final document in correct format for the physician's signature.

Your responsibility for report writing as a medical assistant probably will be somewhat limited. The amount of report writing you do will depend on the degree to which you become involved in the physician's outside activities. Some physicians who engage in research, public speaking, writing articles, and related activities may ask a medical assistant to research periodicals, newspapers, and books for specific information necessary for these activities. Someone who is both a medical assistant and an office manager may be called on to develop a report on office procedures, office equipment, or personnel matters. The basic rules that apply to writing letters are also useful for writing reports, although special rules exist for developing and preparing a report.

Composing at the Computer

Word processing software offers the opportunity to compose at the computer, thus saving an enormous amount of time. The screen can be thought of as a clean sheet of paper on which to write thoughts. As you develop your letters, reports, or other documents, read them for tone and word choice. When you find redundancies, gender bias, overuse or inappropriate use of the passive voice, or overly short or overly long sentences, edit your documents on the screen. Then, print a draft copy for final review and correction. Finally, edit the document on the screen and make final changes before printing the finished copy. Although composing at the computer may be a bit awkward at first, you will soon wonder how you ever found the time to hand write or use the typewriter for rough drafts in the past.

IN YOUR OPINION

1. Do you think that most people write more or fewer letters than they did twenty-five years ago? Why?
2. Can you think of gender-neutral alternatives for these words; man hours, office girl, workmen, mankind, lab girl, manpower?
3. What steps can you take to make sure you are writing at the reader's level?

Step One: Define the Problem and the Audience. Classify the purpose of the communication: informational, request, collection, thank you, or other. Determine the nature and background of the communication and the reader's view of the situation: Has previous correspondence been exchanged? Will the reader be receptive to the document?

Identify the reader by considering education, economic status, marital status (if appropriate), experience, age, attitude, biases, and other factors you consider relevant.

Step Two: Create an Outline. Prepare a brief outline with a one-word identifier that describes the content of each paragraph. The following outline is suggested for a letter advising patients that a new physician has joined the practice.

First paragraph:	Announcement
Second paragraph:	Background
Third paragraph:	Good will

Step Three: Brainstorm Ideas. Jot down thoughts that can be included in each paragraph. Don't worry about the order in which you write them at this stage. The identifiers listed above suggest that the first paragraph of the letter will announce the new physician's name and starting date. The second paragraph describes the physician's medical background. The last paragraph builds good will by explaining how patients will benefit from an additional physician. A brief list of ideas might look like this one:

First paragraph:	Dr. Rogers joining practice August 15
	Available on full-time basis June 26
Second paragraph:	Specialty, Family Practice
	Johns Hopkins University
	Internship, Albert Einstein Medical Center
Third paragraph:	Waiting time reduced for patients
	Taking new patients
	Auxiliary staff increased

Step Four: Put Ideas into Order. Review all the ideas written in Step Three. Choose the best and list them in the order in which they should be presented in the letter.

First paragraph:	Dr. Rogers joining practice
	Available on limited basis beginning June 26
	Full time after August 15
Second paragraph:	Graduated from Johns Hopkins University School of Medicine
	Specialty, Family Practice Internship, Albert Einstein Medical Center
Third paragraph:	Waiting time reduced for established patients
	Taking new patients
	Auxiliary staff increased

Step Five: Write the Paragraphs. The letter is now ready to be written. Construct concise, complete sentences in the order shown in Step Four. Add transitional words as necessary to create a smooth writing style.

FIGURE 10-9 Five-step plan for composing

Sources of Input

The correspondence, memos, and medical reports that medical assistants create and edit on word processors come from a variety of sources, both inside and outside the medical office. Whatever the source, you as a medical assistant will be responsible for organizing and producing the information in the documents so that it is attractive and can be used efficiently. Here are some of the more common forms of information you will keyboard, edit, proofread, and file:

- The physician's dictation
- The physician's notes
- Patient information sheets
- Case histories and other medical reports
- Memos and letters
- Speeches

ROUGH DRAFT INPUT

Hand-written rough draft input is a popular form of document preparation because it can be created at almost any time and in any place. Input from rough draft documents has both advantages and disadvantages.

Advantages
- Documents can be created quickly without concern for appearance
- Many people think best when they use a pencil to add, delete, and cross out
- Medical terminology is usually spelled correctly and accents and dialects are eliminated, which makes the document easier to key

Pitfalls
- Physicians are notorious for their hard-to-read handwriting
- Typed rough draft materials often have been cut and re-taped, making them difficult to follow
- Copy may be sprinkled throughout with correction fluid that is also written over
- Several different type styles can appear in the same document
- Different word processing drafts may exist, causing confusion over which is most current

Tips for Managing Rough Drafts
- Read the entire document to be sure you understand it
- Recopy poor handwriting
- Trace inserted material to its proper location in the document, drawing arrows as needed
- Add missing information, such as an address or title
- Correct spelling and grammar and add punctuation as needed
- Use proofreading marks to clarify editing
- Circle special notes in red
- Add formatting comments or other information that will aid in keying the document
- Make sure you always work with the most recent draft
- Destroy previous revisions

Study the proofreader's marks shown in Figure 10-10 and review the rough draft typed case history in Figure 10-11 to determine the reason for the proofreader's marks.

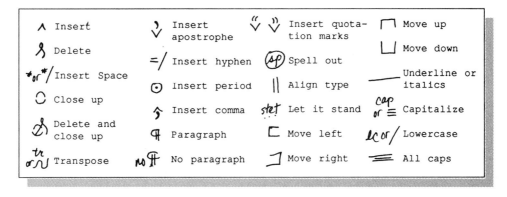

FIGURE 10-10 Proofreader's marks

PATIENT CASE HISTORY

NAME Robert*a* McElroy

PATIENT NUMBER 894

MADELINE HAST, M.D.

DATE August 16, 19—

CHIEF COMPLAINT: This twelve-year-old ~~patient~~ *female* came to my office with ~~his~~ *her*
mother. ~~His~~ *Her* symptoms ~~are~~ *were* headaches, sore throat, and *a cough.*
She had been ∧ coughing for four days. Fever had been present for two
days. A week ago he *s* spent the night with a friend who
has *since* been diagnosed for strep *throat.*

EXAMINATION: Examination shows a generally healthy *female* child who is
developed and nourished well. ~~She~~ weighs *84* ~~64~~ pounds and
5'0" is ~~4~~ feet ~~8~~ inches tall. Her temperature is 101.4
degrees. B.p. is 100/60.
Sp.
Throat, glands and tympanic membranes are clear. Ears
and neck are within limits. Eyes are clear. Rales are
present in the lower chest on respiration. Abdomen is
within normal limits
~~okay~~. The patient is lethargic.

LAB TESTS: None.

DIAGNOSOS: Lower pneumonia.

TREATMENT: Erthromycin, 100 *cc.* ~~cc,~~ 1 teaspoon ~~bid~~ *twice a day* with food
Phenergan VC with codeine, 1 ~~t.bid.~~ *teaspoon twice a day*
Recheck in one week.

REMARKS: This patient appears very umcomfor*t*able.

FAMILY HISTORY: ~~PATIENT IS THE OLDEST~~ of four children. All are in
good general health. The parents are also in good general
health. The maternal grandmother ~~has~~ *suffers from* high blood pressure.

PERSONAL HISTORY: Patient is active. She is fifth grade cheerleader and
also dances. She is successful academically.

_____

Madeline Hast, M.D.

FIGURE 10-11 Proofreading example

Word processing is especially appropriate for a previously keyed rough draft letter that must be edited and sent to a different person.

DICTATION AND TRANSCRIPTION

The threat of medical malpractice lawsuits has forced physicians to document thoroughly all medications, instructions, procedures, treatments, and services for each patient. Many physicians use shorthand and machine dictation and transcription to write their correspondence and medical reports. Machine transcription also has its advantages and disadvantages.

Voice Activated Dictation: Brave New World

Originally, dictation was a process consisting of one person dictating, with another simultaneously writing the spoken words in shorthand and transcribing the document at a later time. Today, it is more common for the physician to dictate into a machine, as described below, for transcription at another time. An exciting development in dictation technology is Voice Activated Dictation. The physician records several hundred words in the Voice Activated system, from which the system learns to recognize the physician's pronunciation. The physician can dictate while, for example, performing a surgical procedure. The system rapidly creates a draft document, which is proofread for errors. Voice activated systems have a good degree of accuracy at recognizing spoken words and they make the dictation process much faster. The medical assistant is freed from the laborious process of transcription and takes on the higher level skill of editing.

Machine Dictation

Some physicians return to their offices after treating each patient to dictate reports and doctor's notes on a desktop dictating unit. Other physicians dictate on a portable dictating machine in the examining room in the patient's presence. This method helps to reduce malpractice claims because (1) the physician dictates the report before any important portion of the visit is forgotten, and (2) the patient knows that a report covering the visit is on file. If there is a discrepancy between the patient's and the physician's understanding of the procedure or treatment, the patient has an opportunity to ask questions after hearing the dictation.

Advantages
- The medical assistant can perform other functions while the physician dictates
- The material can be transcribed later
- Few graduates today have the shorthand skills necessary to write and transcribe medical terminology

Pitfalls
- Dictation from physicians with foreign accents and regional dialects may be difficult to understand
- The transcriber must use medical dictionaries and other reference books to locate spellings and meanings that fit the context of medical documents. (Some software packages have a spell checker.)
- Medical transcription is more difficult than general transcription

Some hints for successful transcription are listed below:

Machine and Transcription Tips
- Use the operator's manual extensively until you learn the machine (Figure 10-12)
- Rely on the indicator slips or the electronic indicator panel of your unit for document length
- Always review the special instructions and comments first
- Follow the rule, "Listen to an earful; then type"
- Do not listen too long before you begin to key
- Play back any material you do not understand; previously dictated material may clarify what comes next
- Punctuate as you go
- If the dictator does not use punctuation, listen for breaks that indicate punctuation
- When you are unsure of punctuation, refer to a punctuation manual after completing the document
- Leave a blank space for medical words you cannot comprehend

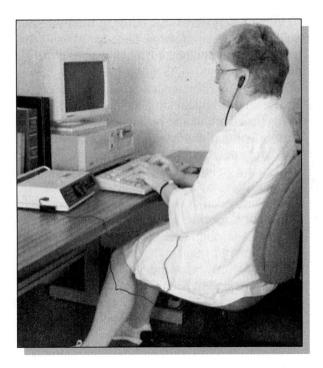

FIGURE 10-12 The dictation-transcription unit shown here has a foot control that starts the machine. When the pedal is released the machine stops.

Medical Terminology

1. Many medical words sound alike but have different meanings, for example, hyperthyroidism and hypothyroidism, or don't sound alike but have the same meaning.

2. Abbreviations are often used. Some should be spelled out, but others should not. Refer to a medical dictionary when in doubt.

3. Latin or Greek beginnings and endings are used to form many medical words. Learn the most commonly used prefixes and suffixes.

4. Many medical words come from Latin or Greek root words. Learn the common roots.

5. Diagnoses and treatments have certain aspects in common. Compare the two when a question exists about a word.

FIGURE 10-13 Medical terminology

- Remember, a medical malpractice lawsuit can be decided on the evidence in a medical report
- Make a list of all notes to ask the doctor at one time rather than repeatedly interrupting

Importance of Medical Terminology

Chapter 1 reviews common medical terminology. If you do not already own a medical dictionary such as *Taber's Cyclopedic Medical Dictionary* or *Dorland's Illustrated Medical Dictionary,* purchase a copy before you begin your first job (or early in your schooling). Even if transcription is not one of your responsibilities, you will use these dictionaries often. Figure 10-13 provides a brief description of medical terminology.

IN YOUR OPINION

1. How could a medical transcriptionist overcome the tedium of routine and consistent keying?

2. Medical transcriptionists often mention poor dictation practices by the originator of a document as a major problem in transcription. What do you think dictators can do to aid transcriptionists? How can transcriptionists facilitate this?

3. Which do you think would be easier—transcription from rough draft or by machine? Explain why.

Word Processing Software

Medical offices frequently use word processing software combined with a letter quality or laser printer to create correspondence and medical reports. The basic word processing features are display, editing, storage, and printing. With these capabilities, the user can create new documents or store standard documents such as form letters, insurance forms, and recall notices and can retrieve them as needed.

WordPerfect and Microsoft Windows are two software packages with many advanced features that make it easy to create professional documents and letter-perfect correspondence. Listed below are some of these time-saving features and how they can be helpful in a medical office:

- A customized medical dictionary containing specific medical terms and physicians' names and used with the spell checker saves valuable time.
- Inserting graphics, charts, and diagrams directly into a document keeps all information together and results in a professional-looking document.
- Word processing "equation editors" enable the use of symbols and other special characters when typing equations and other formulas in a document.
- Using a "database" of patients or physicians and merging it with a form letter results in an automated office correspondence procedure.

FUNCTIONS OF WORD PROCESSING SOFTWARE

Life is much easier for a transcriptionist who has access to an easy-to-use general purpose word processing software package. Most features are standard in the best known programs, but all of them work a little differently, depending on the specific program. Create and Edit are two primary word processing functions.

Creating Text

The software will ask for a document file name and identify the document by that name each time it is recalled for editing, formatting, or printing. The document can be revised and stored under the original name. If both the original version and the revised version will be used, an alternate name can be given to the second version.

Editing Text

Characters, words, sentences, or paragraphs can be added, deleted, changed, or moved within a draft or previously stored document. Some commonly used editing commands are shown in Figure 10-14.

Output

Output refers to the finished product after text is keyed and processed. Output takes many forms, including letters, memos, research articles, insurance forms, completed superbills and ledger cards, medical reports, graphs, charts, computer-output microforms, graphics, and other documents. The user is responsible for formatting the output, although some information will be printed on specially designed forms such as insurance claim forms. However, most of the medical assistant's word processing time is spent formatting correspondence and medical documents. Standard formatting guidelines that can be used on any type of keyboard in addition to illustrations of typical formats are shown in the following section.

FORMATTING WORD PROCESSING CORRESPONDENCE

The term formatting refers to placement of the parts of a letter or medical document. Any formatted communication should be attractive and easy to read. Since letters and internal memorandums account for a large portion of the physician's correspondence, the medical staff should establish standard formats for greatest efficiency. Simple formats are best, especially with electronic equipment. This is because the greatest efficiency comes when a minimum number of keystrokes is required and when standard parts of a document are stored and retrieved as needed. Several procedures for creating an attractive document are appropriate, whether you use a typewriter or word processor to create your documents.

Procedures for Formatting Documents

Several specific formatting suggestions follow. Refer to your WordPerfect or other software manual for short cuts offered by the software.

1. Place your document on the page, as you would place a picture within a frame.
2. Leave plenty of white space in the frame.
3. Center the document on the page.
4. Make sure top, bottom, and side margins are neither too narrow nor too wide. Use the the word count feature in your software's spell check to determine the number of words in your document. The number of words will determine how wide or narrow the margin should be.

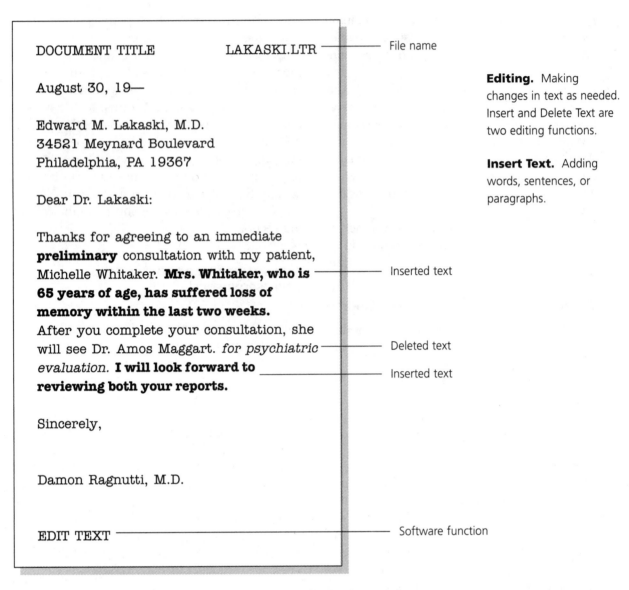

FIGURE 10-14 Edited document showing inserted text in bold and deleted text in italic

Text within the figure:

DOCUMENT TITLE   LAKASKI.LTR ——— File name

August 30, 19—

Edward M. Lakaski, M.D.
34521 Meynard Boulevard
Philadelphia, PA 19367

Dear Dr. Lakaski:

Thanks for agreeing to an immediate
preliminary consultation with my patient,
Michelle Whitaker. **Mrs. Whitaker, who is** ——— Inserted text
65 years of age, has suffered loss of
memory within the last two weeks.
After you complete your consultation, she
will see Dr. Amos Maggart. *for psychiatric* ——— Deleted text
evaluation. **I will look forward to** ——— Inserted text
reviewing both your reports.

Sincerely,

Damon Ragnutti, M.D.

EDIT TEXT ——————————— Software function

Sidebar text:

Editing. Making changes in text as needed. Insert and Delete Text are two editing functions.

Insert Text. Adding words, sentences, or paragraphs.

Block and Modified Block Letter Formats, Open and Mixed Punctuation

The two most common letter formats are block, in which all lines begin at the left margin, and modified block, in which the date and closing lines begin at the center. In both styles, paragraphs may be indented or they may begin at the left margin.

Open and mixed punctuation refers to the punctuation after the salutation and the complimentary close of a letter. When no punctuation appears after these parts, punctuation is said to be "open." When a colon follows the salutation and a comma follows the complimentary close, punctuation is referred to as "mixed."

Figure 10-15 illustrates a block style letter with no paragraph indents and open punctuation. Figure 10-16 illustrates a modified block letter with no paragraph indents and mixed punctuation. Figure 10-17 illustrates a modified block letter with open punctuation and paragraph indents. Block is recommended for letters, especially when electronic equipment is used, because it increases efficiency by reducing keystrokes.

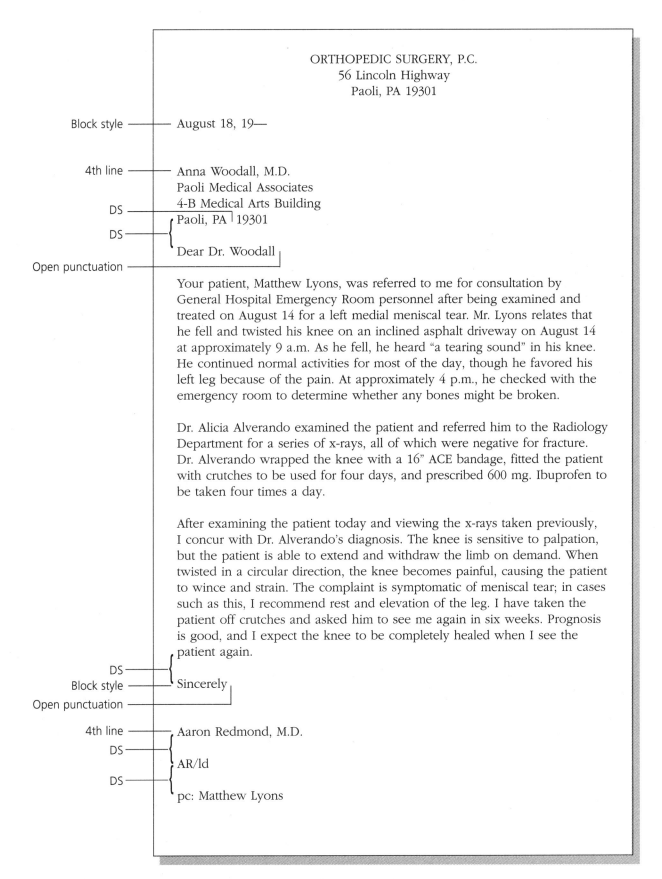

ORTHOPEDIC SURGERY, P.C.
56 Lincoln Highway
Paoli, PA 19301

Block style —— August 18, 19—

4th line —— Anna Woodall, M.D.
Paoli Medical Associates
4-B Medical Arts Building
DS —— Paoli, PA 19301
DS ——
Dear Dr. Woodall

Open punctuation ——

Your patient, Matthew Lyons, was referred to me for consultation by General Hospital Emergency Room personnel after being examined and treated on August 14 for a left medial meniscal tear. Mr. Lyons relates that he fell and twisted his knee on an inclined asphalt driveway on August 14 at approximately 9 a.m. As he fell, he heard "a tearing sound" in his knee. He continued normal activities for most of the day, though he favored his left leg because of the pain. At approximately 4 p.m., he checked with the emergency room to determine whether any bones might be broken.

Dr. Alicia Alverando examined the patient and referred him to the Radiology Department for a series of x-rays, all of which were negative for fracture. Dr. Alverando wrapped the knee with a 16" ACE bandage, fitted the patient with crutches to be used for four days, and prescribed 600 mg. Ibuprofen to be taken four times a day.

After examining the patient today and viewing the x-rays taken previously, I concur with Dr. Alverando's diagnosis. The knee is sensitive to palpation, but the patient is able to extend and withdraw the limb on demand. When twisted in a circular direction, the knee becomes painful, causing the patient to wince and strain. The complaint is symptomatic of meniscal tear; in cases such as this, I recommend rest and elevation of the leg. I have taken the patient off crutches and asked him to see me again in six weeks. Prognosis is good, and I expect the knee to be completely healed when I see the patient again.

DS ——
Block style —— Sincerely
Open punctuation ——

4th line —— Aaron Redmond, M.D.
DS ——
AR/ld
DS ——
pc: Matthew Lyons

FIGURE 10-15 Block style letter with open punctuation

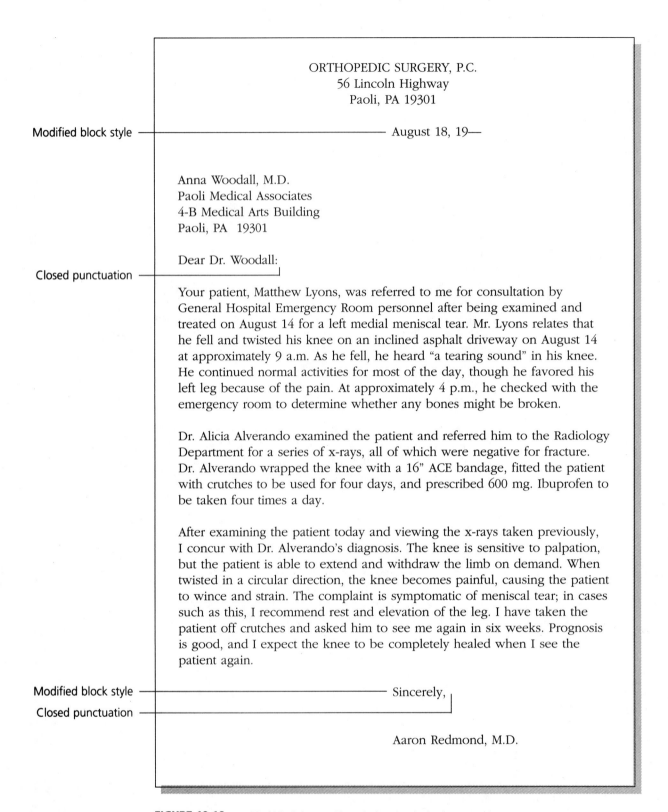

Modified block style ———

ORTHOPEDIC SURGERY, P.C.
56 Lincoln Highway
Paoli, PA 19301

August 18, 19—

Anna Woodall, M.D.
Paoli Medical Associates
4-B Medical Arts Building
Paoli, PA 19301

Closed punctuation ———

Dear Dr. Woodall:

Your patient, Matthew Lyons, was referred to me for consultation by General Hospital Emergency Room personnel after being examined and treated on August 14 for a left medial meniscal tear. Mr. Lyons relates that he fell and twisted his knee on an inclined asphalt driveway on August 14 at approximately 9 a.m. As he fell, he heard "a tearing sound" in his knee. He continued normal activities for most of the day, though he favored his left leg because of the pain. At approximately 4 p.m., he checked with the emergency room to determine whether any bones might be broken.

Dr. Alicia Alverando examined the patient and referred him to the Radiology Department for a series of x-rays, all of which were negative for fracture. Dr. Alverando wrapped the knee with a 16" ACE bandage, fitted the patient with crutches to be used for four days, and prescribed 600 mg. Ibuprofen to be taken four times a day.

After examining the patient today and viewing the x-rays taken previously, I concur with Dr. Alverando's diagnosis. The knee is sensitive to palpation, but the patient is able to extend and withdraw the limb on demand. When twisted in a circular direction, the knee becomes painful, causing the patient to wince and strain. The complaint is symptomatic of meniscal tear; in cases such as this, I recommend rest and elevation of the leg. I have taken the patient off crutches and asked him to see me again in six weeks. Prognosis is good, and I expect the knee to be completely healed when I see the patient again.

Modified block style ———
Closed punctuation ———

Sincerely,

Aaron Redmond, M.D.

FIGURE 10-16 Modified block letter with no indents and mixed punctuation

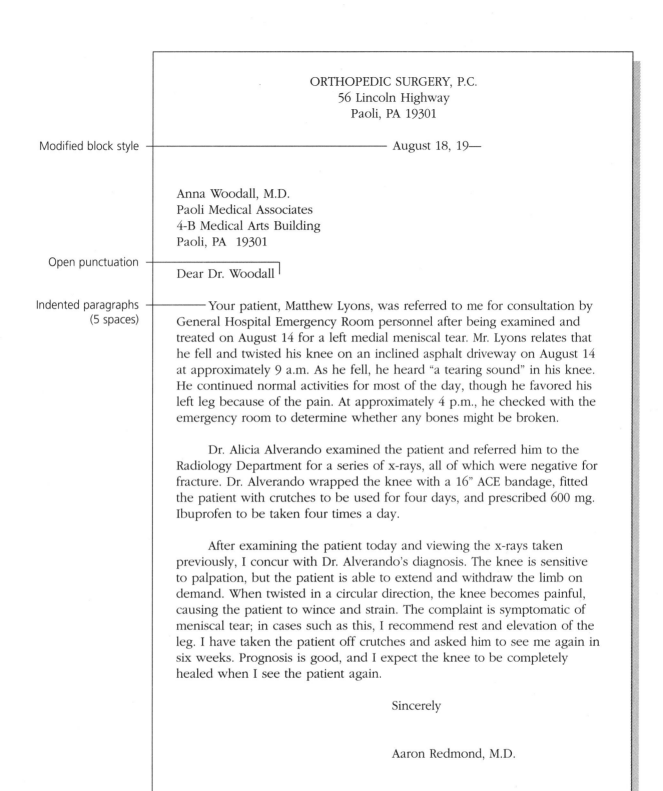

ORTHOPEDIC SURGERY, P.C.
56 Lincoln Highway
Paoli, PA 19301

Modified block style ——————————————— August 18, 19—

Anna Woodall, M.D.
Paoli Medical Associates
4-B Medical Arts Building
Paoli, PA 19301

Open punctuation ——— Dear Dr. Woodall

Indented paragraphs ——— Your patient, Matthew Lyons, was referred to me for consultation by
(5 spaces) General Hospital Emergency Room personnel after being examined and
treated on August 14 for a left medial meniscal tear. Mr. Lyons relates that
he fell and twisted his knee on an inclined asphalt driveway on August 14
at approximately 9 a.m. As he fell, he heard "a tearing sound" in his knee.
He continued normal activities for most of the day, though he favored his
left leg because of the pain. At approximately 4 p.m., he checked with the
emergency room to determine whether any bones might be broken.

Dr. Alicia Alverando examined the patient and referred him to the
Radiology Department for a series of x-rays, all of which were negative for
fracture. Dr. Alverando wrapped the knee with a 16" ACE bandage, fitted
the patient with crutches to be used for four days, and prescribed 600 mg.
Ibuprofen to be taken four times a day.

After examining the patient today and viewing the x-rays taken
previously, I concur with Dr. Alverando's diagnosis. The knee is sensitive
to palpation, but the patient is able to extend and withdraw the limb on
demand. When twisted in a circular direction, the knee becomes painful,
causing the patient to wince and strain. The complaint is symptomatic of
meniscal tear; in cases such as this, I recommend rest and elevation of the
leg. I have taken the patient off crutches and asked him to see me again in
six weeks. Prognosis is good, and I expect the knee to be completely
healed when I see the patient again.

Sincerely

Aaron Redmond, M.D.

FIGURE 10-17 Modified block letter with open punctuation and paragraph indents

Mr. Adam Janus	2	May 5, 19—

FIGURE 10-18 Second-page heading when copy is long

Mr. Adam Janus
Page 2
May 5, 19—

FIGURE 10-19 Second-page heading when copy is short

Second-Page Headings

Second-page headings may be formatted in two ways, depending on the length of the second-page copy. When the copy is long, the heading should be formatted as one horizontal line. If the page needs to appear fuller because the copy is short, the heading should be formatted vertically. In either case, the name of the person to whom the letter is sent comes first, followed by the page number and the date. Both types are illustrated in Figures 10-18 and 10-19.

Stored Letter Parts

Electronic equipment allows parts of documents, such as the date or closing, to be standardized and saved for quick retrieval and output. Figure 10-20 shows a date, salutation, and closing lines that might be stored in a word processor. At the beginning of each day, the numerals in the date can be changed to reflect the current date.

Merged Paragraphs

No discussion of word processing is complete without mentioning a special type of letter created from **merged paragraphs**. This refers to standard paragraphs that are stored in the computer's memory and combined later to form letters or other documents. For example, a medical assistant may be asked to key and save several different paragraphs that can be used in credit

August 18, 19—	(Stored Date)
Dear :	(Stored Salutation. The addressee's name is keyed before the colon. The body of the letter begins two lines below the salutation.)
Sincerely yours,	(Stored Closing Lines. Closing lines are retrieved with two lines added after the body of the letter.)
Aaron Redmond, M.D.	
ms	(Stored Reference Initials. Other lines for carbon copy, photocopy notation, or enclosure are added as needed.)

FIGURE 10-20 Stored letter parts

letters. The paragraphs will differ depending on the delinquency of the patient accounts. By storing several paragraphs on the subject and selecting for each document only those needed, the medical assistant needs to key very little additional information. WordPerfect and other software packages have this capability. A great deal of time can be saved when the medical assistant combines pre-stored paragraphs. Examples of merged paragraphs and a complete letter are shown in Figures 10-21 and 10-22.

In Figure 10-22, paragraphs 1, 4, 7, and 8 are retrieved from memory and then combined and formatted into a form letter. Only the patient's name and address need to be keyed.

MEMORANDUMS

The size of a medical facility determines the number and frequency of memorandums. In a small facility with only one physician and one or two employees, much communication is oral. However, as a practice grows, memorandums become more necessary. Memo headings follow a standard format that can be stored. A standard memorandum format, containing a To, From, Date, and Subject line, is shown in Figure 10-23.

FORMATTING MEDICAL REPORTS

In a private practice, case history/physical examinations and consulting physician reports are

(1) Dear

(2) Your account is past due by 30 days, and we would appreciate your immediate payment. If you have overlooked your account, will you please send a check immediately.

(3) Your account is past due by 60 days, and we have not heard from you. If there is a problem with your account or if you need to discuss your financial situation, please call the matter to our attention.

(4) Your account is past due for more than 90 days and we cannot understand why you have delayed payment. After repeated notices and a request that you call us to explain your problem, we have not heard from you.

(5) You may call me at 555-8954 if there is a problem with your account. We look forward to receiving your payment.

(6) Contact me at 555-8954 if we can explain any portion of your statement that you do not understand. If we do not hear from you, we will expect payment within one month.

(7) We must turn your account over to a collection agency if we do not hear from you within two weeks. Please contact us at 555-8954 before that time in order to set up a payment plan.

(8) Sincerely,

Raymond R. Jackson, M.D.

FIGURE 10-21 Merged paragraphs

Dear

Your account is past due for more than 90 days and we cannot understand why you have delayed payment. After repeated notices and a request that you call us to explain your problem, we have not heard from you.

We must turn your account over to a collection agency if we do not hear from you within two weeks. Please contact us at 555-8954 before that time in order to set up a payment plan.

Sincerely,

Raymond R. Jackson, M.D.

FIGURE 10-22 Letter created from merged paragraphs

the most common medical documents produced. In a hospital, admission summaries, discharge summaries, and laboratory reports account for a large part of output. All of these documents follow a standard format, although it may vary slightly from one practice to another or from one hospital to another.

By storing the appropriate format and using it for each document, output time can be reduced dramatically. Figures 10-24 through 10-27 show typical formats for a case history and physical, consulting physician's report, laboratory report, and hospital discharge summary. Information for a hospital admission contains much of the same information found in the case history and physical. The desktop publishing features of WordPerfect and Windows can be used to create a professional looking report.

To: The Staff
From: Aaron Redmond, M.D.
Date: August 18, 19—

Subject: New Partner

Dr. Marcia Webster will join our practice as a partner on September 24. She is a graduate of Johns Hopkins University School of Medicine with a specialty in Neurology. Dr. Webster completed her internship at the Hospital of the University of Pennsylvania and her residency at Vanderbilt Hospital in Nashville, Tennessee. For the last four years, she has been stationed in Japan where she served in the U.S. Army.

Please join me in welcoming Dr. Webster to our staff. She will depend on you to help her make the adjustment to a new city and a new practice.

FIGURE 10-23 Memo heading aligned at colon indent

PATIENT CASE HISTORY

Name   Nathaniel Watson

Address   924 Maple Lane

Stafford, PA 14860

Patient No. _____

Date of Visit _August 24, 19—_

CHIEF COMPLAINT: This 28-year-old white male complains of headaches that began the day he came out of a halo/jacket after being treated for a fracture of C-6 following a fall from the top of a 20-foot ladder. Patient stepped off the ladder accidentally on April 4, 19—, while painting the gutters of his house. During the fall, he tore a ligament of the liver and jerked his neck so hard that he broke it.

Patient was admitted to General Hospital on April 4 where he underwent emergency surgery for the torn liver ligament and was placed in a halo/jacket. He remained neurologically intact during the six weeks of halo and came out of the halo six weeks ago. He had no headaches during the time he was in the halo, developed them the day he came out of halo, and has suffered with headache pain ever since. He experiences some mild numbness in his arms and occasionally mild neck pain.

EXAMINATION: Neurological examination reveals an alert, cooperative, slightly overweight male with two darkened points over each frontal region where his tongs had been placed.

No spasm in the neck. Range of motion is: 60 degrees, right lateral flexion; 60 degrees, left lateral flexion; 30 degrees, flexion; 30 degrees, extension; 80 degrees, right rotation; 80 degrees, left rotation.

Sensory system is entirely intact, and there is no atrophy or fasciculation of the motor system. Reflexes are entirely intact; head shows no tenderness over the superficial aspect of the greater occipital nerves. Cranial nerves are intact; pupils were equal and reacted well to light.

LAB TESTS: Skull x-rays reveal no osteomyelitis at the tong sites. Cervical spine x-rays reveal a minimal compression fracture of C-7 and a bridge formation between C-6 and C-7. The spine is well aligned, and lumbosacral spine x-rays are within normal limits.

DIAGNOSIS: Status post C-7 compression fracture, now fusing spontaneously to C-6. Neurologically intact. Headaches appear to be a muscular contraction form of headache.

TREATMENT: Treatment will be supportive with liberal use of aspirin recommended. If headaches persist or if patient develops radicular symptoms, he is to see me again for evaluation.

REMARKS: Patient feels he cannot go back to work on either a full-time or part-time basis. I recommend that he take off one more week and return to work on a part-time basis thereafter.

FAMILY HISTORY: Patient is married and the father of four children, ages 1–7, all of whom are in good general health. Father is a paraplegic resulting from an automobile accident; mother is diabetic. The patient has one sister and one brother, both in good general health.

PERSONAL HISTORY: Patient has had no previous accidents or illnesses. He leads an active life and is involved with his children's activities. Since his accident, he has curtailed many of his activities and seems hesitant to resume them for fear of further damaging his neck.

Katherine R. Santiago, M.D.

FIGURE 10-24 Case history and physical report

CONSULTING PHYSICIAN'S REPORT

Neurological Re-evaluation for
NATHANIEL WATSON
February 23, 19—

This patient was referred to me by Katherine R. Santiago, M.D., of Wayne, Pennsylvania, after the patient relocated to my area. I am to recommend a primary care physician and continue to follow the patient on a consulting basis as needed. Dr. Santiago treated the patient for three years following an accident in which he stepped off the top of a 20-foot ladder, breaking his neck and tearing a ligament of the liver. The patient has been taking Sygesic and Parafon Forte regularly. He is taking Elavil on a p.r.n. basis. He had an ENT evaluation in Philadelphia for an ear problem, but he did not learn anything further about his condition. He has a balance problem at night and in the dark. He has neck pain extending into the left shoulder and across the right arm. He works sporadically as a general contractor.

EXAMINATION:

Patient is alert and oriented without impairment of mental function.

Gait and Station: There is no ataxia. Tandem walking is well performed. Romberg sign is not present.

Cerebellar-coordination: There is no tremor, abnormal movement, dysmetria or dysdiadochokinesis. Finger to nose to finger and heel to shin testing are well performed.

Motor System: Strength, tone, and muscle mass are intact in all muscle groups tested. There is no evidence of focal atrophy or fasciculations.

Sensation: Examination reveals a diminished sensation to a pin in the left upper extremity over the shoulder. Touch, position, and vibration are intact Cortical sensation is normal.

Cranial nerves are unchanged from the prior evaluation.

Deep Tendon Reflexes:	BJ	TJ	BR	PJ	AJ	PL
Right:	++	++	++	++	++	flexor
Left:	++	++	++	++	++	flexor

Miscellaneous:

Dorsal lumbar range of mobility is full.

Cervical range of motion is limited to:

Flexion	50 degrees
Extension	35 degrees
Right lateral rotation	30 degrees
Left lateral rotation	30 degrees
Right lateral flexion	20 degrees
Left lateral flexion	15–20 degrees

Impression:

1. Status post cervical fracture.
2. Chronic irritation of the left axillary nerve.
3. Recurrent headaches.
4. Hearing loss, bilateral.

The patient is advised to continue medical management under the primary care of Dr. John S. Camp.

Jackson R. Westfallen, M.D., P.A.
rs

FIGURE 10-25 Consulting physician's report

GENERAL HOSPITAL
PAOLI, PA 19301

DEPARTMENT OF NEUROLOGY Report of Electromyogram

PATIENT'S NAME:	Nathaniel Watson
EMG#:	S507
AGE:	29
DATE:	December 16, 19—
REFERRED BY:	Katherine R. Santiago, M.D.
NERVE CONDUCTION:	Motor and sensory nerve conduction studies were performed in the left upper limb and were within normal limits.
ELECTROMYOGRAPHY:	EMG of the muscles of the left upper extremity and the cervical paraspinals was performed. There were no fibrillations, positive waves or fasciculations. The motor unit potentials were of normal amplitude and duration. The interference patterns were normal.
IMPRESSION:	1) Normal nerve conduction studies in the left upper extremity. 2) No evidence of denervation was found in the muscles sampled.

____

Ashar Ramed, M.D.

FIGURE 10-26 Laboratory report

FORMATTING BUSINESS REPORTS

Word processing is also used for a variety of business reports or manuscripts the physician writes. This activity requires attention to detail and proofreading skill. The attractiveness and accuracy of the report reflect on the medical assistant's ability to organize and manage a project without supervision. Most reports today are edited several times before the final document is distributed. The original may be printed on bond paper with photocopies made for general distribution, or the original may be printed on a master which is used for reproduction with an offset printer. With the advent of desktop publishing, reports generated at a desk can look just like those printed at a professional shop.

Reports must be organized completely before the first word is keyed. Otherwise, the final document will be a hodgepodge of pages that lack a polished appearance. Follow the procedures below as you organize and key reports.

Job Instructions

A job instruction sheet is invaluable for report planners. Every conceivable question that may arise during the report process should be listed and answered. When more than one person keys a report, the job instruction sheet is essential because, without such a guide, each page or section might be formatted differently at the whim of each person keying the document. Figure 10-28 lists some of the basic instructions that apply to every kind of report. The instructions provided apply to a left-bound manuscript only. Add other questions and instructions as they apply to each specific job.

Margin Guide

Word processing software often counts lines as material is keyed. When using typewriters or word processors without line counters, prepare a margin guide to extend 1/2 inch beyond the right margin, so you will be able to count lines as you key.

GENERAL HOSPITAL
PAOLI, PA 19301

DISCHARGE SUMMARY

PATIENT:	Nathaniel Watson
ADMISSION DATE:	April 4, 19—
DISCHARGE DATE:	April 16, 19—
ADMISSION DIAGNOSIS:	Multiple trauma
DISCHARGE DIAGNOSIS:	C-7 Compression Fracture Torn ligament of liver
OPERATIONS/PROCEDURES:	Exploratory laparotomy Ligation of falciform ligament
INFECTIONS:	None
CONDITION ON DISCHARGE:	Improving

BRIEF HISTORY AND PHYSICAL: This patient was admitted to the General Surgery Service on April 4, 19—, and the attending physician was Dr. Francisco Endrile. Patient was transferred to the Orthopedic Unit on April 10, 19—, where the attending physician was Dr. Marguerite Thaxson. This discharge summary will cover the patient's orthopedic care from April 10 to April 16.

The patient is a 28-year-old white male, status post fall from a ladder, 20 feet, sustaining multiple trauma, including neck and shoulder pain. He was admitted to the General Surgery Service where he had an exploratory laparotomy and ligation of the falciform ligament on April 4, 19—. He also sustained a minimally compressed fracture of C-7 and underwent a workup for this injury. He always stayed neurovascularly intact.

PERTINENT LAB AND X-RAY DATA: Tomograms were taken that showed significant combination of the body of C-7, but the posterior elements were intact, and the pieces reduced quite well in extension.

HOSPITAL COURSE: Patient was placed in a halo vest jacket and has remained neurovascularly intact. X-rays in the halo vest show the reduction to be adequate with no subluxation.

DISCHARGE MEDICATIONS AND INSTRUCTIONS: Tylenol with Codeine p.r.n.

DISPOSITION: Home, to be seen in the Spine Clinic in one week.

PROGNOSIS: Good.

_____

Katherine R. Santiago, M.D.

FIGURE 10-27 Discharge summary

1. **Kind of paper**—16-pound bond or less for the rough draft, letterhead quality for the final version.

2. **Size of paper**—8½″ × 11″ unless otherwise instructed.

3. **Number of copies**—original plus one copy, original for author, and copy for medical assistant to file.

4. **Machine to be used**—typewriter, word processor, desktop publisher—word processor, electronic typewriter with memory, or desktop publisher if available.

5. **Color of ribbon to be used**—black; color ribbons add excitement and readability to illustrations, figures, and graphs.

6. **Top and bottom margins for first page**—two-inch top margin; one-inch bottom margin.

7. **Top and bottom margins for all other pages**—one-inch top margin, one-inch bottom margin.

8. **Spacing requirements, single or double**—double, unless otherwise instructed.

9. **Paragraph indentions**—5, 10, 15, or 20 spaces.

10. **Placement of headings and subheadings**

Title of Report, Chapter Title, and Chapter Number	All capitals and centered at top margin. Quadruple space to main heading.
Main Heading	Centered horizontally. Capitals for first letter of major words. Double space to first keyed line.
Subheading One	Flush with left margin. Underlined. Capitals for first letter of major words. Double space to first keyed line.
Subheading Two	Keyed at paragraph indention. Underlined. Capitals for first letter of major words. Double space to first keyed line.

11. **Pagination plan**—page number typed at right margin ½ inch from top of page.

12. **Footnote placement**—superior numbers typed at point of reference; footnotes at end of manuscript.

13. **Placement of illustrations, figures, and graphs**—to be easily read and visually attractive.

14. **Instructions for proofreading**—proof first for accuracy, reading numbers aloud to a second person; proof second for format and inconsistencies in style.

15. **Instructions for collating**—by machine if possible, otherwise collate from bottom up. Combine insets, joggles until perfectly aligned.

16. **Instructions for binding**—permanent binding with eyelets of spiral frame preferable, conservative color.

17. **Instructions for distribution**—based on instructions of author; if mailed, back the pages with sturdy cardboard.

18. **Time frame**—depends on length schedule two days for ten pages—first day to key and proof, second day to edit at keyboard, keyboard, collate, bind, and distribute.

19. **Names and schedule of individuals who will key**—determined by practice policy.

20. **Reference books needed**—general dictionary, medical dictionary, *Physician's Desk Reference* if drug names used widely, thesaurus if editorial decisions to be made, and report style manual.

FIGURE 10-28 Job instruction sheet for report formatting

Title Page

Each report should have a simple, attractive title page. Word processor or desktop publishing programs provide a number of creative type variations for the title page.

Type the title in all capital letters and center it approximately two inches from the top of the page. Center other information vertically and horizontally with the first letter of each word capitalized. WordPerfect and other word processing software offer short cuts in preparing the title page, as well as the table of contents and footnotes discussed below.

Table of Contents

Prepare a table of contents showing main divisions, chapters, and page numbers. Place the title of the division (for example, "Chapter") in all capitals at the left margin and the page numbers at the right margin. Divide division names and page numbers with leaders (. . .). Most word processing programs have a feature that automatically generates a table of contents based on the headings designated in a document—a great time-saver!

Footnotes

The use of electronic equipment has changed techniques of footnoting. Conventional footnotes are numbered in sequence on each page with the reference given at the bottom of the same page. However, it is becoming increasingly popular for all footnotes to be numbered sequentially but referenced only at the end of a manuscript. Refer to a report-writing style manual for the correct method of keying different types of footnotes.

Bibliography

The bibliography is the last item in a report; it contains references for all material cited in the body or used in the research. Bibliographical references are similar in form to footnotes, but the keying pattern is not identical. Refer to a report-writing style manual for the correct method of keying bibliographical entries.

PROOFREADING

No document is complete until it is proofread carefully. Creating a document and using sophisticated software functions are preliminary to proofreading, and a poor proofreader cannot claim to be successful at word processing. Proofreading is not fun, and it is often dismissed or underrated by people who are too impatient to do the job carefully. Proofreading in a medical office is especially important because medical decisions are often based on information found in medical reports.

Documents that go out of the office represent the practice. If mistakes in grammar, punctuation, spelling, format, or content are present, they reflect negatively on the staff. One physician says it this way, "One good proofreader is worth two good typists in my office, and I want to hire people who can find the mistakes I overlook. After all, I'm not supposed to be the proofreader!"

Review these procedures for improving proofreading:

1. Read the document first for content mistakes. Patients' lives may depend on a correct report.
2. Read the document backwards the second time. This will force attention away from the content and allow you to concentrate on spelling, grammar, and punctuation.
3. Read silently with your lips. You may worry about how you look doing this, but that's a small price to pay for a perfect document.
4. Read the finished copy aloud to a partner against the rough draft. There is nothing wrong with admitting that you cannot always find all the mistakes in every document. Reading with a partner is especially valuable when statistical material is involved. Numbers are especially easy to transpose but difficult to find when one proofreads alone.
5. Exchange documents with another medical assistant. "You proofread my documents, and I'll proofread yours" is a workable technique when more than one person keys nonconfidential information.

Spell checking utilities are built into most word processing programs. The spell checker stops at each word that it does not recognize. Look up the questionable word in the dictionary and make corrections. Some programs allow a choice of several suggested spellings listed on the screen.

While spell checker software is helpful for people with a poor spelling background, it is not the perfect solution for documents that include unusual words, foreign words, or abbreviations. Nor can a spell checker distinguish between homonyms (words that sound the same but have different meanings), such as "to," "two," and "too," or "flour" and "flower," or "weather" and "whether." For example, while a common spell checker would include the words "eyes," "ears," "nose," and "throat," it would not recognize the abbreviation "EENT." Special dictionaries or glossary space is available in most programs for adding words that occur frequently in individual offices. Each office adds the words it chooses, and they become a permanent part of the program. Medical spell checker software is available to accompany most programs and is recommended for people who use medical terminology. Punctuation checkers and grammar checkers have been introduced but are not yet as common as spell checkers. Word usage checkers are not yet available, but this software is expected.

IN YOUR OPINION

1. Can you think of some factors not mentioned in the text that make it difficult to read a finished document?
2. What types of letters do you think could most easily be assembled using merged paragraphs?
3. What methods have you found useful in proofreading?

REFERENCES

Humphrey, Doris D., and Kathie Sigler. *The Modern Medical Office: A Reference Manual.* Cincinnati, Ohio: South-Western Publishing Co., 1990.*

Hyden, Janet, Ann Jordan, Mary Helen Steinauer, and Marjorie Jones. *Communicating for Success: An Applied Approach.* Cincinnati, Ohio: South-Western Publishing Co., 1994.

Johnson, Joan, Marie Whitaker, and Marcus Wayne Johnson. *Computerized Medical Office Management.* Albany, New York: Delmar Publishers, 1994.

Oliverio, John, William Pasewark, and Bonnie White. *The Office: Procedures and Technology.* Cincinnati, Ohio: South-Western Publishing Co., 1993.

Tessier, Claudia, and Sally C. Pitman. *Style Guide for Medical Transcription.* Modesto, California: American Association for Medical Transcription, 1985.

*Currently published by Delmar Publishers.

Chapter Activities

PERFORMANCE BASED ACTIVITIES

1. Your pediatric practice is celebrating its fifth birthday. Write a letter inviting Randy Markham, aged 6, to the office birthday party. Write a second invitation letter to Randy's father. Key and print your letters in an appropriate format and include the letterhead information as shown below. (DACUM 2.3, 3.1, 3.4)

Boys 'N Girls Health World
Pediatric Practice
17 Ranchero Drive, Boulder, CO 80302

---

2. One member of the office staff has been absent without an excuse three times in the last month. Write a note warning of possible consequences of this behavior. Keep your note positive in tone. Key and print in an appropriate format, using the form below.

Cedarcrest Oncology Clinic

TO:

FROM:

DATE:

SUBJECT:

(DACUM 1.1, 3.1, 3.3, 3.4)

3. Exchange drafts of the letters in Nos. 1 and 2 with a classmate. Proofread each other's letters and mark with the correct proofreader's marks. Turn in the corrected draft with your finished letters. (DACUM 3.1)

4. Key the following information in acceptable case history form, using the format below. (DACUM 3.1, 3.3, 3.5)

Patient's Name, Lance Bradley
123-B Nathan Court
Wayne, Pa 19087-0000
Date of Visit: 6/18/—

Chief Complaint: This seven-year-old black male was brought to my office by his grandfather. About 9:45 a.m. today the patient was sliding down a slide and cut his right foot on a brick at the base of the slide. Examination: Patient is alert but in pain. There is an approximate 2.5 cm. laceration of the right foot, post/lateral aspect, with full ROM of toes and ankle. Skin is pink, warm, and dry. His temperature is 100°F, pulse 104, respiration 16. Lab Tests: None. Diagnosis: 1 in. × 1/4 in. laceration of right foot.

Treatment: Betadine Surgical Scrub. Normal Saline irrigation. 1% Lidocaine. Five No. 5.0 nylon sutures. Dry sterile dressing, 3 in. Kling bandage. Remarks: None. Family History: Patient is an only child. The father suffers from emphysema. The mother is in apparent good health. There is a family history of early heart disease and hypertension. Personal History: Patient is an active second grade student with a wide variety of outdoor interests. He plays soccer, football, T-ball, and softball. His development is normal.

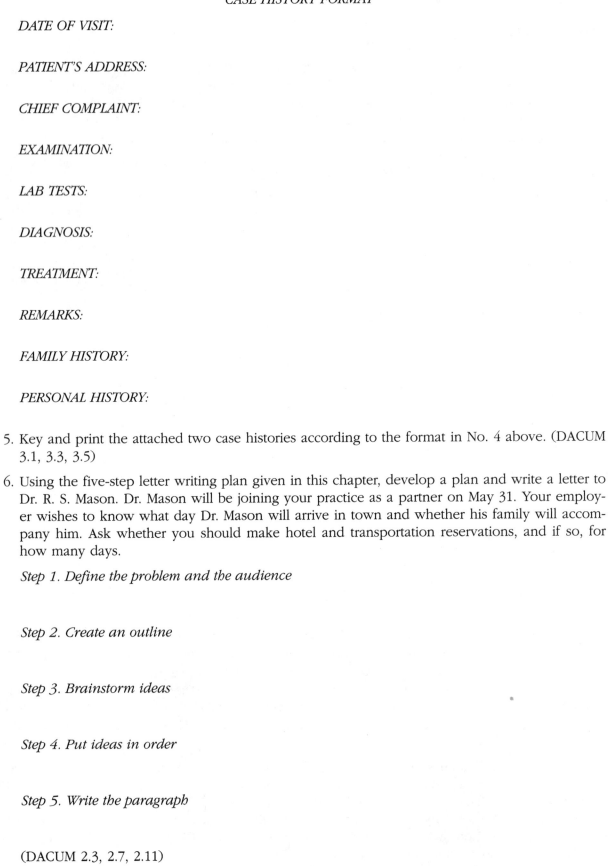

CASE HISTORY FORMAT

DATE OF VISIT:

PATIENT'S ADDRESS:

CHIEF COMPLAINT:

EXAMINATION:

LAB TESTS:

DIAGNOSIS:

TREATMENT:

REMARKS:

FAMILY HISTORY:

PERSONAL HISTORY:

5. Key and print the attached two case histories according to the format in No. 4 above. (DACUM 3.1, 3.3, 3.5)

6. Using the five-step letter writing plan given in this chapter, develop a plan and write a letter to Dr. R. S. Mason. Dr. Mason will be joining your practice as a partner on May 31. Your employer wishes to know what day Dr. Mason will arrive in town and whether his family will accompany him. Ask whether you should make hotel and transportation reservations, and if so, for how many days.

Step 1. Define the problem and the audience

Step 2. Create an outline

Step 3. Brainstorm ideas

Step 4. Put ideas in order

Step 5. Write the paragraph

(DACUM 2.3, 2.7, 2.11)

EXPANDING YOUR THINKING

1. Using a dictionary or thesaurus if necessary, list at least five other choices for each of the following over-used words. You may also use the software thesaurus found in WordPerfect and other packages.

   interesting _____

   important _____

   nice _____

2. Which word processing functions reviewed in this chapter would be used in each of the following situations:

   a. To number the pages of a document?

   _____

   _____

   b. To change the phrase, "Dr. Maurice Gallagher," to "Maurice Gallagher, M.D.," everywhere it appears in a document?

   _____

   _____

   c. To save a document?

   _____

   _____

   d. To send a holiday greeting to all patients?

   _____

   _____

   e. To find a word you want to change within a document?

   _____

   _____

   f. To combine part of a case history with a letter to a consulting physician?

   _____

   _____

   g. To align the right margin of a case history?

   _____

   _____

   h. To transfer a paragraph from the end of a letter to the beginning?

   _____

   _____

Chapter 11

Professional Activities and Travel Arrangements

LARAMIE, WYOMING

Arranging travel for the physicians in our group practice is one of the tasks I most enjoy. My objective in arranging travel is to make sure that the travelers don't have any nasty surprises, such as finding out that they have a four-hour layover before a connecting flight or arriving to discover that their rooms are not available.

When Dr. Carberry was invited to present a paper at a conference in India, I found her an around-the-world fare that was cheaper than flying to New Delhi and back, and it included a side trip in Europe! She said that the weekend in Rome was a wonderful way to relax from the stress of the conference. I also called the Department of State to check on travel and health advisories for the countries she would be passing through.

In addition to arranging her travel, I did much of the background research for Dr. Carberry's paper. I made several calls to professional associations, which sent me a lot of material, and I supplemented it with articles I pulled up from our on-line network. I highlighted and arranged the material by topic to save her time. Dr. Carberry appreciated all the information I was able to develop.

Julie Henry
Medical Assistant

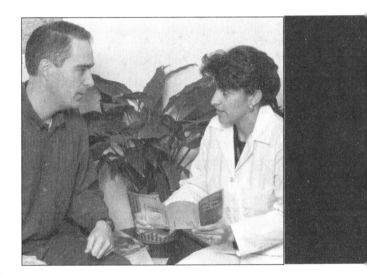

PERFORMANCE BASED COMPETENCIES

After completing this chapter, you should be able to:

1. Manage the physician's travel schedule. (DACUM 3.7)
2. Locate resources and information for patients and employers. (DACUM 3.6)
3. Provide annotated background materials for the physician's research papers and speeches. (DACUM 2.7, 2.11)
4. Orient patients to office policies and procedures. (DACUM 7.1)

5. Instruct patients with special needs. (DACUM 7.2)
6. Teach patients methods of health promotion and disease prevention. (DACUM 7.3)
7. Orient and train coworkers. (DACUM 7.4)

HEALTHSPEAK

Association Organization that advocates special interests through information or lobbying.

Bibliography List of books or articles about a subject, including the author, title, publisher, date, and page of the information.

Business class Flight class that offers more amenities than coach, but fewer than first.

Direct flight Flight that connects two cities without a plane change.

Itinerary Schedule of travel, including departure and arrival times, flight numbers, lodging, and telephone numbers.

Literature search Review of published sources at the library or by computer to find articles on a specified topic.

Non-stop Flight that connects two cities without making intermediate stops.

Objective The intent of the process.

Orient To provide an informational overview.

Process Activity that includes input, modification or change to the input, and output; input can include people, materials, or information.

Secondary research Study of sources already published.

The Physician's Professional Activities

As in many fields today, physicians have access to a great deal of information. Obtaining information is not a problem; however, getting exactly the information needed and nothing more can be a challenge. Because the physician engages in many professional activities, your role as a medical assistant often will be to track down vital pieces of information without burying your office in paper.

Physicians have many opportunities to take active leadership roles in their communities. Following is a partial list of such activities, adapted from materials of the National Association of Community Health Centers (NACHC), Department of Health Professional and Clinical Affairs.

- Marketing and public relations
- Civic affairs and public speaking
- Publication of research and other articles
- Training at professional forums
- Professional linkages with foundations, federal agencies, and research centers
- Recruitment and retention activities for health professionals
- Health policy monitoring and development
- Clinical trials with developers of health care products, such as pharmaceutical companies
- Advisory functions and technical assistance
- Disseminating resource information

Most of these activities involve information gathering and analysis. As a medical assistant, you may be asked to help the physician get started on one of these projects by conducting a preliminary literature search and screening.

Medical and general periodicals are indexed. Although indices are printed and kept in the public and college libraries, it is much quicker to search literature by means of a database. If the practice's computers do not have networking capabilities to link with Prodigy, the Source, or other available networks, any large library allows database search. The library may do the search, or the medical assistant may be able to do it. The library may or may not charge a fee.

Most searches are conducted by entering key words, such as "anorexia" and "eating disorders." The computer lists names of articles that contain these words and the source of each article. The user may choose which selections to print and, in some cases, can print a summary of the article or the whole article. If key words that are too general, such as "psychology," or "respiratory" are entered, too many references to be scanned effectively will be produced. If the references are too vast, a more specific word must be substituted.

Professional organizations are among the best sources for specialized data. Figure 11-1 is a partial list of professional organizations from

American Academy of Pediatrics

American Managed Care and Review Association

American Medical Association

American Medical Student Association

American Public Health Association

Association of American Dental Schools

Association for Health Services Research

Healthy Mothers, Healthy Babies Coalition

National Organization for Fetal Alcohol Syndrome

Nurse Practitioners in Reproductive Health

Society for Adolescent Medicine

FIGURE 11-1 Sample professional organizations

the NACHC Professional Linkages list. These are only a few of the thousands of associations worldwide representing medical specialties, practices, demographic groups, and types of illness and injury. Some of these associations may even provide speaker support kits with slides, graphs, and tapes to accompany a presentation. Federal agencies such as the following produce research and publications. Contact them for additional information:

Health Care Finance Administration
Public Health Office
    Office of Health Promotion and Disease
      Prevention
    Office of Minority Health
    National Vaccine Program
    Health Resources and Services
      Administration
      Bureau of Primary Health Care
      Bureau of Health Professions
      Bureau of Maternal and Child Health
    Centers for Disease Control and
      Prevention

The list goes on and on! You can see why it is a challenge to find the one piece of information that you want.

After you conduct a preliminary search and receive materials from periodicals, agencies, and associations, you should organize your information using the following steps.

1. Remove duplicate information
2. Organize information by topic
3. Put information in logical order
4. Highlight and mark materials so that the physician can quickly and easily review it when developing the speech or article

Doing research is an art and a science. Your proficiency in developing good sources of data and transforming that data into usable information will enhance your value in any medical practice.

IN YOUR OPINION

1. How could you organize materials on the subject of smoking-related diseases for a presentation to a high school group? What audiovisual aids would improve the presentation?
2. What are some of the search words and combinations of search words you could use to conduct a database search for a paper on good eating habits for the elderly?
3. Name six possible sources for research on bulimia.

The Medical Assistant's Professional Activities

One of the medical assistant's most important public relations activities will be teaching, training, orientation, and instruction of patients or coworkers. Special skills are needed to do an effective job.

TRAINING COWORKERS

A big difference exists between knowing how to do something and being able to train someone else to do it. The medical staff should know how their activities fit into the whole process so that they can understand the consequences of their actions on others (Figure 11-2). Following are some tips on becoming an effective trainer.

1. Explain the purpose or objective of the process.

"Our goal in answering the phones is to give callers prompt, courteous, consistent, service so that they receive a good impression of our professionalism."

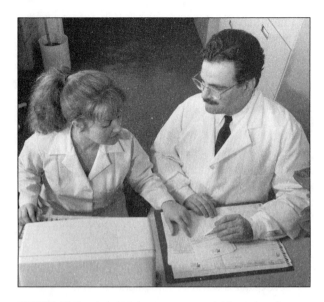

FIGURE 11-2 When training someone, explaining why a function or process is done can be as important as showing them how it is done.

Compare this instruction that does not include an explanation.

> "Answer the phone by saying, 'Dr. Rugger's office.'"

2. Explain how this process fits into the whole system.

> "After we log the checks, we forward them to Carole. She photocopies the checks, deposits the checks in the bank, and returns the photocopies to us so that we can attach them to the patient file. That way, if there is a question about payment, we can refer to the patient file."

Compare that explanation with this one.

> "When we get checks, we write the number in this book and then put them in this basket."

3. Break the training process down into steps, and document each step. Processes with many steps, a great deal of backtracking, and several exceptions are bad processes and will be difficult to learn. Often, trainees are blamed for mistakes when it is the process that is at fault. For example, a medical assistant might say to a trainee:

> "We keep all patient files except for Dr. Mammet's in a central storage area. Dr. Mammet likes to keep his patient files in his office. Also, all our Medicaid patients' records are separated and filed in this blue filing cabinet, except for the patients who are not U.S. citizens. Those records go in here. Dr. Revere is doing a study of sexually transmitted diseases, so all the files of patients with those diagnoses go to her first before filing."

It would be difficult for anyone, especially a trainee, to remember all this detail.

If a procedure is not written down, the medical assistant and trainee should document the steps. This will make subsequent training easier and more consistent.

4. Remember that people learn in different ways. Most people learn best with a combination of show and tell and lots of practice. Successful trainers use this technique along with support and encouragement.

5. Listen carefully to the person's questions. Develop different ways of explaining the same thing; repeating the original explanation will not improve the person's understanding. Do not be afraid to say, "I don't know, but I'll find out." Explain *why* a trainee must do something, not just *how*. People are more likely to make correct decisions if they understand the intent of the process.

IN YOUR OPINION

1. Think of a time when you were taught well how to do something. What made the instruction good?
2. Think of a time when you were poorly instructed. Describe it, and analyze what made it bad.
3. What are the ways in which you learn best?

PATIENT INSTRUCTION

Patient instruction is an extremely valuable and rewarding activity. Often a doctor's office is the place where people discover major changes are about to occur in their lives and learn how to manage them. A mother with a newborn, a patient with heart disease trying to diet and exercise properly, a diabetic child learning to inject insulin, a teenager adjusting to adolescence, a widowed spouse; all these people can benefit from information about their circumstances.

Attention to clear, concise patient instructions and information in the language and at the level of patient understanding can make the difference between a good and excellent level of service.

Research provides the following information about patient learning.

- Most people learn best when they need to know, as when they are hospitalized.
- Patients who understand a medical procedure will be more cooperative.
- Explanation of prescribed treatment encourages compliance with directions.
- Patients cannot be expected to understand and remember the reasons for health problems and details of treatment procedures after one explanation, especially in situations of high emotional impact.
- Patients may be reluctant to ask questions of the physician, especially if the doctor appears to be rushed.
- Health education material is more likely to be used if it is easily available.

Providing Patient Literature

Pamphlets and brochures that explain illnesses and treatments are invaluable, and each practice should keep a supply. The literature distributed or made available in the waiting room may include general topics such as nutrition, but should also include the major issues for the patients of the practice. A psychiatrist's office might offer brochures on depression, obsessive-compulsive disorders, anxiety, and stress. An obstetrician might display pamphlets on breast feeding, sex during and after pregnancy, back pain, and changing nutritional needs.

In most cases, it will not be necessary for you as a medical assistant to develop these materials yourself. In the case of procedures unique to your office, of course, you will need orientation materials. But for materials related to medical conditions, refer to the list of professional associations in the section on physicians' professional activities or research the associations appro-

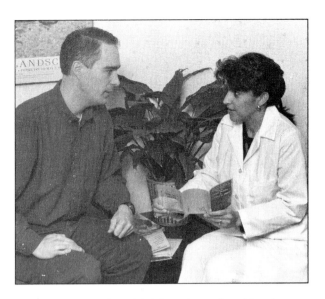

FIGURE 11-3 Clearly explain information and provide written instructions in the language and at the level of patient understanding.

priate to your practice. You will find a great deal of information available at nominal cost.

The best method for explaining information to patients follows the simple format described below.

1. Sit with the patient in a private area free of distractions
2. Explain the contents of the pamphlet in a clear tone of voice (Figure 11-3)
3. Be patient
4. Pause frequently to see if the patient has a question or seems distracted or confused
5. Be attentive to questions and concerns
6. Give the patient a copy of the brochure
7. Encourage patients to call you if they have questions

Keep a follow-up list of such patients and call them a few days after their visits. This will not only impress them with the quality of your service, but may forestall problems and the need for another visit. A "tickler" file may be used for this purpose.

Managing Travel

Physicians do not travel as often as business executives; however, they may attend medical conventions and take other selected trips. As a medical assistant, you may be asked to make reservations for these trips by telephone through a private travel agency or directly with the airline, hotel, rental car agency, or other travel organization. The following discussion provides reference information about options you should consider when creating a travel plan for the physician.

TRAVEL AGENCIES

A travel agent (1) researches the physician's destination and provides brochures about the area to be visited, (2) arranges for air and ground transportation, (3) develops highway routes for automobile travel, (4) creates an itinerary, (5) arranges for lodging in one or several locations, and (6) makes local entertainment and sightseeing suggestions. After a travel agent delivers tickets, check the tickets against the itinerary carefully. A good travel agent will keep the physician's seating preferences for air travel, credit card number, and frequent flyer numbers on file. If a travel agent makes errors or fails to provide you with consistent, complete information about travel choices, investigate other travel suppliers.

AIRLINE TRAVEL

All major airlines have toll-free 800 numbers. If you know that only one or two carriers provide service on the route needed, you may wish to contact the airline yourself instead of working with a travel agent. Several of the general computer databases such as Internet also include airline information, and airline reservations can be developed and scheduled through the database.

The two simplest ways to reduce the cost of air travel are to book ahead a week or more and to plan a Saturday overnight stay. The travel agent may suggest intermediate stops as a way to reduce costs, but the money saved is rarely worth the time loss and aggravation.

Several classes of service are available to airline passengers: first, business, and coach are the most common choices. The features of each of these classes are explained below.

- First class: Offers wider seats, more leg room, better food, and complimentary alcoholic beverages. There is no charge for movies if they are offered.
- Business class: Not offered by every airline or on every flight; most common for international or lengthy flights. Offers wider seats and more leg room than coach.
- Coach class: Up to 50 percent the cost of first class. Can be uncomfortably crowded when the flight is full. Experienced travelers usually specify an aisle seat so that they can stand or move more easily.

A page from the *Official Airline Guide* is shown in Figure 11-4. Departure times are listed according to the time in the departure city, and arrival times are listed according to the time in the destination city. For example, a physician leaving New York at 10:05 A.M. arrives in California at about 9:30 A.M., even though the trip requires almost five hours' flying time. Since the flier travels across three time zones, the clock moves backward during the flight. This time difference accounts for the "jet lag" that travelers suffer when they fly long distances.

SHIP

Physicians take cruises for both personal and business reasons. Continuing education requirements for license renewal can often be met through a work/pleasure cruise that offers a medical seminar or conference as part of the travel package. Often, these special trips are advertised to physicians through a sponsoring university, and the medical assistant's responsibility for scheduling is minimal. A medical assistant responsible for arranging such a trip may use a travel agent.

TRAIN

Train travel is more attractive in some parts of the country than others. For example, physicians living in the Northeast often make short train commutes among Washington, New York, and their home cities to relieve the frustration of traffic congestion. Travel agents can plan train travel.

AUTOMOBILE

A physician may wish to rent a car for in-town travel after flying to a destination. Automobiles for use anywhere in the world can be rented

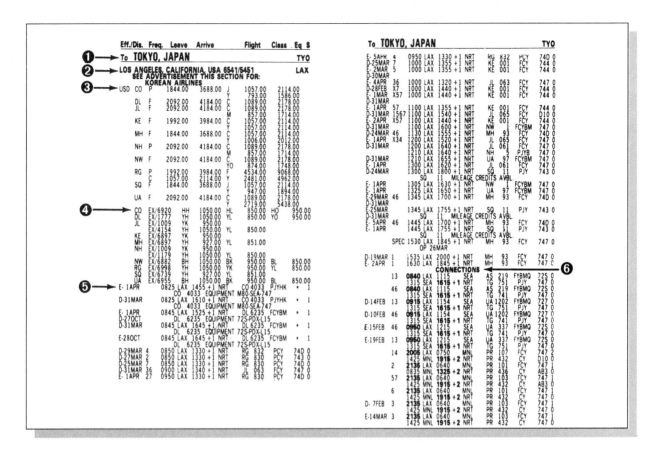

FIGURE 11-4 Sample international flight schedule (Courtesy of the Official Airline Guides, Inc., copyright 1990)

through a local rental-car franchise, such as Hertz or Avis, or through a travel agent. Auto rental companies all have 800 numbers. Be sure to ask about special weekend rates, upgrades, and other "deals." Membership in the rental company's preferred customer club will assure the traveler quick service on arrival and departure. When the physician prefers to use an automobile for taking a long trip, you can ask a travel agent to provide a route guide and highway map. The physician may also subscribe to the American Automobile Association (AAA), a nationwide network that provides assistance to travelers. AAA will provide route guides, as well.

LODGING

Medical conferences are usually held in hotels with appropriate accommodations, and the sponsoring organization contracts for a large number of rooms in the hotel to be used by conference participants. The advertisement for the convention frequently includes a room reservation, which the medical assistant mails. A required deposit for one night's lodging can be made by check or credit card.

Lodging for trips unrelated to conferences can be arranged through a travel agent, the hotel or motel to be used, or the local franchise of a hotel or motel chain. A written confirmation of all room reservations should be requested and included with the physician's itinerary. Major hotel chains have 800 numbers for reservations at locations worldwide.

Several types of information are required before a reservation for lodging can be made. These requirements are listed below:

Type of Room—One room or a suite

Type of Accommodations—Twin beds, standard bed, or king-sized bed

Date and Time of Arrival—Arrivals after 6 p.m. require a deposit in advance for one night's lodging.

This guarantee can be charged by telephone to the physician's credit card. Guarantees are not refundable.

Length of Time Room Is Needed—One night, two nights, or longer

TRAVEL FUNDS

Costs associated with a physician's trip are closely monitored for income tax purposes. A travel advance request that allows funds to be drawn from the practice's business account can be completed before the trip, or the physician may use personal funds during the trip. The physician would then complete a travel expense form for reimbursement from the practice account upon return.

When funds are advanced, the medical assistant completes a travel advance form, and the bookkeeper or accountant prepares a check. The medical assistant may cash the check and give the money to the physician with the itinerary. After the physician returns and provides the receipts, the medical assistant records all expenses including those for meals, lodging, transportation, tips, cash, and miscellaneous items on a travel expense form and turns it over to the accountant with all receipts. The extra paperwork is necessary in order to account properly for all funds at income tax time. A travel advance form is shown in Figure 11-5, and a travel expense form is shown in Figure 11-6.

INTERNATIONAL TRAVEL

Several items must be considered when a physician takes a foreign trip. A travel agency should always arrange for international travel, since agents are experienced in planning such trips and often know shortcuts or can offer specific advice about entering individual countries.

Passport

The physician must acquire or renew a passport before entering any foreign country, except for Canada, Bermuda, the West Indies, Mexico, and a few others. In these countries, proof of U.S. citizenship is required.

To obtain a passport, an individual needs a completed application (which may be obtained from the post office), proof of U.S. citizenship, proof of identification with a personal signature, two photographs taken within the last six months by a passport photographer, and the passport fee. The Department of State requires as proof of citizenship a birth certificate with a raised seal; photocopies are not acceptable. It is a good idea to call ahead of time to verify acceptable documentation. A previously expired passport and naturalization papers are other acceptable forms of proof of citizenship. Applications for a passport can be obtained from a travel agency; processing takes about two weeks, but renewals can be prepared in twenty-four to forty-eight hours.

Some foreign countries grant visa permission for individuals to enter. Usually, the visa appears as a stamped notation on the passport and designates the country to be entered and the amount of time approved. A travel agent can advise which countries require a visa.

Vaccinations

A travel agent or the Department of Health can provide information regarding vaccinations needed for visiting specific countries or recommended health precautions. Vaccinations are rarely required anymore, but typhoid vaccination, gamma globulin, current tetanus, or malaria suppressant may be recommended.

PREPARING AN ITINERARY

The medical assistant should prepare a complete, concise itinerary before each trip. The travel agent will do this if an agency is used. The physician's spouse and business associates should receive extra copies, and the medical

TRAVELER'S NAME _____ DATE _____
NAME OF PRACTICE _____
PURPOSE OF TRAVEL _____
DEPARTURE TRAVEL TO _____ DATE ____
RETURN TRAVEL FROM _____ DATE ____
AMOUNT OF ADVANCE _____
SIGNATURE _____

FIGURE 11-5 Travel advance form

Travel Expense Statement

NAME Anderson Marcus Adam   SOC. SEC. NO. 238-54-1345

TITLE Physician   TRAVEL DATES FROM April 1 TO 3, 19--

PURPOSE OF TRIP Medical Equipment Show

DATES	SPEEDOMETER READING Out / In	LOCATION/POINTS VISITED	DETAILS OF SUBSISTENCE (Attach receipts of items $25 or more)				TOTAL	Do Not Use This Space FOR ACCT. DEPT.
			Breakfast	Lunch	Dinner	Lodging		
6/1		Nashville/Chicago		12.50	32.80	148.00	193.30	
6/2		Chicago	8.00			148.00	156.00	
6/3		Chicago/Nashville	6.75	10.50	136.90		154.15	

NOTE: This statement must be submitted within 10 days of last date of travel for reimbursement

DISTANCE TRAVELLED _____ KILOMETERS @ _____ CENTS A KILOMETER
(Must be supported by automobile travel record above.)

COMMON CARRIER: __X__ Taxi: _____ Limousine: __X__ Airline X _____ Train   42.00 / 328.00

MISCELLANEOUS EXPENSES: (telephone, postage, etc.):
Total here, itemize below   15.75

GRAND TOTAL OF TRAVEL EXPENSES   889.20

List all miscellaneous expenses:

Explanation ——— Telephone calls ——————— Amount ___ 15.75

Explanation ————————————————————— Amount _____

I certify that the above statements are true and I have incurred the described expenses in the discharge of my official duties for **NORTHSIDE MEDICAL CENTER, P.C.**

SIGNATURE ——————————— APPROVED ——————————— DATE ———————————

FIGURE 11-6 Travel expense form

assistant should keep one in case the physician must be contacted during the trip. The itinerary shows travel times and destinations, meeting times, and lodging where the doctor will stay. Telephone, FAX, and telex numbers as well as any appointments should also be included as a part of the trip. A travel agent will prepare an itinerary as a routine service.

The medical assistant should type the itinerary in neat, readable form, fold and insert it in a packet with the physician's airline ticket. All confirmations and notes about the trip should be stapled to the itinerary. An itinerary is shown in Figure 11-7.

```
                    Itinerary for Adam Anderson
                         Chicago, Illinois
                          April 1-3, 19—

Sunday, June 1     Nashville to Chicago

                   8:40 a.m.      Leave Nashville on American Airlines flight #234. Snack on
                                  flight.

                   10:16 a.m.     Arrive at Chicago O'Hare Airport Room reservation at
                                  Marriott Downtown (Confirmation attached)

                   12:00 noon     Meet Dr. Allen Rorbach in Marriott dining room

                   3:00 p.m.      Registration for Midwest Medical Equipment Show Grand
                                  Lobby

Monday, June 2     9 a.m.–5 p.m.  Midwest Medical Equipment Show
                                  Grand Ballroom

                   3:00 p.m.      Computer Software Associates presentation in Meeting Room G

Tuesday, June 3    Chicago to Nashville

                   9 a.m.–5 p.m.  Midwest Medical Equipment Show continued

                   10:00 a.m.     Creative Recordkeeping Corporation presentation in Meeting
                                  Room C

                   5:00 p.m.      Dinner with Drs. Cecil, Anthony, Matz. Reservations in
                                  Golden Inn at airport

                   7:50 p.m.      Leave Chicago O'Hare Airport United Airlines flight #692

                   9:08 p.m.      Arrive Nashville. 9:30 p.m. Reservation with Davis Limousine
                                  Service to your home.
```

FIGURE 11-7 Itinerary

IN YOUR OPINION

1. What are the most important reasons for physicians to travel?
2. What are some travel pitfalls that can be avoided by careful planning?
3. Which of the physician's travel preferences should you know to make planning easier and more effective?

REFERENCES

Greenberger, Martin, and Puffer, James. *From Telemedicine to Healthcom, Facilitating Health Communication for the Older Person,* December 1987.

Hoch, Robert A. National Association of Community Health Centers Department of Health Professional and Clinical Affairs, *Opportunities for Physician Leadership in NACHC,* Meeting Notes, May 5, 1993.

Humphrey, Doris, and Kathie Sigler. *The Modern Medical Office: A Reference Manual.* Cincinnati, Ohio: South-Western Publishing Co., 1990.*

National Association of Community Health Centers Department of Health Professional and Clinical Affairs, *Program Fact Sheets,* June 8, 1993.

Oliverio, John, William Pasewark, and Bonnie White. *The Office: Procedures and Technology.* Cincinnati, Ohio: South-Western Publishing Co., 1993.

*Currently published by Delmar Publishers.

Chapter Activities

PERFORMANCE BASED ACTIVITIES

1. Using 800 numbers, develop information for a trip that includes the following information. Do not actually make a reservation. You do not want to pay for it.

   a. a flight to New York City, Chicago or Los Angeles

   b. a stay for three nights at a Marriott, Hilton, or Sheraton

   c. travel to Burlington, VT (from New York City), Milwaukee (from Chicago), or Las Vegas (from Los Angeles) for the weekend by plane or car

   Make an itinerary and list costs of air, hotels, and rental cars.

   AIR:

   Carrier: _____

   Flight Number: _____

   Departure Time: _____

   Arrival Time: _____

   Cost: _____

   HOTEL:

   Name of hotel: _____

   Cost: _____

   Description of accommodations: _____

   Directions from airport: _____

   TRAVEL TO SECONDARY CITY:

   Method: _____

   Cost: _____

   (DACUM 3.7)

2. At your local library, conduct a search on one of these topics: teen pregnancy, breast cancer, AIDS prevention, or another topic approved by your instructor. Compose a bibliography and obtain copies of at least five articles, pamphlets, books or other published information. Find the names, addresses, and phone numbers of at least two organizations or associations that can provide information on the topic. Save your work for a Portfolio item.

   Research checklist:
   * reference librarian
   * periodical index (book)
   * card index for books
   * book index database
   * periodical database
   * pamphlet file
   * *Encyclopedia of Associations*—ask the librarian

   (DACUM 3.6)

3. Using your bibliography from No. 2, prepare an outline for a presentation on your selected topic. Highlight the material and name charts and graphs that could most effectively support the presentation. Save your work for a Portfolio item. (DACUM 2.7, 2.11)

4. At your mentoring practice, develop a written procedure for a common office process that currently exists only in the "medical assistant's head." List the steps in the process or present as a diagram. (DACUM 7.1, 7.4)

EXPANDING YOUR THINKING

1. Interview someone at your mentoring practice about giving instructions. Write a short paper describing how patients are instructed and informed concerning one of the following:

   a. A chronic illness such as asthma, kidney disease, diabetes, or arthritis

   b. An acute illness or injury such as a heart attack, stroke, amputation, or bone fracture

   c. A major life change such as pregnancy, adolescence, menopause, or aging

   d. A psychological condition such as depression or anxiety

   e. Addiction, alcoholism, or obesity

2. Choose one of the following situations and compile a list of questions you would ask if you were a patient in one of these circumstances:

   a. Your sister-in-law is pregnant and a cocaine addict

   b. Your father has bleeding ulcers

   c. Your mother is scheduled for heart bypass surgery

   d. You have just been diagnosed with breast cancer

   e. Your brother has been diagnosed with a genetic disorder and you are planning to have children.

3. Interview five people who travel frequently. Ask each to describe their worst travel experience. Make a list of the responses and note how many times each factor was mentioned if several people list the same cause, such as "flight cancelled due to snowstorm." As a class, compile all of your lists and present the results in a chart or graph.

Chapter 12

Managing Medical Records

TAOS, NEW MEXICO

For several years, I worked with patients in a clinic. Two years ago, my employer sent me to a course to learn the most up-to-date ways of managing medical records, and I quickly became fascinated by the complexity and challenge of this field. As I am thorough and detail-oriented, this job fits my natural strengths. I'm now the supervisor of two medical records specialists.

If our clinic does not maintain accurate, complete, and timely records, we may not be reimbursed by an insurance company. That reduces our practice's income and, ultimately, my salary!

When we receive doctors' notes, we immediately scan them to make sure the proper level of detail is included. If not, we check with the physicians while the cases are still fresh in their minds. Our records management team has saved the practice money and delay by staying on top of this task. Personally, I expect to take increasingly responsible positions in the medical records field.

Wilma Leaphorn
Medical Records Supervisor

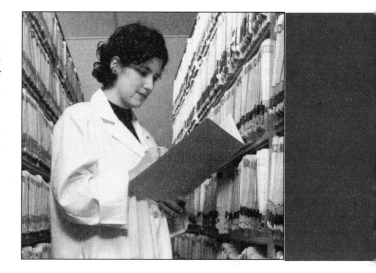

PERFORMANCE BASED COMPETENCIES

After completing this chapter, you should be able to:

1. Create preliminary medical records. (DACUM 4.6)
2. Maintain medical records. (DACUM 3.3)
3. Determine needs for documentation and reporting. (DACUM 5.2)
4. Identify each type of document stored in a typical medical record. (DACUM 4.6)

Blood tests Analysis of blood to determine whether infection is present, excessive urea is evident, or glucose or other substances are present in too high or too low a concentration.

Case history Analysis of the patient's complaint, examination results, lab results, diagnosis, prescribed treatment, and family and personal history.

Closed files Medical records of patients who are no longer under the physician's care because they have moved, changed doctors, or died.

Doctor's notes, or progress notes Doctor's comments that are added to the medical record each time the patient is treated.

Electrocardiogram Graphic illustration of the heart's activity.

Inactive files Medical records of patients who have not visited the physician for an extended period.

Laboratory request Test to be administered and the name of the attending physician.

Pathology and cytopathology Field of laboratory testing that shows the results of studies of body tissue and body cells.

Patient health questionnaire Questions about the patient's previous health and surgical history and family history.

Patient information form Completed by a patient immediately upon arriving at the medical office for the initial visit.

Problem-oriented medical record Patient's complaints identified in list form.

Shingling Method of filing small reports.

SOAP Method of reporting patient's diagnosis and treatment plan: subjective examination (S), objective test results (O), doctor's assessment (A), and treatment plan (P).

Source-oriented medical record Information grouped according to its source.

Urinalysis Routine laboratory test of urine often requested by physicians.

X-rays, CAT scans, and ultrasound Diagnostic tests to determine whether any unusual medical condition, such as a tissue mass, is present in the body.

A medical record is a permanent document giving a complete account of a person's illness or injury and the services rendered by medical professionals. Usually, the medical record contains the patient's medical history, results of physical examinations, doctor's notes, laboratory reports, prescriptions, medical instructions, and other relevant medical information.

Recently, the level of detail required on medical records has increased. If records are not clear and legible, or if they do not accurately reflect actual proceedings, the practice may not be fully reimbursed by insurance companies or other third-party providers. Complete accurate records also protect the practice against malpractice claims. Medical assistants who understand record-keeping requirements and actively seek missing information enhance the financial security of the practice.

Medical records benefit the patient, the physician, and the public. They are used for research, insurance claims, and legal actions. The government and insurance companies use medical records to evaluate the quality and cost of medical and surgical procedures in different parts of the country. For the patient, the medical record serves as a quick reference to aid the physician with diagnosis and treatment. An accurate, up-to-date record allows a physician to tell at a glance what previous conditions, illnesses, or allergies to medication may contribute to the patient's present problem and what future treatment is appropriate. For example, a medical record showing that a patient is allergic to penicillin alerts the physician to prescribe a sulfa drug or other antibiotic, instead of a penicillin-based drug, for a bacterial infection.

Complete medical records can protect the physician from liability during medical malpractice claims by outlining the course of treatment the physician prescribed for an illness or accident. A lawsuit can turn in a physician's favor if the medical record shows documentation of proper treatment or, in contrast, can turn against a physician when documentation is not present or incomplete. For example, if a physician is being sued for malpractice because a patient believes that her baby was delivered too early by cesarean section, the physician can show sonogram results proving that the actual delivery date was warranted by the sonogram.

Medical records serve the public because researchers can perform statistical analyses of data contained in them. Researchers may discover from a confidential analysis of many patients' medical records a common factor or factors present in many or all patients who suffer from the same medical problem. For example, information from medical records helped scientists conclude that Reye's syndrome, a rare childhood disease of the liver and central nervous system, develops while a child is recovering from a mild viral illness, such as chicken pox or influenza, or from taking aspirin after a viral illness. Several recent treatments for acquired immunodeficiency syndrome (AIDS) are based on analyses of the medical records of previous AIDS patients.

Trends and Issues in Medical Record Keeping

Case histories and documentation of medical examinations are becoming more complex and detailed because of the requirements of insurance companies. The fees insurance companies pay are determined by the *Current Procedural Terminology* (CPT) code assigned to the treatment or procedure and the *International Classification of Diseases* (ICD) code assigned to the diagnosis. The medical record must precisely match the CPT and ICD codes submitted. Medical office assistants are required to collect, sort, store, and retrieve records in an organized way. In Chapter 14 you will learn about CPT and ICD codes and the requirements for each.

Hospitals, physicians, insurance companies, and government agencies each have their own formats and data requirements for medical records. The medical assistant wastes a great deal of time when information has to be reformatted to match the requirements of each agency. The chance for error is also increased. Standardization of medical record formats would also make it much easier to automate and share data from physician's office to hospital to laboratory. Organizations such as the Joint Commission on Accreditation in Oakbrook, Illinois, are advocating standardization of formats for medical records as one way to manage the cost and complexity of medical record keeping.

Many barriers to standardization exist. The greatest barrier is the modification or replacement cost almost every medical practice, hospital, insurance company, and health agency in the country would incur.

Standardization would simplify the use of modern medical telecommunications systems that link databases in different locations. Many health organizations, such as the Hospital of the University of Illinois, already store their medical records in house on an optical disk system through the use of an optical character recognition scanner, as discussed in Chapter 8. Once standardization issues have been resolved, databases such as this can be shared.

The problems of fully automating medical records nationwide, or even worldwide, are policy issues, not technological issues. For example, if all records are in a computer, how does the physician "sign" them? Most states presently prohibit "electronic signatures" and would have to change their laws to permit this practice. Technology is available for each physician to "sign" an electronic document with a voice-activated code or password when laws permit their use.

Another legal barrier to full automation is protection of records from undocumented changes. Anyone who has worked with word processing software knows how easy it is to change text. To change a medical record, however, one cannot simply open the file and change a patient's height from 6' 1" to 5' 10", or age from 22 to 42. Changes and corrections must be made by adding notes to the record, never by changing or deleting information already recorded. Therefore, to meet legal requirements, software for medical record keeping must include security measures that prevent the edit of previously entered materials in order to meet legal requirements. These and other issues have created a demand for consultants who specialize in medical record keeping.

Creating a Medical Record

A medical record is kept for each patient under a physician's care. The first time the patient visits the doctor, you as the medical assistant will create the record based on interview information the patient supplies. Each time the patient returns you will update the record by adding medical reports, test results, and other data as necessary in an organized manner. Most medical offices continue to maintain traditional paper records. Over the next decade, however, more sophisticated medical records software will likely come into existence, and more physicians will automate their systems.

COLOR CODING THE FOLDER

The first step in creating a paper medical record is to prepare a folder to hold the medical information. Commercial color-coded labels placed on the folder tab to form color patterns are widely used on medical record folders. When folders are filed alphabetically on a shelf, large patterns of color blocks are created (Figure 12-1). An out-of-place file breaks the color pattern, making incorrectly filed records easy to detect. One formula for coding, the TAB AlphaCode system, is shown in Figure 12-2.

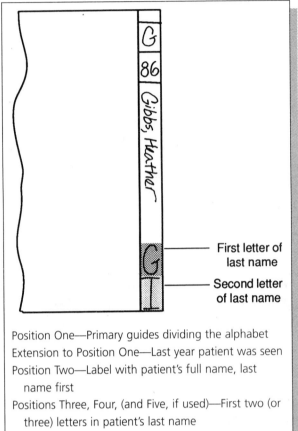

First letter of last name

Second letter of last name

Position One—Primary guides dividing the alphabet

Extension to Position One—Last year patient was seen

Position Two—Label with patient's full name, last name first

Positions Three, Four, (and Five, if used)—First two (or three) letters in patient's last name

FIGURE 12-2 TAB AlphaCode system

A partial color coding chart is shown in Figure 12-3. Notice that combinations of letters form color patterns. In the name Caton, for example, the "C" is represented by orange and the "a" by brown. Folders for other patients whose names start with "Ca" also show orange and brown in positions three and four. If a folder showing orange and blue in the third and fourth positions (representing "Ce") is filed incorrectly with the "Ca" folders, it is easily visible because the color pattern is interrupted. A colored strip can be used in position two to separate folders according to primary physician when more than one physician shares an office. For example, a green strip may represent all the patients for Physician No. 1, and a red strip may represent all the patients for Physician No. 2.

In the same way that different colors can represent letters of the alphabet, different colors

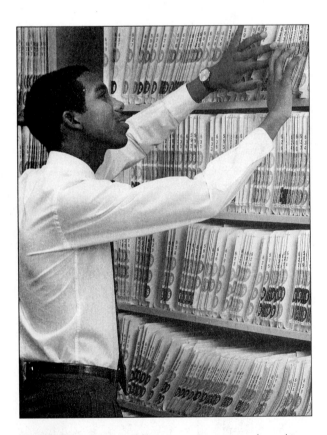

FIGURE 12-1 Open-shelf filing systems are commonly used to store color-coded medical records.

Letter Represented	Color
A	Brown
B	Yellow
C	Orange
D	Light Blue
E	Blue
F	Pink
G	Green
H	Purple
I	Grey
J	Red

FIGURE 12-3 Partial color coding chart

represent the numbers zero through nine in a numeric system. Patient numbers are color-coded in positions one through five, creating large blocks of color when folders are filed correctly. Refer to *Medical Filing* by Terese Claeys, published by Delmar Publishers, for a discussion of serial, terminal digit coding of records. Some medical offices use color codes to identify the year a patient last came to the office. For example, patients who were seen in 1995 might have red color codes on their records.

CONTENTS OF THE MEDICAL RECORD

The medical record contains various forms and reports, some completed by the patient and others completed by the physician. Initially, the medical record includes two questionnaires completed by the patient: the patient information form and the patient health questionnaire. It also includes a history and physical form that the physician completes during an interview with the patient. Laboratory reports, examination findings, consulting reports, and other medical documents are added during the course of treatment. Several typical forms are discussed and illustrated in the next section. (See Figures 12-4 through 12-11.)

Patient-Completed Forms

Patient Information Form The patient is asked to arrive early for the first visit to complete a patient information form such as that in Figure 12-4. It includes the name, address, and telephone number of the patient; the name, address, and telephone number of the person responsible for payment (if different from the patient); all insurance company names and policy numbers; and other information needed to set up an accounting record for the patient. The patient information form often is taped to the left side of the folder where it is visible each time insurance information is needed.

Patient Health Questionnaire The patient health questionnaire, as shown in Figure 12-5, asks questions about the patient's previous health and surgical history and the patient's family history, both personal and medical. This information gives the physician an overview of factors that may influence or help determine current treatment.

Physician-Completed Forms

Case History The physician may dictate the case history for the medical assistant to transcribe after the patient's initial visit (Figure 12-6). The case history describes (1) the patient's complaint or physical problem, (2) the results of the physical examination, (3) the results of lab tests, (4) the diagnosis, (5) the prescribed treatment, (6) any pertinent additional remarks, (7) a family history, and (8) a personal history.

Doctor's Notes Doctor's notes, or progress notes, are added to the medical record each time the patient is treated (Figure 12-7). Comments about the condition, diagnosis, and treatment are listed as well as prescription information, telephone consultations, and other related information. The person who writes the notes, usually the physician, initials them.

Laboratory Request

A laboratory request indicating the name of the test to be administered and the name of the attending physician is completed when a test is required. A copy is stored in the medical record (Figure 12-8).

PATIENT INFORMATION

Please Print Clearly   DATE *SEPT. 9, 19__*

NAME *NATHAN LEE*   AGE *45* SEX *M*

12/7/41   ☐ SINGLE   ☐ MARRIED   ☐ WIDOWED   ☒ DIVORCED
BIRTH DATE

ADDRESS *1071 FULTON DR.*

CITY *ATLANTA*   STATE *GEORGIA*   ZIP *30312-1768*

PHONE *555-0542*   OCCUPATION *SALES REPRESENTATIVE*

EMPLOYED BY *FEZCO, INC.*

CITY *ATLANTA*   STATE *GEORGIA*   ZIP *30316-9502*

SPOUSE'S NAME *NA*

EMPLOYED BY *NA*

CITY *NA*   STATE *NA*   ZIP *NA*

PHONE *NA*   OCCUPATION *NA*

REFERRED BY *DR. ABNER DOWARKSIK*

MEDICAL INSURANCE? ☒ YES ☐ NO   SURGICAL? ☒ YES ☐ NO

MEDICAL INSURANCE GROUP NO. *GA66951*   CERTIFICATE NO. *475*

COMPANY *STONE MOUNTAIN GENERAL*

SURGICAL INSURANCE GROUP NO. *1765*   CERTIFICATE NO. *818*

COMPANY *UNITED SURGICAL PLAN*

NAME *NATHAN LEE*
(PERSON RESPONSIBLE FOR PAYMENT)

ADDRESS *1071 FULTON DR.*

CITY *ATLANTA*   STATE *GEORGIA*   ZIP *30312-1768*

FIGURE 12-4 Patient information form

Laboratory reports are often small and irregular in size; therefore, they can be easily lost if not permanently secured to the folder. Shingling is a method of affixing small reports in chronological order to a standard size sheet of paper. The earliest report is taped to the bottom of the sheet of paper, the second earliest report is taped on top of the first about one inch above the bottom, and so on up the page. Shingled laboratory reports are shown in Figure 12-9.

Typical Laboratory Tests

Urinalysis A urinalysis is a routine laboratory test often requested by physicians. From urine tests, physicians can determine whether infec-

tion is present in the body, as well as a variety of other conditions. A urinalysis report is shown in Figure 12-10.

Electrocardiogram An electrocardiogram (EKG), a graphic illustration of the heart's activity, is used to test heart conditions (Figure 12-11). Taken at intervals such as every six months or every year, EKGs are compared to determine whether a change in heart activity has occurred since the last test.

Blood Test Blood tests reveal whether infection is present in the body, urea is elevated in the blood, or glucose or other substances are pre-

PATIENT'S NAME	Marvin Connelly

ADDRESS *610 Shady Lane*   INSURANCE *Metropolitan*   DATE *3/4/--*

TEL. NO. *242-4261*   REFERRED BY *John Lazarus*   OCCUPATION *Carpenter*   AGE *29*   SEX *M*   S (M) W. D.

FAMILY HISTORY: FATHER *Deceased*   MOTHER *Healthy*   BROTHERS *1*   SISTERS *2*

CANCER _____ TUBERCULOSIS _____ INSANITY _____ DIABETES *Father* HEART DISEASE _____ RHEUMATISM _____

GOUT _____ GOITER _____ OBESITY *Father* NEPHRITIS _____ EPILEPSY _____ OTHER _____

PAST HISTORY: DIPHTHERIA _____ MEASLES ✓ MUMPS ✓ SCARLET FEVER _____ SMALL POX _____ INFANTILE PARALYSIS _____

TYPHOID _____ PNEUMONIA _____ INFECTIONS _____ GONORRHEA _____ SYPHILIS _____ TONSILLITIS ✓ OPERATIONS *None*

MENSTRUAL: ONSET _____ PERIODICITY _____ TYPE _____ DURATION _____ PAIN _____ L.M.P. _____

MARITAL: MISCARRIAGES _____ ABORTIONS _____ CHILDREN _____ STERILITY _____

HABITS: ALCOHOL *Moderate* TOBACCO *N/A* DRUGS *N/A* COFFEE *2 cups/day* MEALS *heavy* WATER *3 cups/day*

SLEEP *7 hrs./night* BOWEL MOVEMENTS *Regular* EXERCISE *Light* AMUSEMENTS *Bowling*

PRESENT AILMENT *Back pain, especially painful when lying down. Pain started about 1 week ago in lower back — has moved upward*

PHYSICAL EXAMINATION: TEMP. *99.2* PULSE *100* RESP. *16* B.P. *130/90* HEIGHT *6'1"* WEIGHT *195*

SKIN *Normal* MUCOUS MEMBRANE *Normal* EYES *Normal limits* EARS *no redness or drainage* NOSE *Normal* MOUTH *Normal*

NECK *Supple* CHEST *Normal* LUNGS *Bilateral breath sounds* HEART *Normal tones* ABDOMEN *Soft* RECTUM *Normal*

VAGINA _____ GENITALS _____ EXTREMITIES _____ OTHER _____

LABORATORY FINDINGS: *X-ray normal*

DIAGNOSIS: *Back strain*

TREATMENT: *Heat, rest*

REMARKS: _____

| DATE | | | SUBSEQUENT VISITS AND FINDINGS | CASE NO. |
MO.	DAY	YR.		
12	20	--	*Laceration of third finger left-hand p.i.p. joint.*	
			Good movement, no tendon damage.	
			3. 5-0 prolene sutures	

FIGURE 12-5 Patient health questionnaire

sent in too high or too low a concentration in the blood (Figure 12-12).

Radiology Report X-rays, CAT scans, and ultrasound examinations are diagnostic tests analyzed by radiologists to determine whether any unusual medical condition, such as a tissue mass, is present in the body. The radiologist prepares a report of the findings for the medical record (Figure 12-13); the actual x-rays are stored in another location because they are large and bulky.

```
PATIENT CASE HISTORY                                    Patient No.  839


 Name    Edgar Strindberg                            Date of Visit   4/14/--

 Address   5168 Placid Run Lane

           Atlanta, GA  30312-1865


 CHIEF COMPLAINT:      This 57-year-old male came to my office complaining of
                       mild to slightly severe chest pains.  He is taking Tylenol
                       II for pain, but no other pain-relieving medication.

                       Patient is alert and oriented.  He stated that approxi-
                       mately two weeks ago he began feeling a tightness across
                       his chest, equating it with the feeling of a tourniquet
                       wrapped around his chest.

 EXAMINATION:          Routine examination reveals a well-developed, well-nour-
                       ished male in apparent good health.  The patient is
                       slightly overweight; he should lose 10-15 pounds to be
                       within the normal range.  Blood pressure was slightly
                       above normal--145/90.

 LAB TESTS:            Chest X ray revealed heart scar tissue plus evidence of
                       inflammation of chest cavity lining.  An EKG revealed an
                       irregular heartbeat rate of 128 and evidence of old myo-
                       cardial infarction.  A two-hour blood sugar test was also
                       performed--180, indicating hyperglycemia.

 DIAGNOSIS:            1.  Unstable arteriosclerotic heart disease, old myocar-
                           dial infarction, and recent heart irregularity
                       2.  Type II hyperglycemia
                       3.  Essential hypertension
                       4.  Probable pleurisy

 TREATMENT:            Ampicillin, 500 mg. q.i.d., by mouth
                       Recheck in two weeks

 REMARKS:              Patient may continue working, but he must take regular
                       breaks for rest.

 FAMILY HISTORY:       Patient is married and has four children, ages 7-16.
                       The youngest child, age 7, is mentally handicapped.
                       Father is living and retired; he has suffered from two
                       heart attacks in the past five years.  Mother deceased
                       in automobile accident 15 years ago.  The patient has
                       two brothers, ages 52 and 49, both healthy.

 PERSONAL HISTORY:     Patient has led an active life.  He considers himself to
                       be a "workaholic."  The patient suffered from a mild
                       heart attack two years ago.  He seems emotionally stable
                       and secure and has had no other major illnesses since
                       childhood.

                            John H. Sparks, M.D.
```

FIGURE 12-6 Case history

Pathology and Cytopathology Report Pathology and cytopathology reports are prepared to show the results of studies of body tissue and body cells. A Pap smear is an example of a cyto-pathology report (Figure 12-14).

IN YOUR OPINION

1. Why should medical forms be standardized nation-wide?

2. How would you handle the transition from the present system of individualized medical formats to a standard system?

3. How does coding with color help the medical assistant?

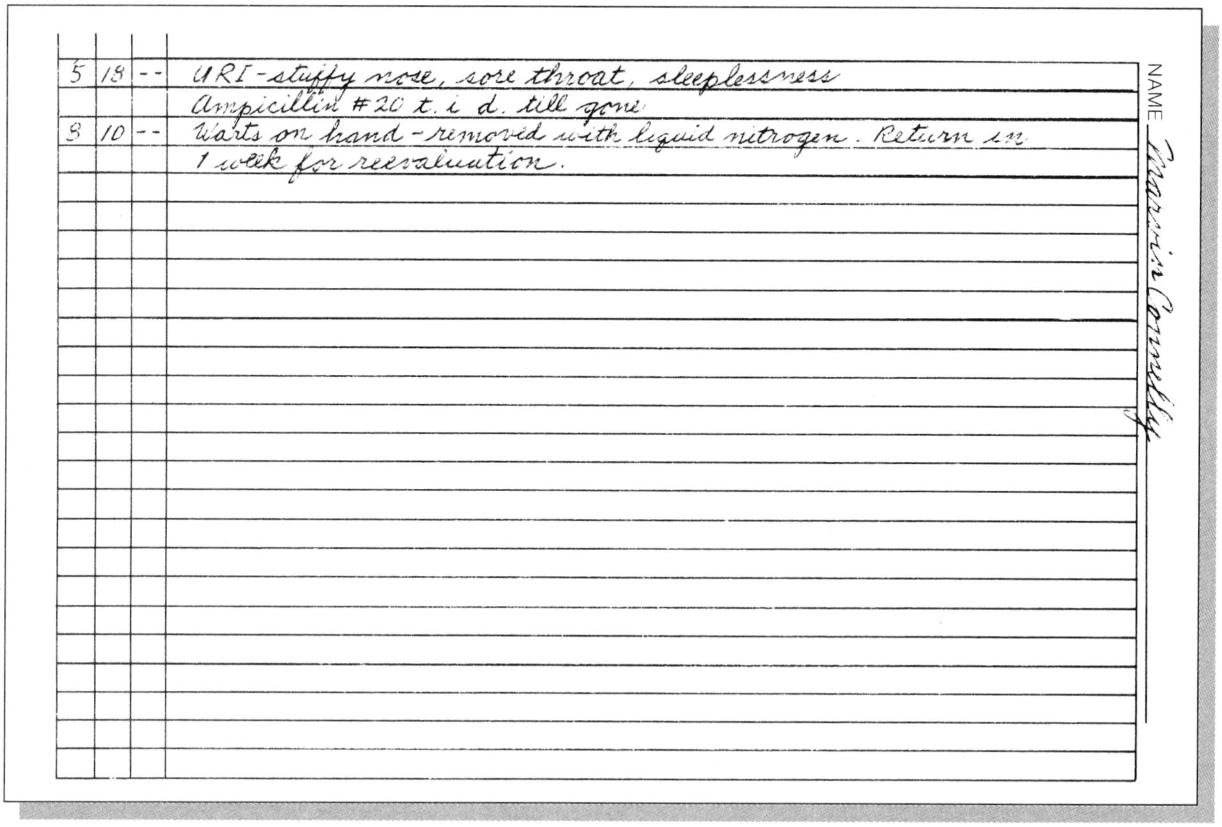

5 18 -- URI - stuffy nose, sore throat, sleeplessness
Ampicillin #20 t. i. d. till gone
8 10 -- Warts on hand - removed with liquid nitrogen. Return in 1 week for reevaluation.

NAME Marcia Connelly

FIGURE 12-7 Doctor's notes

Problem-Oriented and Source-Oriented Medical Records

Two different formats are used for recording information in the patient's medical record. The problem-oriented medical record, developed in the 1970s, identifies the patient's complaints in a problem list. The source-oriented medical record groups information according to its source; for example, from laboratories, examinations, nurse's or doctor's notes, consulting physicians, and other sources.

PROBLEM-ORIENTED MEDICAL RECORD

The problem-oriented medical record (POMR) came into use as a way to organize medical information in an orderly and easy-to-understand manner. In a POMR, the patient's complaints are seen as a series of problems, which are identified from the initial case history, the physical examination, and the results of diagnostic tests and procedures. Each problem is given a number, which is used when referring to the treatments and procedures the physician performs to correct the problem. Each time the patient returns for treatment of a recurring problem, the reference number for the problem is written before the doctor's notes about the visit. If more than one problem is identified, the number of each problem is listed, along with the treatment and procedures. If a patient describes a new complaint, it is added to the problem list and given its own number. The problem list is stored in a prominent location in the medical record so that anyone reviewing the record can locate it quickly.

The POMR is most useful in settings where several different people must refer to records. For example, in an ambulatory clinic staffed by several physicians on a rotating basis, a patient

LABORATORY REQUEST

John H. Sparks, M.D.   555-0078
8504 Capricorn Drive
Atlanta, GA 30033-7775

Date ___4/16/-- ___

To ___Rachel Morgan___
___Briarcliff Labs___

Re ___Susanne Snoffer___

Please perform the following tests:
- ☐ Culture of _____
- ☐ C S F for _____
- ☐ Feces for _____
- ☐ E K G _____
- ☐ B M R _____
- ☐ Pregnancy _____
- ☑ Urinalysis _____
- ☐ H P N _____
- ☑ Blood Sugar _____
- ☐ R H Factor & Blood Type _____
- ☐ SED Rate _____
- ☑ W B C & Diff _____
- ☐ R B C & H G D _____
- ☐ Other _____

John H. Sparks, M.D.
Signature

FIGURE 12-8 Laboratory request

may see a different physician on each visit. With the POMR method, the physician can quickly scan the charts to review the patient's progress.

The doctor's notes for a POMR follow an established formula called SOAP. After the physician identifies and numbers the problem, the doctor's notes are organized and dictated using the initials S-O-A-P, which stand for Subjective, Objective, Assessment, and Plan. Figure 12-15 explains the SOAP formula, and Figure 12-16 shows a problem-oriented medical record.

SOURCE-ORIENTED MEDICAL RECORD

The source-oriented medical record (SOMR) stores similar forms and reports together. For example, all laboratory reports are shingled and stored in one section; all consultation reports are stored in another; and all doctor's notes, nurse's notes, consulting reports and other reports are grouped according to their source and stored in separate locations in the folder. When a specific report is needed, the physician must flip through the entire medical record to find it. As a result, the SOMR format means that the physician must look through the folder several times during a patient's visit to obtain all the necessary information from various sources.

Database Management

Databases of paper medical records are standard in most medical practices today. Offices that do use medical record software tend to store only a capsule portion of each record on disk and continue to maintain paper files as well.

PAPER DATABASES

Most offices that use traditional paper medical records store them on open shelves and in file cabinets. As a medical assistant, you will use either an alphabetic or a numeric filing method for filing records.

Active Files
Open-shelf filing cabinets with stationary or pull-out open shelves are commonly used for storing active files. The folder tabs, which extend beyond the side of the folders, show the caption or name of the folder (Figure 12-17). Three-, four-, and five-position folders with color coding make retrieval of records easy and fast.

Inactive and Closed Files
When a patient has not visited the physician for an extended period, the medical record is moved to the inactive files. Most physicians consider a patient to be inactive after two to three

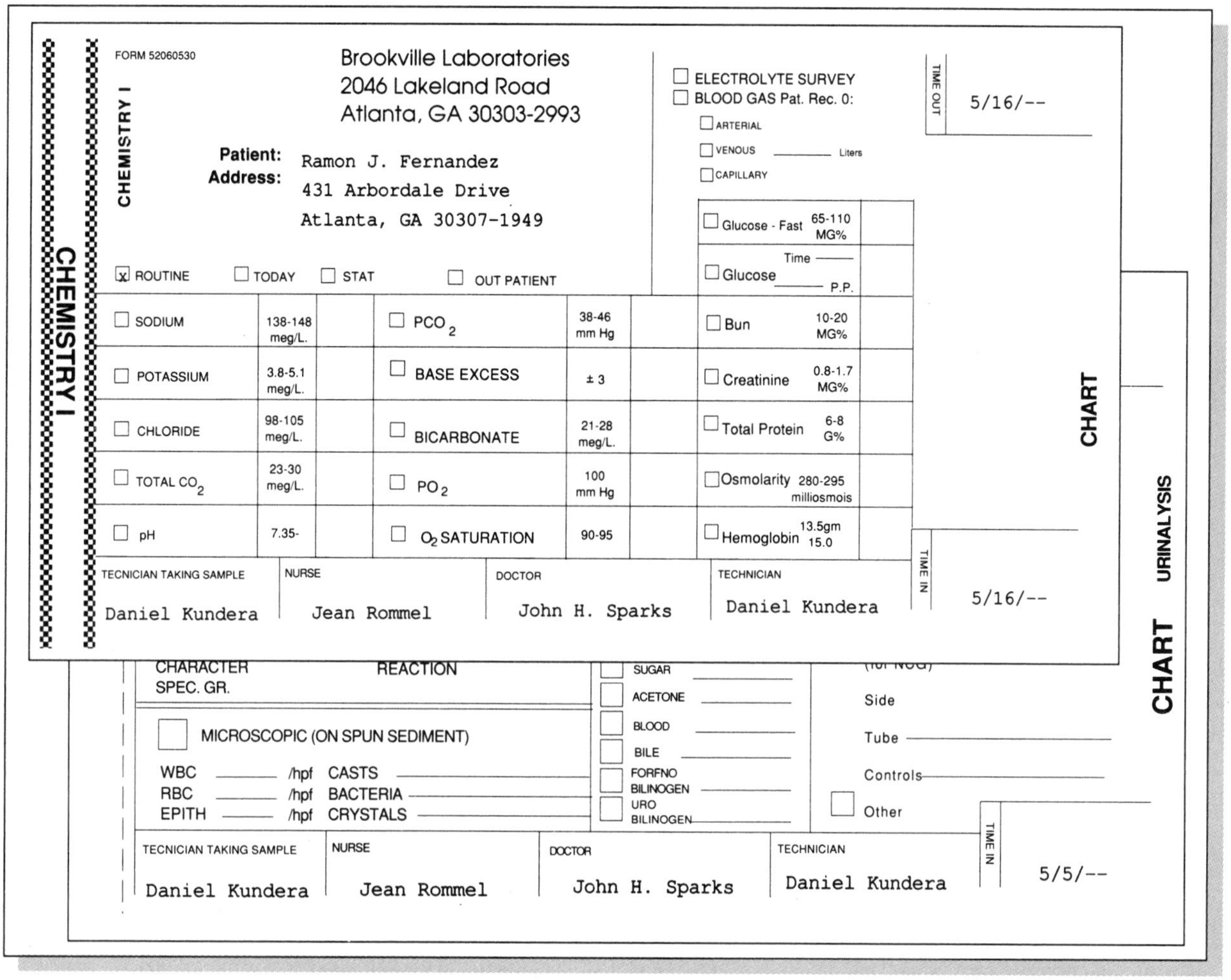

FIGURE 12-9 Shingled laboratory reports

years. Inactive files are usually stored in an out-of-the-way location to conserve space for active files.

Closed files contain the medical records of patients who are no longer under the physician's care because they have moved, changed doctors, or died. Since malpractice suits may be filed several years after the disputed treatment, inactive files and closed files are kept indefinitely. The laws of each state specify how long after a disputed action a claim can be made. The statute of limitations in a state determines how long medical records must be kept and the number of years that may pass before a claimant may no longer file a suit.

Microfiche or microfilm is often used to store inactive and closed records. Since a sheet of microfiche is about the size of a 3" × 5" card and holds 96 pages of information, records for several patients can be filmed on one microfiche sheet and stored in less space than would be necessary for conventional records.

Miscellaneous Correspondence

Letters, memos, reports, and other documents not directly related to patients are filed alphabetically in individual folders according to subject in a separate file labeled "Miscellaneous Correspondence." Follow these procedures for filing material in the Miscellaneous Correspondence file.

1. Clip together all correspondence by subject and arrange it in chronological order with the most recent in front.

FORM 52140530

Brookville Laboratories
2046 Lakeland Road
Atlanta, GA 30303-2993

TIME OUT 5/6/--

URINALYSIS

Patient: Rosa Marcus
Address: 6124 Bluehill Lane
Atlanta, GA 30324-3849

HOW COLLECTED ☐ VOIDED ☐ MID-STREAM ☐ CATH
FOR CYSTOSCOPY PATIENTS ☐ BLADDER ☐ RIGHT KIDNEY ☐ LEFT KIDNEY
PERIOD OF SPECIMEN ☐ SINGLE ☐ 24 HRS HRS
TIME SPECIMEN COLLECTION ENDED HR./MIN DATE

x ROUTINE | TODAY | STAT | OUTPATIENT

[x] ROUTINE URINALYSIS
ROUTINE VOLS. ______ COLOR ______
CHARACTER ______ REACTION 7.0
SPEC. GR. 1.025

☐ MICROSCOPIC (ON SPUN SEDIMENT)
WBC 10-20 /hpf CASTS ______
RBC 0-3 /hpf BACTERIA 2+
EPITH mod /hpf CRYSTALS ______

☐ ALBUMIN 1+
☐ SUGAR 2+
☐ ACETONE 2+
☐ BLOOD 0
☐ BILE 0
☐ FORFNO BILINOGEN
☐ URO BILINOGEN

☐ Pregnancy test (for NCG)
Side ______
Tube ______
Controls ______
☐ Other

TECNICIAN TAKING SAMPLE: Mary Angus
NURSE: Jacob Smith
DOCTOR: John H. Sparks
TECHNICIAN: Nelda Ashbaugh
TIME IN 5/6/--

URINALYSIS CHART

FIGURE 12-10 Urinalysis report

2. Prepare an individual folder for a single subject when more than five items are clipped together.
3. Transfer these materials to a folder.
4. File the new folder alphabetically with the other individual folders in the Miscellaneous Correspondence file.
5. File the remaining materials alphabetically by subject in a folder. Store the folder at the back of the individual folders.

COMPUTERIZED DATABASES

With a computer, it is easy to develop a database of patients, drugs, diagnoses, procedures, diseases, or any other category of information the physician wishes to monitor. Using Search and Sort commands, physicians can search the data in their patients' medical records for almost any information they desire. For example, one practice in Kentucky was able to search its computer database quickly for patients in whom intrauterine devices (IUDs) were inserted when medical research indicated that IUDs were not as safe as previously thought. The practice also searched the files for the names of all children treated by the physicians and sent notices to parents about a new vaccine for the prevention of meningitis.

Using a database is quite easy. After the data is entered, information can be sorted and printed out according to name, patient number, code, birth date, insurance company name, or any other common factor. If a research project is undertaken about a disease, the database can be searched for the names of all patients who have the disease. A database search of patient names is shown in Figure 12-18. The figure shows a partial list of patients whose names start with A–C.

IN YOUR OPINION

1. Does a POMR or SOMR make more sense to you? Why?
2. Can security be more easily maintained for paper records or computerized records?
3. What things should a medical assistant check when receiving a file back from a physician after a patient's visit?

ELECTROCARDIOGRAM

DIAGNOSIS ________ DIGITALIS ________ QUINDINE ________ OTHER ________

ATR.RATE ________ VENT. 57 ORS .10 OT ________ PR .16

DESCRIPTION:

INTERPRETATION:

SINUS BRADYCARDIA; OTHERWISE NORMAL RECORD

Brookville Laboratories
2046 Lakeland Road
Atlanta, GA 30303-2993

Patient: George Anders
Address: 427 Collins Ave.
Atlanta, GA 30326-8823

AXIS ________ RHYTHM ________

EKG NO. 411 DATE 5/6/-- TIME 10:00

LEADS 1 2 3 AVR AVL AVF V1 V2 V3 V4 V5 V6 CAL. 1MV

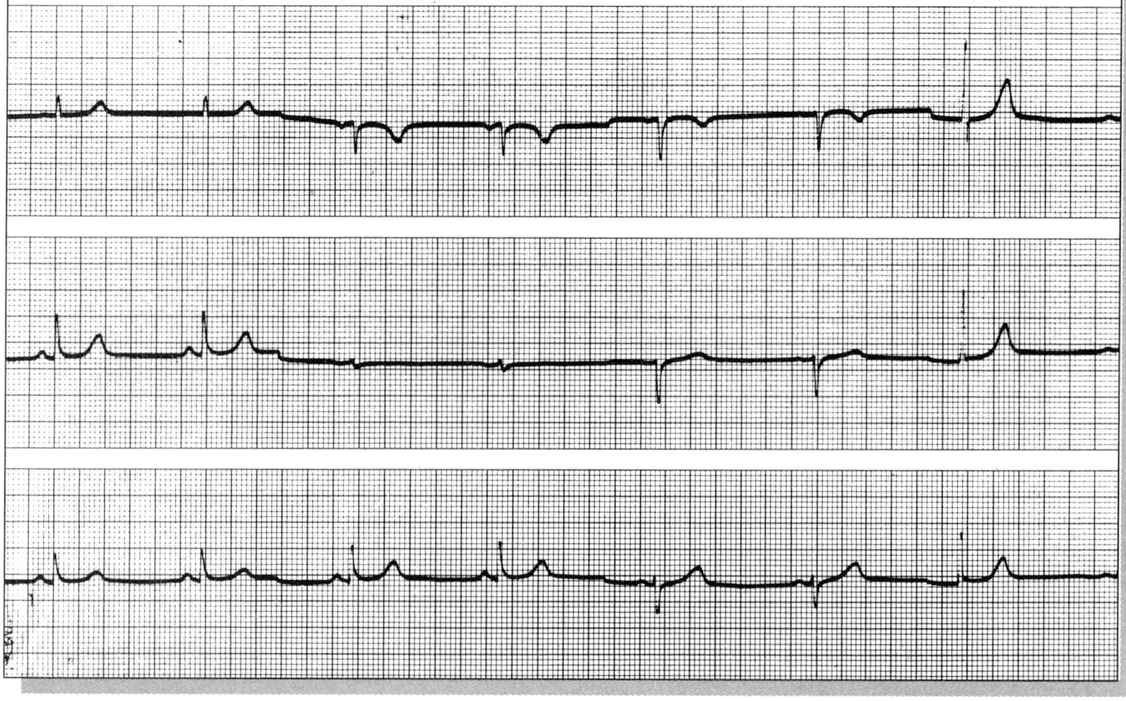

FIGURE 12-11 Electrocardiogram

HEMATOLOGY FORM 9212094

☒ CBC ☐ Hgh ☐ RBC ☐ Hct ☐ WBC ☐ CELL INDICES RBC & HEMATOCRIT

REMARK CLINICAL DX. ☐ OUTPATIENT ☒ ROUTINE ☐ OR in AM ☐ EMERGENCY

HEMATOLOGY

	DATE								
YEAR --	NORMAL VALUES COUPER COUNTER	M 7.8± 3 F 7.8± 3	M 5.4± 0.8 F 4.8± 0.6	M 16.£± 2 F 14.£± 2	M 4‡± 5 F 4‡± 9	M 87± 7 F 9£± 9	M 29± 2 F 29± 2	M 34± 2 F 34± 2
MONTH 5	NORMAL VALUES WINTROBE	M 7.£± 3 F 7.8± 3	M 5.4± 0.8 F 4.8± 0.6	M 1£± 2 F 14± 2	M 4‡± 5 F 4‡± 9	M 87± 5 F 87± 9	M 2£± 2 F 29± 2	M 34± 2 F 34± 2
	TEST	WBC x 10[3]	RCB X 10[6]	HGB gm	HCT %	MCV %	MCH %	MCHC %
DAY 6				12.0	36.0			

NURSE Jacob Smith

REPORTED BY Mary Angus

DATE 5/6/--

TECH TAKING SAMPLE Nelda Ashbaugh

☒ DIFFERENTIAL

POLY	STAB	LYMPH	MONO	EOS	BABO	BLAST CELLS	MYELOCYTES	METAMYELOCYTES	NABC 100 WBC	ANISOCITOSIS	POIKILOCYTOSIS
3	66	28	2	1							

☐ SED RATE ☐ CSR ☐ PLATELET ☐ RETIC

NOTES

Brookville Laboratories
2046 Lakeland Road
Atlanta, GA 30303-2993

Patient: Rosa Marcus
Address: 6124 Bluehill Lane
Atlanta, GA 30324-3849

HEMATOLOGY CHART

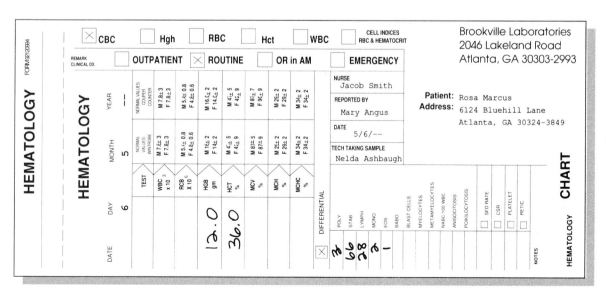

FIGURE 12-12 Blood test report

DEPARTMENT OF RADIOLOGY

NUCLEAR MEDICINE REPORT

Patient's Name   Jennifer Alexander
Hosp. No.
Room No.
Ref. Physician

Date   3/15/--

Nuclear
Medicine No.: 005375

Pregnant:

Examination:	Isotropic Compound:	Dose:	Ancillary Studies:
Thyroid Scan I 131 Uptake	Sodium I 131		

The patient has had a thyroidectomy for hyperthyroidism. A 24-hour radioactive iodine uptake is .08% reflecting the surgical removal of the thyroid.
A small area of functioning thyroid tissue is seen to the right of the midline probably in the region of the upper pole of the thyroid. There is no evidence of activity in the lower left midline neck in the region of the palpable nodule.

Dr. Sabina Gwyn

NUCLEAR MEDICINE REPORT

FIGURE 12-13 Radiology report

Rules for Filing

Medical records, ledger cards, general correspondence, research reports, tax records, and magazine articles related to the physician's specialty are typical documents that you will file in a medical office. The alphabetic and numeric filing methods are commonly used for filing patient records; the alphabetic, numeric, geographic, and subject methods are used for other materials.

ALPHABETIC INDEXING

The alphabet is basic to all four methods of filing: alphabetic, numeric, subject, and geographic. Several standard rules apply for filing by the alphabetic method.

Standards for Alphabetic Filing

Rule 1: Order of Indexing Units For filing purposes, the parts of an individual's name are called **indexing units.** The surname, or last

Brookville Laboratories
2046 Lakeland Road
Atlanta, GA 30303-2993

Patient: Rosa Marcus Age 45
Address: 6124 Bluehill Lane
Atlanta, GA 30324-3849

METROPOLITAN HOSPITAL
ATLANTA, GA

CYTOLOGY

☒ GENITAL
☒ CERVICAL
☐ VAGINAL
☐ MATURITY INDEX
☐ LAB USE ONLY

☐ NON GENITAL
☐ SPUTUM ☐ GASTRIC
☐ URINE ☐ SMALL INT.
☐ BREAST ☐ LARGE INT.
☐ PLEURAL ☐ OTHER
☐ PERITONEAL
☐ BRON. WASH
☐ BRON. BRUSH
☐ C S F
☐ ESOPH

CLINICAL INFORMATION:
LAST MENSTRUAL PERIOD:
6/31/--

PREVIOUS SMEARS ________ 19 ____
DIAGNOSIS NEGATIVE
PREGNANT ☐ YES ☒ NO
YEARS POSTMENOPAUSAL

CONSULTATION REPORT:
☐ UNSATISFACTORY
☒ NEGATIVE
☐ NO ENDOCERVICALS
☐ ATYPICAL BENIGN
☐ DYSPLASIA
☐ POSITIVE
☐ IN SITU
☐ INVASIVE
☐ OTHER

REMARKS:

Date: 6/24/--

CYTOTECHNOLOGIST

PATHOLOGIST

CHART COPY

FIGURE 12-14 Pathology and cytopathology report

name, is identified as the first indexing unit; the first name or initial is identified as the second unit; and the middle name or initial is identified as the third unit. For example, you would index the name *Samuel Arthur Clark* like this: *Clark* (first unit); *Samuel* (second unit); and *Arthur* (third unit).

Rule 2: Names of Businesses Names of businesses, institutions, and organizations are indexed in the order in which the name is written. Abbreviations such as *Co.*, *Inc.*, and *Ltd.* are also indexed as written. Therefore, the business name *Clinical Supply Company* would be alphabetized exactly as it is written, using *Clinical* as the first indexing unit.

Rule 3: Symbols and Coordinating Words Symbols and coordinating words like *a, an, and, the, in, of, #,* and *&*, that are part of a name are also considered as indexing units. For example, you would index the business name *Palmer & Palmer Labs* like this: *Palmer* (first unit); *and* (second unit); *Palmer* (third unit); and *Labs* (fourth unit). Notice that *&* is written out as *and*.

S	**Subjective**	Information based on the patient's feelings and symptoms (feels bad, no energy, headaches). The examiner writes the subjective analysis in the patient's own words and includes the chief complaint or reason for the visit.
O	**Objective**	Information based on the results of diagnostic tests and procedures. These are symptoms that can be seen or proved (bruises, high blood pressure, fever).
A	**Assessment**	Diagnosis of the problem based on subjective and objective data.
P	**Plan**	Manner in which the problem will be managed. The plan usually consists of three parts: (1) Medical management, including medication, diet, and therapy; (2) diagnostic follow-up, including x-rays and additional lab tests; and (3) patient education, including reinforcement of the physician's instructions by the medical assistant.

FIGURE 12-15 SOAP formula used in doctor's notes

PROGRESS NOTES

Patient's Name *Michael Brandy*   Page *1*

Date	Problem Number	S-O-A-P
		S: Subjective
		O: Objective
		A: Assessment
		P: Plan
9/14/--	1	S: Stuffy nose, sore throat, sleeplessness
		O: Fever 101 degrees, throat red
		A: URI
		P: Ampicillin #20, t.i.d. till gone; plenty of rest,
		plenty of fluids, well-balanced diet.
1/10	2	S: Headaches, sneezing, sore throat in AM
		O: Eyes red, nose stuffy, dark circles under eyes
		A: Seasonal allergies
		P: Seldane, #280, mg. t.i.d. till gone

FIGURE 12-16 Problem-oriented medical record

In addition, if a business name begins with *The,* that word becomes the last indexing unit. For example, the name *The Sands Ambulance Service* would follow this system: *Sands* (first unit); *Ambulance* (second unit); *Service* (third unit); and *The* (last unit).

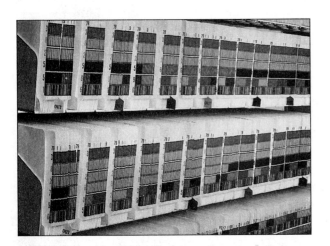

FIGURE 12-17 Color-coded labels of folder tabs are widely used to make incorrectly filed records easier to detect.

Rule 4: Initials and Abbreviations Initials and abbreviations of business and personal names are indexed as written. Hyphens, periods, or parentheses are ignored in the indexing order. For example, in the name *A B C Radiology Co.,* *ABC* is treated as one indexing unit, and in the name *C & D Drug Co., C and D* are treated as three separate indexing units.

Rule 5: Possessives The apostrophe is not considered when indexing possessives. Therefore, *Harper's* is indexed as *Harpers* and *Manns'* is indexed as *Manns.*

Rule 6: Titles A person's title is considered as the last indexing unit. For example, you would consider the title *Dr.* in the name *Dr. Ester Diaz* as the last indexing unit. However, if a title appears with the last name only, you index the name and title as written. To illustrate, with the name *Professor Mendel, Professor* would be the first indexing unit, and *Mendel* would be the second unit.

A - B				
Albertine, Glenn	1-1-366	Bea, Won	1-1-173
Acosta, Ansel	1-1-168	Beach, John	1-1-174
Ade, John E.	1-1-11	Becker, Helen	1-1-1
Aguilar, C.A.	1-1-233	Bender, Burel	1-1-175
Anderson, Terry	1-1-65	Berm, Bertha	1-1-252
Anthony, Mark	1-1-275	Berryhill, Lon Jr.	1-1-320
Applestein, Beatrice	1-1-90	Best, Kermit	1-1-176
Armboy, Gil	1-1-413	Blythowitz, Hazel P.	1-1-336
Ash, Maureen	1-1-412	Bradford, Lauren	1-1-203
Ashbrook, Betty J.	1-1-39	Braude, Jacob	1-1-91
Bagby, Colleen	1-1-414	Buser, Seth	1-1-230
Bancroft, Iris	1-1-305	Bullerdick, Lloyd	1-1-92
Basham, Arville O.	1-1-61	Burton, Eric	1-1-434
Bazam, Jose	1-1-172	Busch, Nancy	1-1-435

C - D				
Caeser, Julie	1-1-274	Crum, Ralph	1-1-108
Carrington, Dennis	1-1-306	Csaba, Szabo	1-1-110
Carter, Samuel	1-1-209	Dalby, Reni	1-1-440
Carvalho, Donald	1-1-31	Daniels, Anthony	1-1-200
Chan, Hubert	1-1-436	Daniels, Godfrey	1-1-352
Cheeks, Ethel G.	1-1-337	Daniels, Susan F.	1-1-199
Cloud, Vanessa M.	1-1-218	Davis, Melvin	1-1-28
Cole, Winifred	1-1-416	Del Pino, Mario	1-1-49
Combs, Calvin	1-1-190	Delite, Ernest	1-1-105
Conklin, Sally	1-1-415	Dent, Julius	1-1-104
Connors, James	1-1-237	Dills, Eric	1-1-88
Cook, Steve	1-1-202	Dines, Eddy	1-1-179
Coons, Ann	1-1-437	Doggs, James	1-1-140
Cose, Wallace	1-1-115	Dorman, Nora	1-1-442
Cox, Gaile	1-1-84	Doris, George	1-1-236

FIGURE 12-18 Patient names sorted by alphabet

Rule 7: Married Women A married woman's name is indexed as used, whether she continues to be known by her maiden name or by her husband's name. Some married women use their husbands' last names and their own first names, and middle names or initials. Others use their husbands' last names, first names, and middle names or initials. In either case, the last name is the first indexing unit; the first name is the second unit; the middle name or initial is the third unit; and the title *Mrs.* or *Ms.* is the last unit. Therefore, the name *Mrs. Alice Marie Lunkin* is indexed like this: *Lunkin* (first indexing unit); *Alice* (second unit); *Marie* (third unit); and *Mrs.* (last unit).

If a married woman uses a combination of her own last name and her husband's last name, you should consider the compound name as one indexing unit. For example, in the name

Ms. Althea Sanders- Smith, the first indexing unit is *SandersSmith.* Notice that the hyphen is omitted. When a married woman is known by more than one name, all forms of the name are cross-referenced.

Rule 8: Foreign Language Prefixes A foreign language prefix is considered to be a part of the business name or personal name that follows it. Capitalization or spacing between the prefix and the root word does not influence the indexing order. Examples of foreign language prefixes include *De, Di, Du, L', Las, O', Van,* and *Van Der.* Therefore, you would consider the surname *Di George* as one indexing unit, *DiGeorge.* Similarly, you would index the business name *William Van Hook Optical Co.* like this: *William* (first unit); *VanHook* (second unit); *Optical* (third unit); and *Co.* (last unit).

Rule 9: Identical Names When several names of individuals or businesses are the same, you must use the address for filing. Addresses are indexed alphabetically first by city, then by state (if the city name is duplicated), then by street name and address or building number. Addresses and building numbers are indexed in ascending order, meaning that the numbers go from smaller to larger.

In the same way, the seniority designations *Junior* (Jr.) and *Senior* (Sr.) are considered in alphabetic order. The seniority designations II, III, and IV are put into numeric order. Therefore, *Francisco Toros II*'s name would be listed before *Francisco Toros III.*

Rule 10: Numerals in Business Names A numeral that is part of a business name is written as a single word and indexed as a single unit. For example, *9th Avenue Garage* is filed as *9* (first unit); *Avenue* (second unit); and *Garage* (third unit). In addition, all Arabic numerals and Roman numerals are filed sequentially before alphabetic characters.

Rule 11: Organizations and Institutions Names of organizations and institutions are indexed exactly as they are written. For example, *National Association of Radiologists* is filed like this: *National* (first unit); *Association* (second unit); *of* (third unit); and *Radiologists* (last unit).

Rule 12: Separated Single Words Separate parts of words that the dictionary treats as a single word are indexed as written in the business name. Therefore, if the word is separated in the business name, it should be indexed as separate units. For example, even though the word *interstate* is normally considered one word, for the name *Inter State Listing Service, Inter* and *State* would be treated as separate words.

Rule 13: Compound Names Parts of compound business names separated by a space are indexed as individual units. Hyphens are disregarded and the parts are considered as a single unit. Forms of the word *Saint,* such as *San* and *Sainte,* are considered prefixes and are indexed as part of the names that follow. (See Rule 8.)

Rule 14: Coined Words, Unusual Words Coined or unusual words are indexed as written and hyphens are disregarded. For example, the first word of *Shur-Fit Optical* is indexed as *ShurFit.*

Rule 15: Government Names All government agencies, both domestic (in the United States) and foreign, are indexed according to political divisions. Sometimes the words *United States Government* are understood to be part of a name but are not written in the name. They should always be considered as Units 1, 2, and 3 for filing purposes. The name of the government body is indexed first (country, state, city) and is followed by the other units in descending order of importance (department, bureau, division, agency.) The words *Bureau of, Department of, County of,* etc., are eliminated unless they are needed for clarity.

For example, the name *State of Georgia Department of Human Resources* would be indexed exactly as it is written. But the name *U.S. Department of Health and Human Services* would be indexed like this: *United States Government* (first, second, and third units), followed by *Health and Human Services, Department of.*

CROSS-REFERENCING

A cross-reference card is used when a name might be indexed in more than one way. Foreign names, names of married women, unusual business names, hyphenated names, multiple business names, abbreviated or single letter names, and names that may be spelled several ways are examples of situations in which a cross-reference card should be made. The original card lists the name that is the most likely means of identification. A second, and perhaps a third card is used to show other names by which the individual, firm, or agency might be identified.

ALPHABETIC FILING GUIDES AND TABS

Primary file guides made of heavy cardboard or plastic are used to identify the broad categories of a file. In an alphabetic file, primary guides usually divide the alphabet into twenty-six sections, one for each letter of the alphabet. The primary guides are placed in the first position of the file shelf (at the top) or file drawer (at the far left). Secondary guides subdivide the alphabet into smaller parts; for example, the primary guide *A* may be subdivided into *Aa–Al* and *Am–Az*. These are placed in second position of the file shelf or drawer. File folders with their individual captions often are placed in third position. For the medical office that wishes to further subdivide folders, guides are available for fourth and fifth positions. File dividers can also be color-coded, thus reducing the need for some of the secondary guides used in the past.

Procedures for Alphabetic Filing

Follow these procedures to assure easy retrieval of materials filed by alphabetic method:

1. Code the document by underlining the indexing units or by writing the code name in the upper right corner.
2. Cross-reference the document as needed.
3. Locate the correct alphabetic guides in the filing system.
4. File the document and any cross-references in the filing system.
5. Retrieve the file folder as needed.

NUMERIC FILING

Numeric filing is a method of filing by number instead of by letter. The numeric method is used in many medical offices to maintain the confidentiality of patient records. A number on a folder tab does not reveal a patient's identity as easily or as directly as the person's name does. In large medical centers and hospitals with many folders, the numeric method is used to make files easier to retrieve.

The Accession Book or Patient Identification Ledger

The **accession book** or **patient identification ledger** provides a consecutive record of the numbers and names of all patients. When a new patient visits the medical office, the next available number in the accession book is assigned to that patient, and the person's name is written beside the number. This number identifies the patient and is written on each paper associated

with the patient before the paper is filed. For example, lab reports, case histories, letters, or other documents that refer to the patient are coded with the patient's number.

Numeric procedures can also be used in subject and geographic filing systems. Subjects or geographic names are assigned a number; then a list is maintained for each folder name and its identifying number.

Alphabetic Card File

An alphabetic card file containing a card for each patient is an essential part of numeric and alphabetic filing systems. Each card lists the patient's full name, address, telephone number, and patient number. Alphabetic cards are stored in a rotary card holder, a card tray, or a card box in alphabetic order according to the patient's last name. When a patient's folder must be retrieved, the patient's card can be located, the patient number identified from the card, and the folder matching the number in the patient files can be located.

In addition, most medical offices maintain a separate file for miscellaneous alphabetic cards. These cards list the names, addresses, and telephone numbers of hospitals, ambulance services, police, research organizations, professional organizations, suppliers, and other physicians.

Numeric File Guides and Tabs

Numeric file guides break numeric files into manageable sections. Folders may be divided into number groups of 1–99, 100–199, 200–299, and so on. Secondary guides placed in second position may be used to subdivide the numbers further. The tabs of individual folders are usually shown in third position. Fourth- and fifth-position folders are available for medical offices requiring them. To maintain confidentiality, the folder tab usually lists only the patient's number, although in some offices the patient's name is also listed. Folders are stored in ascending order with the smallest number in the front.

Miscellaneous Correspondence File

When a numeric system is used for filing medical records, an alphabetic correspondence file is usually maintained for materials not related to patients. These materials contain general information pertaining to the practice, professional organizations, or research. The alphabetic caption on each folder identifies the contents. A separate folder labeled *Miscellaneous* or *Miscellaneous Correspondence* is stored at the back of the file or shelf to hold miscellaneous materials or correspondence involving fewer than five items about a single subject. When five related items accumulate, the medical assistant should prepare a new folder with an appropriate tab caption and then merge it in alphabetic order with the other folders. This is different than with a patient file, which must be made up immediately.

Procedures for Numeric Filing

Follow these procedures when a new patient visits a medical office that uses numeric filing:

1. Assign the next unused number in the accession book to the patient.
2. Complete an alphabetic card for the patient.
3. Prepare a file folder listing the patient number on the tab.
4. Store the folders in ascending order with the other patient folders.

Follow these procedures to retrieve a file:

1. Locate the patient's name in the alphabetic card file and identify the patient's number.
2. Look for the patient's number on the folder tabs of the medical records. Remove the appropriate medical record from the files.
3. Return the folder to the files when there is no further need for it.

SUBJECT FILING

Subject filing is a method of filing by subject titles instead of by individuals' names. Subject titles are used in medical offices to identify diseases, research, treatments, drugs, and other areas of interest to the physician. For example, a physician researching children's diseases may use the titles *Diabetes, Muscular Dystrophy, Heart Disease,* or others. Letters, memos, research reports, and other items from many different sources are stored in the folders.

The business-related activities of a medical office also lend themselves to subject filing. For example, a medical office may have folder tabs labeled *Medicare, Medicaid, Workers' Compen-*

sation, Blue Cross/Blue Shield, or others. Usually subject files are stored alphabetically; however, a number may be assigned to each subject so the folders can be filed by the numeric method.

Materials filed by subject often need to be cross-referenced because all individuals do not think in the same terms. For example, a letter about research on skin disease might be filed by the subject title *Skin Disease* and cross-referenced under the letter writer's name.

GEOGRAPHIC FILING

Geographic filing is a method of filing by geographic area instead of by a person's name or by a subject. Often geographic and subject methods are used together. Although most medical offices do not use geographic files, they are useful in medical research centers to identify regions of the country in which research is being conducted. For example, the geographic method might be used to identify states or regions in which research into allergies is being conducted. Geographic materials may be stored by the alphabetic or numeric methods.

Cross-referencing is also important to the geographic system. This is because all individuals who use the materials may not think in terms of the same geographic areas.

RESEARCH FILES

Medical research is filed according to either the subject or geographic methods. Research about allergies, for example, might be filed according to the name of the allergy, such as *hay fever* or *poison ivy,* or according to the geographic areas of the country where the allergy is found. Sometimes both the subject and geographic methods are used in a research file. Whichever method is used, the categories are arranged in alphabetic order.

The Medical Assistant's Role in Record Keeping

Managing a system of medical records that meets medical, administrative, ethical, and legal requirements is a very important task. If you are

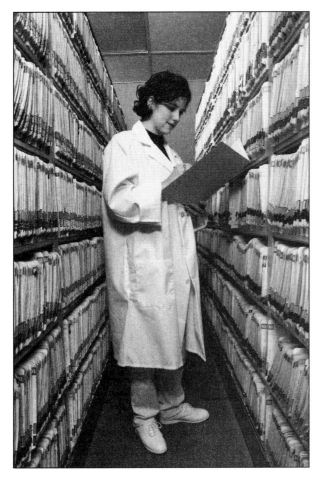

FIGURE 12-19 Maintaining complete, accurate and up-to-date medical records is an important task.

the medical assistant entrusted with this responsibility, you must conscientiously maintain complete, accurate, and up-to-date records (Figure 12-19). Follow these procedures for managing patients' records:

1. Chart or file all information about patients every day.
2. Show all new information to the physician for reading and initialing.
3. Shingle records less than 8.5" × 11".
4. File all materials in the correct file.
5. Place correspondence about patients in their medical records and unrelated correspondence in the *Miscellaneous Correspondence* file.

IN YOUR OPINION

1. Why is it important to understand filing rules before using a computer database?
2. Why is cross-referencing essential?
3. How do the filing needs of a general practice and a research institution differ?

REFERENCES

Becklin, Karonne, and Edith Sunnarborg. *Medical Office Procedures.* New York: Glencoe, 1992.

Claeys, Terese. *Medical Filing.* Cincinnati, Ohio: South-Western Publishing Co., 1993.*

Gartee, Richard, and Doris D. Humphrey. *The Medical Manager.* Cincinnati, Ohio: South-Western Publishing Co., 1995.*

Humphrey, Doris D., and Kathie Sigler. T*he Modern Medical Office: A Reference Manual.* Cincinnati, Ohio: South-Western Publishing Co., 1990.*

U.S. Department of Labor, Bureau of Labor Statistics. *Occupational Outlook Handbook.* Washington: U.S. Government Printing Office, 1993.

*Currently published by Delmar Publishers.

Chapter Activities

PERFORMANCE BASED ACTIVITIES

1. Refer to the sample color coding system in Figure 12-3. On 3" × 5" cards, color code the names of the following patients. Use colored markers to produce the colors needed. Then file the cards in correct alphabetic order.

   a. *Jeff Ramsey Hight*

   b. *Cynthia Givens*

   c. *Mrs. William (Marian) Highers*

   d. *Gregory Eaton, Jr.*

   e. *Samuel Higgens*

   f. *Tara Handley*

   g. *Melinda Headley*

   h. *Saratina Handley*

   i. *Tina Hardley*

   j. *Gregory Eaton, Sr.*

   (DACUM 3.1, 3.3)

2. Using the format in Figure 12-15, rewrite the information from the following case to show how the physician would record it in a problem-oriented medical record.

   Bernard Richards visited the doctor complaining of a twisted ankle suffered in a fall. The ankle hurt when the patient walked on it and was sore to the touch. It was also swollen. X-rays revealed that the patient's ankle had a hairline fracture; simple fracture. The doctor prescribed Ibuprofen, 600 mg. #28. One tablet 4 times daily with meals; bed rest; crutches for walking. The patient is to return in four days for a cast after swelling is reduced.

   (DACUM 2.7, 2.10, 4.14, 5.2)

3. Summarize an article from a recent medical periodical about trends in medical record keeping. (DACUM 1.8, 2.7, 2.11)

4. Contact your mentor and a medical assistant from one other practice. Ask them to share their greatest problems in maintaining medical records. Compare and write a summary of their answers. (DACUM 1.1, 1.4, 2.1, 2.6)

EXPANDING YOUR THINKING

1. Keeping in mind the type of information maintained today in paper medical records and the type of information stored in computerized medical records, indicate with a "P" or "C" the following items most likely to be found in a paper record or computerized record where stored.

Information

   a. *The names of all children given a particular drug.*

   b. *The insurance policy numbers of several patients.*

   c. *A patient's blood pressure reading from the previous visit.*

   d. *The results of a urine test.*

   e. *The ZIP codes of all patients.*

   f. *A letter to a consulting physician about a specific patient.*

2. What three groups of people are served by medical records? How is each served?

3. Describe three ways in which a computerized database can be used in a medical office.

   Content of Database   *Need for Database*

   1. _____

   2. _____

   3. _____

4. How does color coding help in locating a medical record?

5. Review a typical medical record with your mentor. Ask your mentor to explain the organization and placement of materials in the record. Then explain the organization in a chart or short paper.

6. Explain the organization of a problem-oriented medical record and a source-oriented medical record.

7. What type of database is most often found in medical offices today? Why is this kind of database popular?

8. What is the medical assistant's role in maintaining medical records?

9. How is the storage of active and inactive files different?

Portfolio Assessment

1. With a team of two classmates, select one common medical office software application, such as scheduling, billing, word processing, or clinical record keeping. Research the software from at least three of the following: computer magazines, medical journals, university research centers, computer sales representatives, medical office personnel, or other sources. Give a panel presentation of the advantages and disadvantages of adding this application to a medical office's operation. Your presentation should cover costs, implementation time, office disruption, and ultimate rewards. Audiotape or videotape your presentation. (DACUM 1.1, 1.5, 1.6, 1.8, 2.3, 2.6, 3.4)

2. With your team, create a plan for implementing the software application you researched in No. 1 for a group practice. Assume a staff of three physicians, four medical assistants, four nurses, a lab assistant, and a financial person. Include details for steps such as the following:

   Research   Planning
   Purchasing   Installing
   Training   Pilot testing
   Data gathering   Data input
   Measurement of results

   (DACUM 1.5, 1.8, 2.3, 2.7, 2.11, 3.4, 6.2, 6.6, 6.10)

3. Using the material gathered in Chapter 11, Performance Based Activities Nos. 2 and 3, work with two or three other students to develop an informational brochure on one of your topics. Target a special group such as patients or high school students. Produce the brochure on word processing or desktop publishing software, if possible, and use simple graphics. (DACUM 1.5, 2.3, 2.7, 3.1)

4. After investigating the procedures used at your mentoring practice, prepare an outline for training staff in one of the following: telephone answering, call routing, or message taking. Use a format that is simple and clear for trainees learning the process. (DACUM 1.1, 1.6, 2.3, 2.7)

Computers and Financial Management in the Medical Office

You have already learned that computers are used in medical offices for scheduling appointments, creating documents, communicating electronically, maintaining records, sorting and storing data, patient testing and monitoring, and repetitive calculation. In the process of automating office functions, medical assistants are discovering additional ways that computers can increase income, creativity, and office morale. These are accomplished primarily through eliminating or reducing time-consuming, repetitive tasks.

In Part IV, you will learn how computers are used in financial applications such as accounting, insurance claims, and billing. You will also learn traditional methods for handling these important tasks. After reading these chapters you will have completed all the material related to office management, and you should have a good understanding of the importance of the computer as a tool in your career as a medical assistant.

Chapter 13

Pegboard Accounting and Computerized Practice Management

CAPE GIRARDEAU, MISSOURI

Pegboard accounting is my primary responsibility at Walker Cardiology Associates, Inc. Although we are changing to a computerized accounting system soon, I wouldn't give up the experience I've gained from managing the pegboard accounting system this past year. There's no question that I'll understand the computer system better and more quickly after learning a manual accounting system first.

Each day I work with many superbills and ledger cards and with the daily log. I post patient accounts, record payments from insurance companies and individuals, write checks, manage petty cash, and handle a variety of other financial transactions. In addition, Dr. Cortez and Dr. Raleigh ask every few days about the practice's financial standing compared to last year. They also like to know how their individual fees are producing income for the practice. Keeping up with all this is a big task, but doing it well gives me a sense of accomplishment. When I first started working here, I couldn't even balance my own checkbook!

Next week, I'm attending a seminar to learn how to move from a pegboard system to a computerized accounting system. The doctors chose me to attend the seminar because they have confidence in my ability to manage the transition. I'm really pleased because there are several medical assistants in the office who have worked here much longer than I have.

Amanda Dufresne
Medical Assistant

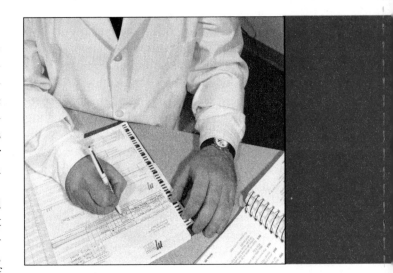

PERFORMANCE BASED COMPETENCIES

After completing this chapter, you should be able to:

1. Use pegboard bookkeeping system. (DACUM 8.1)
2. Execute beginning and ending activities for patient transactions in the office and at the hospital. (DACUM 8.4)
3. Prepare summary reports of cumulative financial activity for the current accounting period. (DACUM 8.6)
4. Complete deposit slips, check registers, checks, petty cash logs, and other required financial forms. (DACUM 8.1, 8.5)
5. Match the components of a manual system with the corresponding screens of a computer system. (DACUM 3.4)

HEALTHSPEAK

Current Procedural Terminology (CPT) Industry coding standard recognized by most insurance companies and widely used in medical offices to identify procedures and services performed.

Daily log The day's summary of patient transactions.

ICD codes Diagnosis codes from the *International Classification of Diseases,* Ninth Edition, used to identify the patient's medical problem.

Ledger card Chronological listing of one family's financial activity with the practice.

Pegboard accounting Traditional method of maintaining accounts, named for the flat writing board on which accounting papers are prepared.

Practice analysis Overview of procedures and treatments provided and income derived during a specified period.

Proof of posting Verification of the calculation of columns in the daily log.

Superbill Patient charge slip or receipt listing the typical examinations, procedures, treatments, and services a patient might have during one visit.

Pegboard Accounting

As a medical assistant, you may be asked to maintain the patient accounts. This function is very important because the financial success of the practice depends on accurate and timely record keeping. If you are asked to handle patient accounts, you must have a good understanding of bookkeeping, a mind for details, and the ability to complete tasks on time.

The traditional method of maintaining accounts is called pegboard accounting. It is named for the flat writing board with attached pegs on which accounting papers are prepared. Pegboard accounting is relatively simple and very efficient when handled by a medical assistant with good handwriting and a keen mind. With the introduction of computers in medical offices, computerized accounting has replaced many pegboard systems. Nevertheless, a background in pegboard accounting is helpful even when a computerized system is used because it provides the basis for understanding the process by which the computer manages patient financial activities.

Pegboard accounting refers to a simple "write-it-once" method of record keeping. Carbonized or no-carbon-required accounting papers are placed on top of one another, so that any charge or payment posted one time with a hard-tipped ball point pen will imprint on all sheets beneath the original. Posting to several records in one writing reduces the probability of error and saves valuable employee time.

As a medical assistant, you will spend a large portion of the day using the pegboard accounting system, for it is one of the most important responsibilities in a medical office. The size of the practice determines which medical assistant is assigned to pegboard accounting. In a one- or two-physician practice, a medical assistant may be asked to greet patients and also handle pegboard accounting activities, whereas in a large group practice, one medical assistant's entire day may be spent managing pegboard accounting or entering charges into a computer. Refer to Figure 13-1.

COMPONENTS OF PEGBOARD ACCOUNTING SYSTEMS

Pegboard accounting systems are available from most medical office supply companies. Although these systems vary slightly according to the manufacturer, all of them consist of the actual writing board and three basic components: (1) the superbill, (2) the ledger card, and (3) the daily log. In addition, a check register or cash disbursement component accompanies most systems. A typical pegboard is a hard writing board with pegs along the side or top. At the beginning of each day, a daily log is placed over the pegs to prepare for the first patient.

As the patient arrives and registers, the medical assistant retrieves the person's ledger card from the file and places it on top of the daily log. The assistant places a pad of sequentially numbered superbills on the pegs. With the set of three items in place on the pegs, the medical assistant writes the date, the patient's name, the previous balance, and the account number, if used, on the superbill. All of this information will automatically be posted through the carbon to the ledger card and daily log beneath. This process is repeated each time a patient registers for an appointment.

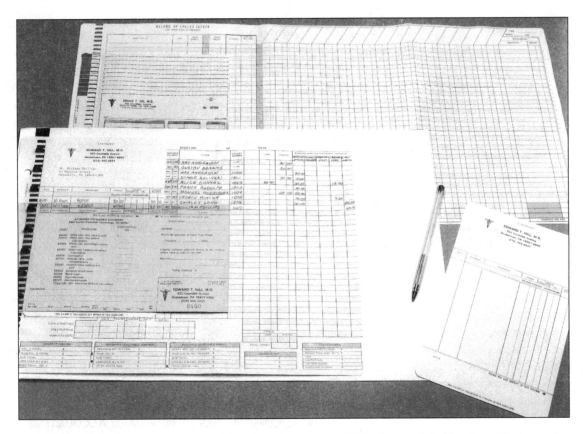

FIGURE 13-1 Pegboard accounting is one of the most important responsibilities in a medical office. A good background in pegboard accounting is useful to the medical assistant even when a computerized system is used.

At the end of the day, the daily log lists transactions for all patients seen during the day. The ledger cards are up to date and a superbill showing all charges and payments has been given to each patient. The bank deposits and day totals can also be developed.

Superbill or Receipt

The superbill, also known as a patient charge slip or a receipt, lists all the typical examinations, procedures, treatments, and services that a patient might have during one visit. Codes that identify each procedure and service performed by the medical staff are also printed on the superbill. *Current Procedural Terminology,* 4th Edition, (CPT-4), developed by the American Medical Association, is an industry coding standard recognized by most insurance companies and widely used in medical offices. Superbills are individualized by specialty. The services and procedures codes shown for a family physician

are different from the listings for a urologist, cardiologist, or other specialist. ICD-9 (*International Classification of Diseases, 9th Edition*) diagnosis codes are also printed on superbills in some offices, since Medicare and some insurance providers require these codes to document claims.

A comprehensive superbill that serves as an Attending Physician's Statement can be used to document an insurance claim or as evidence for the health maintenance organization (HMO). When accompanied by a partially completed claim form, it will be accepted in place of the fully completed form, saving time for both the patient and the medical assistant.

After a patient's name and other information are written on a superbill, the superbill is clipped to the medical record and follows the patient from the time of registration until after the examination is completed. During the examination, the physician marks (✓) or circles the appropriate code on the superbill to indicate the procedure or treatment performed and designates when the patient should return for a follow-up appointment. When the examination is complete, the physician gives the superbill to the patient, nurse, or medical assistant. The medical assistant then calculates the charges.

Using the fee schedule previously established by the physician, the medical assistant writes the charge for each service on the blank line beside the code number. The superbill is replaced in its original position on top of the daily log, then the ledger card is inserted between the superbill and daily log. As the charges, payments, adjustments, and the current balance are recorded in the proper columns of the superbill, the information is posted simultaneously to the ledger card and daily log beneath.

Ledger Card

The ledger card is a summary of one family's account with the practice and lists chronologically all financial activity for the account over a period of time. The name and address of the person responsible for the account and an account number, if used, are keyed at the top of the ledger card. Each time a family member visits the physician, the medical assistant retrieves the ledger card from the ledger card file and inserts it between the superbill and daily log on the pegboard. The assistant records information about the visit on a new line of the card. When all the lines of a ledger card are filled, a new ledger card is stapled to the first so there is no break in the chronological listings.

A new patient does not have an existing ledger card. Therefore, the medical assistant must prepare a new ledger card before beginning pegboard accounting activities. Chapter 12 contains information about creating a patient file, including instructions for preparing a ledger card. The new ledger card is then used just like an existing one.

The following information is automatically recorded on a ledger card when a superbill is completed: (1) the date of service, (2) the patient's name, (3) the professional service rendered, (4) the charge, (5) any payment or adjustment credits, and (6) the new balance. The

family's last name should also be recorded since the name of the person responsible for the account may be different from other members' names, especially in blended families.

The medical assistant also records payments made by mail and charges for hospital visits on the ledger card, although these are not usually recorded on a separate superbill. Information for posting mail payments and hospital charges is provided later in this chapter.

In some small offices, the ledger card is also used as a billing statement, and the word "Statement" appears at the top of the card instead of the word "Ledger Card." At the end of the billing period, a photocopy of the card is made and mailed to the responsible person. More often, however, payment is required at the time of the visit, or a computerized statement is developed and mailed by the physician's billing service.

Daily Log

The daily log is a summary of the medical office's daily financial activity; therefore a separate log will be started every morning. During the day, as each superbill is aligned over the daily log and completed, information is transferred automatically to the daily log. In addition, mail payments and hospital charges are transferred to the daily log when they are recorded on the ledger card. At the end of each day, the daily log shows a complete picture of all charges, payments and adjustments, and outstanding balances for each patient. After each column is totaled, a summary of the day's financial activity is provided.

Completing Patient Transactions

Patient financial transactions are divided into two categories: (1) those that take place at the time of the patient's visit to the physician's office, and (2) those that are made by mail or that are the result of a hospital visit. Although all three pegboard elements are used for an office visit, only the ledger card and daily log are required for recording mail payments and hospital visits.

TRANSACTION AT THE TIME OF A VISIT

Although most people have health insurance and file claims for reimbursement of their charges, the patient is ultimately responsible for the account. Some physicians require their patients to pay for services at the time of the visits; other physicians allow patients to charge all or a portion of their fees (Figure 13-2). When the office requires payment at the time of service, it is important to state this policy on a sign at the registration desk. Otherwise, some patients may not be prepared to pay, leading to embarrassment for everyone. If a practice accepts charge cards, this information should also be posted. See the following instructions for an overview of the beginning activities of a patient's financial transaction cycle.

Pegboard accounting provides an orderly, simple way of maintaining a patient's account. When a patient registers after arriving at the medical office, the medical assistant will start **beginning activities**. Following the examination, the medical assistant will perform **ending activities** to complete the transaction cycle.

Procedures for Beginning Patient Transactions

1. At the beginning of each day, attach a new daily log to the accounting pegboard.
2. Place the writing line of the first patient's superbill over the first blank line of the daily log. Make certain the headings on the superbill are aligned correctly with the headings on the daily log.
3. Write (1) the date, (2) the name of the patient, (3) the account's previous balance from the ledger card, (4) the name of the person responsible for paying the account, and (5) the account number, if used. (In Step 3, if there is no previous balance, draw a line or write "0" in the Previous Balance column.)
4. Clip the superbill to the front of the patient's medical record. Put the medical record in a standard location where the nurse or medical assistant can find it and deliver it to the physician.
5. When the next patient arrives, place the writing line of a new superbill on the next blank line of the daily log and follow Steps 3 and 4. Continue preparing superbills in this manner for all patients.

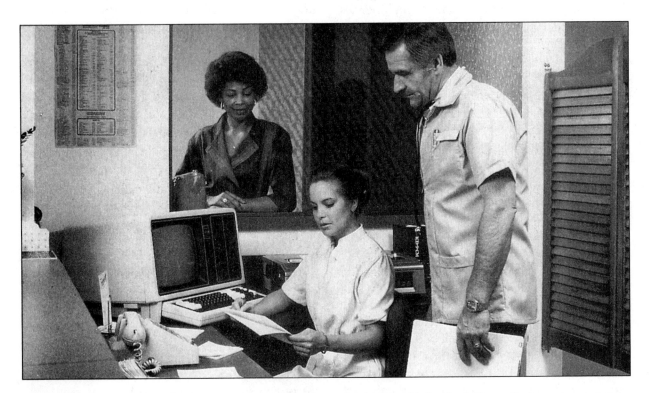

FIGURE 13-2 In some medical offices, patients must pay for services at the time of a visit; in other offices, patients can charge all or a portion of their fees.

When the patient, nurse, or medical assistant returns with the superbill after the examination, complete the following steps.

Procedures for Ending Patient Transactions
1. Review the procedures marked on the superbill by the physician or nurse. Write the predetermined fees your practice charges for these procedures on the blank line beside the procedure code. Total all the fees.
2. Place the patient's ledger card in the correct position on the daily log. Place the first blank line of the ledger card over the line of the daily log that lists the patient's name.
3. Place the writing line of the superbill over the writing line of the ledger card. Align the columns of the superbill with the columns of the ledger card.
4. In the Charges column at the top of the superbill, write the total of all fees.
5. In the Credits section at the top of the superbill, write the amount of payment that was made as well as any adjustments for previous overcharges.
6. Find the Current Balance by following these steps:
   a. Subtract today's Credits from today's Charges.
   b. Add the remainder, if there is one, to the Previous Balance.
   c. Write the Current Balance in the correct column. If the Current Balance is zero, write "0" or draw a line through the Current Balance column.
7. Separate the office copy of the superbill and place it in a special drawer where it will be kept for the person who maintains the physician's accounts.
8. Give the remaining copy of the superbill to the patient. The superbill serves as a statement of any remaining balance and as documentation for an insurance claim.
9. File the ledger card in the ledger card file.

PAYMENTS BY MAIL

A medical office that bills patients on a regular cycle receives many checks or money orders by mail. Sometimes, though not often, patients may also pay by cash at the office. In either case, the payment must be recorded on the ledger card and the daily log, bringing both the patient's financial record and the daily log up to date. A superbill is not necessary since no new service was performed. Except for cash payments, a receipt is not necessary since the canceled check serves as a valid receipt. Some superbills have a tear-off receipt portion.

Record all payments on the day they are received. To do this, retrieve the patient's ledger card from the ledger card file and place it on the daily log so that the first blank line of the daily log and the first blank line of the ledger card align.

Procedures for Recording Payments
1. Write the date.
2. Write "Mail Payment—Check" in the Description column if the payment is a personal check. If the payment is from an insurance company, write the name of the carrier.
3. Write the amount of payment in the Payment column.
4. Subtract the payment from the Current Balance.
5. Write the new balance in the Current Balance column.

Insurance companies sometimes combine payments for several patients in one check. When this occurs, refer to the explanation attached to the check and determine each account name or number and the amount that should be credited. Retrieve the ledger cards for each family's account and post them individually.

CHARGES FOR HOSPITAL VISITS

The method of recording a physician's daily visits to hospitalized patients varies. However, one of three methods is generally used: (1) daily recording to the ledger card and daily log, (2) at discharge with a superbill, and (3) at discharge with no superbill. Refer to Figure 13-3.

Daily Recording
Some medical offices record hospital visits each day on the patient's ledger card and on the daily log, but they do not use a daily superbill. At the time of the patient's discharge from the hospital, the office prepares a superbill showing total

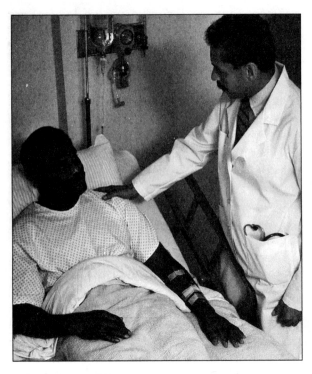

FIGURE 13-3 Some patient financial transactions are the result of a physician's hospital visit.

IN YOUR OPINION

1. What questions might a new medical assistant have about pegboard accounting?
2. Which of the three methods for recording hospital visits seems most efficient?
3. What training would help medical assistants who plan to handle pegboard accounting activities?

charges for hospital visits and mails it to the patient. With this method, the superbill replaces a routine statement. It is not used in combination with the ledger card and daily log.

At Discharge with a Superbill

Some medical offices maintain a list showing the dates of admittance for all hospitalized patients. As each patient is released from the hospital, total charges for the physician's daily visits are recorded on all three components of the pegboard accounting system by the write-it-once method. Then the superbill is mailed to replace a routine statement.

At Discharge with No Superbill

With the third method, total charges for the physician's daily hospital visits are recorded on the ledger card and daily log when the patient is discharged. A routine statement is then mailed during the normal billing cycle. With this method, a superbill is never used, and the patient's charges are not billed at the end of hospitalization unless the date coincides with the patient's routine cycle billing.

Supplemental Daily Log Information and Analyses

In addition to showing the daily summary of patient transactions, a daily log provides space for other financial data. Almost all systems provide a cross check of posting, an accounts receivable tally, and a cash tally. These are called proof of posting, accounts receivable control, and cash control. Depending on the manufacturer of the pegboard system, some or all of the following information may also be included: cash receipts summary, check summary, week-to-date summary, month-to-date summary, or year-to-date summary. Other special features individualized for the practice may include (1) columns for analyzing charges according to type of service or procedure and (2) columns for listing each physician's financial activity.

DAILY TOTALS AND MONTH-TO-DATE

A typical daily log will require daily totals for each column (for example, for Charges, Payments, Adjustments, Current Balance, and Previous Balance). To calculate month-to-date totals, transfer the month-to-date totals from each day and write them in the Previous Page section. Then calculate new month-to-date charges by adding Totals This Page to Previous Page Totals. Using a different daily log design with additional space, week-to-date totals can also be calculated for practices requiring this information.

PROOF OF POSTING

Proof of posting is important because it verifies the addition, subtraction, and calculations of each column. If the posting is done correctly at each transaction, the total of the Proof of Posting box should equal the total of Current Balance.

ACCOUNTS RECEIVABLE CONTROL

Accounts receivable provide a good measure of a practice's financial health because they show the amount of money its patients owe. When accounts receivable are too large, cash flow is low and the practice may have difficulty paying its bills. In this event, the practice must make a greater effort to collect a portion of the outstanding balances. Collection procedures are discussed in Chapter 15.

DAILY CASH PAID-OUTS

From time to time, the office will need cash for minor office expenses. A petty cash fund of $50 to $75 is usually set aside for this purpose. When money from petty cash is spent, a note should be made on the daily log indicating the amount and the purpose of the payment. Always keep receipts from purchases for tax purposes.

CASH CONTROL

Maintaining a daily summary of cash collected and paid out is important, since cash that is unaccounted for can disrupt the office's financial records (Figure 13-4). All cash over the amount kept in the petty cash fund should be deposited in the bank each day. Individuals handling cash should be bonded. Ask your insurance carrier how you can become bonded; this is usually a matter of paying an additional insurance premium.

BUSINESS ANALYSIS SUMMARIES

Some daily logs provide space for business analysis summaries, allowing for a breakdown of fees according to service or procedure performed or according to the service's provider. For example, the information that was transferred from the patient's superbills and the columns where the transactions are broken down according to the provider of the service could be reviewed. (Each transaction is probably listed under one of the physician's names.) In a

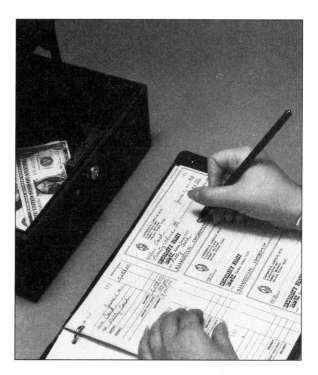

FIGURE 13-4 A petty cash fund is usually set aside for the purpose of using cash for minor office expenses.

group practice, this information provides a quick means of analyzing each physician's contribution to the practice in terms of daily fees. The breakdown can also show other summaries; for example, a summary of the services provided each day, including office visits, periodic examinations, laboratory, allergy injections, x-rays, surgery, and diagnostic services.

Daily Deposits

All checks and all cash in excess of the petty cash fund should be deposited in the bank each day. They should be endorsed "For Deposit Only" as soon as they are received. Some daily logs provide a space for listing checks for deposit; however, the bank at which the office has an account may provide a form. Use the following procedures when preparing a deposit slip.

Procedures for Preparing Deposit Slips
1. Count the currency and coins and compare the tally with the total from the Cash column of the daily log. Record the total amount of

cash to be deposited in the Cash column of the bank deposit slip (for example, $85).

2. Write the receipt number from the patient's superbill for the first check to be listed. When there is no superbill, write the name of the company or individual on whose account the check is drawn. Some physicians prefer to identify checks by the name of the person on whose account the check was drawn.

3. Write the American Banking Association (ABA) number that identifies the bank on which each check is drawn in the next column of the form. This number is usually printed in the upper right corner of checks and is the top number of a two-part number divided by a horizontal line.

4. Write the amount of each check.

5. Total the Cash and Checks column of the deposit slip. Compare this total with the Credits section from the daily log. If adjustments are shown for any patients, subtract them from the Credit section before the comparison is made, since adjustments are credits that do not involve an exchange of money. For example, an adjustment for an overcharge would not be included on the deposit slip.

Paying Office Accounts

One of your duties as a medical assistant may be to write checks on the medical office accounts. Although practice varies and some physicians employ an accountant to write checks and maintain accounts, in many small offices this responsibility belongs to the medical assistant. With a pegboard, a check register sheet, and padded checks with a carbonized writing strip on the back, you will find that the "write-it-once" system of pegboard accounting provides a simple manner of paying accounts and maintaining a current record.

CHECK REGISTER AND CHECKS

A check register is a record of checks issued that provides the following information: (1) the date of the check, (2) the number of the check, (3)

the name of the account being paid (the payee), and (4) the amount of the check. In addition, space is usually provided for listing bank deposits and showing a current bank balance. The check register sheet, which is similar to the daily log, has holes down the sides or across the top that fit over the pegs of a pegboard. When padded checks with a special carbonized strip are placed on top of the check register, the writing line of the first check aligns with the first blank line of the check register. Information written on the check is automatically transferred to the check register.

BUSINESS EXPENSE ANALYSIS

Check registers often provide additional space for maintaining an analysis of office expenses. In a typical pegboard with check register, space is provided for eleven accounts, including (1) building lease, (2) automobile lease, (3) equipment lease, (4) medical supplies, (5) office supplies, (6) professional development expenses, (7) travel, (8) insurance premiums, (9) janitorial service, (10) utilities, and (11) telephone. Categories vary according to the amount of accounting handled by the medical assistant and may also include payroll, taxes, and other expenses.

Check Register

Check register activities can be divided into two categories: writing checks and allocating payments to an office account. Before either of these functions can be completed, however, the pegboard must be prepared.

Procedures for Using a Check Register

1. Replace the daily log with a check register sheet. Position the holes in the sheet over the pegs of the pegboard.

2. Write the ending bank balance for the previous day (for example, $2,643.37).

3. If the check register is new, write the headings for the practice's accounts.

4. Place the packet of checks over the pegs so the Pay to the Order Of line of the first check aligns with the first blank line of the check register.

Writing Checks

If you are responsible for writing checks, you must have a mind for detail and a clear understanding of the importance of maintaining current accounts. If creditors are not paid on time, if payments are made improperly, or if office accounts are confused, the physician suffers embarrassment and ill will of the people who are owed money.

Procedures for Writing Checks

1. Flip the pad of checks to the left so only the smallest numbered check lies across the check register.
2. Write in full the amount of the check on the Pay line.
3. Write the name of the payee on the Pay to the Order Of line.
4. Write the date and the check number in the appropriate boxes.
5. Write the amount of the check.
6. Subtract the amount of the check from the Balance Brought Forward line. If any deposits were made since the last check was written, add the deposit. Write the new balance forward.

Balance Forward and Allocation of Payments

The medical assistant should determine the business account to which the payment should be allocated after each check is written and record the amount of the check in the proper column. The medical assistant must then calculate a new bank balance forward. If the company name does not identify the type of account being paid, the medical assistant may then refer to the invoice for which the check was written.

IN YOUR OPINION

1. Which software application discussed in previous chapters is most applicable to the kinds of transactions discussed above? Why?
2. What are several benefits to a practice of analyzing each doctor's production?
3. What are the advantages and disadvantages of a single individual handling all financial transactions?

Computerized Account Management

 Patient account management is the most widely used computer application in medical offices. Account management software is used to prepare the patient charge slip or superbill, develop medical reports, complete billing statements, and prepare insurance claim forms. Computerized management of patient accounts can save a medical practice thousands of dollars a year by eliminating costly human errors, accelerating the collection process, and handling routine clerical and accounting activities. With account management software, medical office employees are relieved of routine, time-consuming activities such as posting, billing, and collection. As a medical assistant, you may be asked to use the computer's account management software as part of your daily responsibilities. Several medical software programs are in use in medical offices today. The figures on the following pages come from one popular package, *The Medical Manager*.

PATIENT ACCOUNTS

A software management program offers many advantages in managing patient accounts. The program automatically creates a patient charge slip at the time of each patient's visit and calculates the charges after the physician's examination. The management program also creates and updates the ledger card; adds new names to the list of patients and to the daily log; and transfers data to produce insurance forms, statements, a list of checks received each day, and deposit slips. In addition, the program automatically ages accounts at each billing cycle and creates billing statements. As a result, when patient accounts are computerized, practice collections usually increase.

On a patient's first visit to the medical office, the individual is asked to complete a personal information form. This includes the name and address of the person responsible for payment of the account, the name and address of the responsible person's insurance company, and the policy number. Other information, such as whether the account should receive credit messages and finance charges is also entered into the computer. All of this information can be entered quite quickly. After this initial information, charges, payments, and adjustments will be entered as they occur during the course of the patient's care.

 Figure 13-5 shows an information form completed by the patient during the first office visit. Figure 13-6 shows the first patient information screen after this information has been entered in *The Medical Manager*. Several other screens will be required to enter all the patient's information.

DAILY ACTIVITIES

The computer is also useful for managing an office's daily activities. Each day several activities must be completed to ensure that the practice operates efficiently. These activities include (1) preparing a daily list of appointments; (2) completing a charge slip, a ledger card, and a portion of the daily log for each patient; and (3) preparing a daily cash and check register.

The Daily List of Appointments

Medical offices that are computerized usually have programs to handle appointment scheduling. Such a program can generate a daily list of appointments automatically. If scheduling software is not available, the medical assistant will prepare a daily list of appointments at the end of each day or at the beginning of each morning, and distribute it to all staff members who work with patients. It is easy to compile the daily list by simply entering the names from the appointment book in the computer. When the medical assistant enters the first patient's name, the computer supplies the account number, if used, the name or identification number of the physician, and the balance due on the account. After the medical assistant enters the appointment time and reason for the visit for the first patient, the computer is ready for the next patient's information to be entered. When the medical assistant has entered all of the day's appointments, a list of the appointments for each physician or a master list showing appointments for several physicians in a practice can be print-

ed. If appointment scheduling is competely computerized, the computer will generate a daily list of appointments automatically, which eliminates the need for the above procedure.

Computerized Patient Charge Slip

When a patient arrives for treatment, the name the medical assistant enters in the computer and a patient charge slip prints automatically. This slip, sometimes called a superbill, is attached to the medical record and taken to the examination room. Following the examination, the physician or nurse circles the treatment or treatment code and enters only nonstandard fees, if applicable. Next, the charge slip is returned to the medical assistant, who enters the diagnosis codes and procedure codes in the computer. By matching procedures codes to the preset fee schedule stored in the computer's memory, the program calculates the day's charges. After payments or credits are entered in the system, the program will calculate an ending balance. Finally, a copy of the completed patient charge slip is presented to the patient as a receipt. This slip gives information about the patient's account and serves as a reminder of any overdue balance. A computerized patient charge slip is shown in Figure 13-7.

Computerized Patient Ledger

The computerized patient ledger contains personal information about each patient; including the name, address, and telephone number, the person responsible for payment, and all insurance carriers. The ledger also lists all previous office visits and the procedures, procedure codes, charges, payments, and adjustments for each visit. Most account management software can be customized to meet the special needs of an individual medical office.

As information is entered from the circled patient charge slip, the computer automatically updates the ledger by adding a description of each procedure and procedure code and each diagnosis and diagnosis code. It automatically posts the charges and calculates the balance after credits and adjustments are entered.

The ledger may be viewed on the computer screen, or printed out at any time. If a patient calls with a question regarding an account, the

Patient No: 10

Doctor: Carrington, #3
Bill Type: 11
Extended Info: Yes

Patient Registration Form

Sydney Carrington and Associates - 34 Sycamore Street - Madison, CA 95653   TODAY'S DATE: _1/10/89_

Carlson	Steven	W	(916) 988-3293	(916) 988-6495
RESPONSIBLE PARTY LAST NAME	FIRST NAME	MI	(AREA CODE) HOME PHONE	(AREA CODE) WORK PHONE

3456 West Palm #34
MAILING ADDRESS

345-65-3434   M   11/16/20
SOCIAL SECURITY NUMBER   SEX M/F   DATE OF BIRTH

_____
STREET ADDRESS (IF DIFFERENT)

Hite Telecommunications Co. (Retired)
EMPLOYER NAME

Madison	CA	95653
CITY	STATE	ZIP CODE

87 S Main Street
EMPLOYER ADDRESS

Leland Groves, M.D.
REFERRED BY:

Floral City CA 90083   (916) 988-6495
EMPLOYER (CITY, STATE, & ZIP)   PHONE

IF YOU HAVE DEPENDENTS WHO ARE ALSO BEING SEEN AS PATIENTS, PLEASE FILL IN:

Sharon A. Carlson
FIRST DEPENDENT'S NAME

_____
SECOND DEPENDENT'S NAME

3/13/25	F	Wife	643-86-5639
DATE OF BIRTH	SEX	RELATIONSHIP	SOC. SECURITY #

DATE OF BIRTH	SEX	RELATIONSHIP	SOC. SECURITY #

Madison County Hospital   (916) 436-5910
EMPLOYER OR SCHOOL   PHONE

_____   _____
EMPLOYER OR SCHOOL   PHONE

234 Lincoln Rd Madison CA 95651
ADDRESS OF EMPLOYER OR SCHOOL

_____
ADDRESS OF EMPLOYER OR SCHOOL

INSURANCE INFORMATION: (YOU DO NOT NEED TO FILL IN ADDRESS IF YOUR INSURANCE IS MEDICARE, MEDICAID, CHAMPUS, OR BC/BS)

Pan American Health Ins
NAME OF PRIMARY INSURANCE COMPANY

9876-086546
IDENTIFICATION #

Madison County Hospital
GROUP NAME AND/OR #

4567 Newberry Rd	Los Angeles	CA	98706	
ADDRESS	CITY	STATE	ZIP CODE	PHONE

Sharon A. Carlson
INSURED PERSON'S NAME (IF DIFFERENT FROM THE RESPONSIBLE PARTY)

_____
ADDRESS (IF DIFFERENT)   CITY   STATE   ZIP

643-86-5639	(916) 436-5910	Husband	
SOCIAL SECURITY #	PHONE	WHAT IS THE RESPONSIBLE PARTY'S RELATIONSHIP TO THE INSURED?	

SECONDARY INSURANCE

I also have Medicare - 34563434A
Epsilon Life & Casualty
NAME OF SECONDARY INSURANCE COMPANY

M5A876587665
IDENTIFICATION #

_____
GROUP NAME AND/OR #

P.O. Box 189	Macon	CA	98706	(415) 456-7654
ADDRESS	CITY	STATE	ZIP CODE	PHONE

Steven W. Carlson
INSURED PERSON'S NAME (IF DIFFERENT FROM THE RESPONSIBLE PARTY)

_____
ADDRESS (IF DIFFERENT)   CITY   STATE   ZIP

345-65-3434	(916) 988-3293	Self	
SOCIAL SECURITY #	PHONE	WHAT IS THE RELATIONSHIP TO THE INSURED?	

FIGURE 13-5 Patient registration form (Adapted from Gartee and Humphrey, *The Medical Manager, Student Edition, Version 5.3,* copyright 1995, Delmar Publishers)

Guarantor: Carlson   Account #: 18

* Guarantor's Information *

First name: Steven   M.I.: W   Home Phone #: (916) 988-3293

Street Address1: 3456 West Palm #34   Work Phone #: (916) 988-6495

Street Address2:   Date of Birth: 11/16/28   pc: N

City: Madison   State: CA   Social Sec. #: 345-65-3434

Zip Code: 95653   Sex (M/F): M   Patient ID #:

* Account Information *

Account Date: 01/10/—   Ref Dr #:2 Leland W Groves M.D.

# of Dependents: 1   Doctor #: 3 Sydney Carrington, M.D.

# of Ins Plans: 3   Status: 1 Active

Extended Info Level: 2 Full   Bill Type: 11   Class:

                               Note #: 8   WP ID: WP18.8

[   ]

Discount %: 0   Budget Pmt: 0.00

FIGURE 13-6 Computerized information form (First Screen) (Adapted from Gartee and Humphrey, *The Medical Manager, Student Edition, Version 5.3,* copyright 1995, Delmar Publishers)

| VICTORIA McHUGH, M.D. 102 FREDERICKS RD. NEW YORK, NY 10012-0000 | STATEMENT DATE 08/29/-- PATIENT NUMBER 113 PREVIOUS BALANCE $0.00 | | OFFICE PHONE: (404) 555-0078 |

DATE	CODE	DESCRIPTION	AMOUNT
02/12/--	00000	BALANCE FORWARD	23.00
02/16/--	71020	CHEST X RAY, 2 VIEWS	40.00
03/14/--	81000	URINALYSIS	20.00
04/22/--	85022	CBC	12.50
06/13/--	99221	INIT. HOSP. EXAM, EXTENSIVE	75.00
07/05/--	93040	RHYTHM STRIP	17.00
07/26/--	93000	ELECTROCARDIOGRAM	35.00
08/29/--	PMT	PERSONAL CHECK	-93.65 CR
		BALANCE DUE	$128.85

STATEMENT DATE 08/29/--	
CURRENT	0.00
OVER 30-DAYS:	52.00
OVER 60-DAYS:	75.00
OVER 90-DAYS:	1.85
BALANCE DUE	$128.85

THANK YOU FOR YOUR PAYMENT.

113

| OFFICE CLOSED SEPTEMBER 5TH. NEW CHARGES HAVE BEEN SENT TO YOUR INSURANCE CARRIER(S). | VICTORIA McHUGH, M.D. 102 FREDERICKS RD. NEW YORK, NY 10012-0000 | LINDA B. HAYLEY 532 5TH STREET ATLANTA, GA 30033-2385 |

FIGURE 13-7 Computerized patient bill (From Claeys, *Medical Filing,* copyright 1993, Delmar Publishers)

```
                        PATIENT LEDGER
                        ================

    Patient #218          WALRATH, MARY              Date:  06/24/--
                          206 COL. DE WEES DRIVE
                          WAYNE, PA  19087           PHONE: (404) 555-6123

             Insured #1                    Insured #2

             SAME                          WALRATH, FRANCIS
                                           206 COL. DE WEES DRIVE
                                           WAYNE, PA  19087

    Insurance #1:  PRUDENTIAL    Policy #:  987654321    Group #:  987700
    Insurance #2:  BLUE CROSS    Policy #:  321654907    Group #:  123456987

    =================================================================

    01/26/--    59400    TOTAL OBSTETRICAL CARE              1200.00
    01/26/--    99202    INTERMEDIATE EXAM, NEW PT.            30.00
    01/26/--    88150    PAPANICOLAOU SMEAR                    18.50
    01/26/--    PMT        DEPOSIT OB CARE                   -250.00
    02/18/--    PMT        Insur. Pmt.   01/26/-- 90015       -20.00
    02/18/--    ADJ        Adj. Cat. #1 01/26/-- 90015        -10.00
    02/25/--    85022    CBC                                   12.50
    02/25/--    99212    LIMITED EXAM, ESTAB. PT.              15.00
    02/25/--    PMT        Cash Pmt.   01/26/-- 94000         -75.00
    04/26/--    85022    CBC                                   12.50
    04/26/--    99212    LIMITED EXAM, ESTAB. PT.              15.00
    04/26/--    76805    DIAGNOSTIC ULTRASOUND                 55.00
    04/26/--    88150    PAPANICOLAOU SMEAR                    18.50
                                                          ------------
                        Balance for MARY WALRATH          $1,022.00
```

FIGURE 13-8 Computerized patient ledger card (From Claeys, *Medical Filing,* copyright 1993, Delmar Publishers)

medical assistant can call up the ledger on the screen by entering the patient's name. When a correction is needed it can be made on the screen and stored. Figure 13-8 shows a posted ledger account produced by computer.

Computerized Daily Log

The daily log is generated from information posted to accounts each day. At the end of the day, the computer can produce a daily log that reports payments, charges, and adjustments by patient name and account number. These reports usually show the total number of patients seen each day, as well as the day's total billings, collections, and adjustments. You can also post broken appointments and "no-shows," so they can be printed on the daily log. Including these appointments explains the broken sequential numbering on the patient charge slips. The daily log can be customized according to the financial reporting needs of a practice, whether it is run

by a single physician or by a large group. A daily log produced by computer is shown in Figure 13-9.

Cash and Check Register

In addition to the capabilities already discussed, the computer can also be used to make a daily listing of all cash and checks received. The program searches through all the transactions completed for each patient during the day and calculates the amount of cash received and the amount paid by check. Then a check register showing each check number, the American Banking Association number, the amount of the check, and the patient's name and account number can be printed. A check register can be printed for one physician or for several physicians in a practice. The check register can be attached to a bank deposit slip, thereby requiring no further manual work. A check register is shown in Figure 13-10.

Sydney Carrington, M.D. (3)

Account	Patient Name	Dt Post	Type	Dates of Service	Dept	Voucher	[to Vchr Total] Proc Code	Units	Pri/Sec		Ail	St	Amount
10.0	Carlson, Steven	01/10/—	CHG	01/10/—	0	1050	99214	1	2/	5	N	2	50.00
10.1	Carlson, Sharon	01/10/—	CHG	01/10/—	0	1051	99213	1	7/	0	N	2	40.00
34.0	Dudley, Wayne	01/10/—	CHG	01/10/—	0	1053	99215	1	6/	0	N	2	85.00
34.0	Dudley, Wayne	01/10/—	CHG	01/10/—	0	1053	76499	1	6/	0	N	2	150.00
34.0	Dudley, Wayne	01/10/—	CHG	01/10/—	0	1053	81000	1	6/	0	N	2	8.00
34.0	Dudley, Wayne	01/10/—	CHG	01/10/—	0	1053	85014	1	6/	0	N	2	18.00
34.0	Dudley, Wayne	01/10/—	CHG	01/10/—	0	1053	93000	1	6/	0	N	2	57.00
110.0	Evans, Patrlcia	01/10/—	CHG	01/10/—	0	1056	99214	1	5/	0	Y	2	50.00
110.0	Evans, Patrlcia	01/10/—	CHG	01/10/—	0	1056	71020	1	5/	0	Y	2	125.00
110.0	Evans, Patrlcia	01/10/—	CHG	01/10/—	0	1056	76088	1	5/	0	Y	2	58.00
21.2	Edwards, Andrea	01/10/—	CHG	01/10/—	0	1057	99213	1	5/	0	Y	2	40.00
21.2	Edwards, Andrea	01/10/—	CHG	01/10/—	0	1057	81000	1	5/	0	Y	2	8.00
21.2	Edwards, Andrea	01/10/—	CHG	01/10/—	0	1057	85014	1	5/	0	Y	2	18.00

Summary for: Sydney Carrington, M.D.

Item Description	Today 01/10/—	Period-to-Date 01/01/— – 01/10/—	Year-to-Date 01/01/— – 01/10/—
Total Charges	707.00	707.00	707.00
Total Receipts	0.00	0.00	0.00
Total Adjustments	0.00	0.00	0.00
Accounts Receivable	707.00	707.00	707.00
Total # Procedures	13	13	13
Service Charges	0.00	. . . .	. . . .
Tax Charges	0.00	. . . .	. . . .
Deposit Amount	0.00`	. . . .	. . . .

FIGURE 13-9 Daily log report (Adapted from Gartee and Humphrey, *The Medical Manager, Student Edition, Version 5.3,* copyright 1995, Delmar Publishers)

PRACTICE MANAGEMENT

The financial success of a medical practice depends on accurate, up-to-date records and analyses. Computer systems allow the medical office to develop a wide variety of reports in a minimum amount of time. For example, these reports can show how physician and staff time is spent, what procedures are used most often, and how income is generated from the practice. Since each computer system can generate different kinds of reports, the software manual for a particular system provides information to allow a practice to take advantage of what it offers. Several practice management reports are discussed in the next section.

Practice Analysis

A practice analysis provides a quick overview of the procedures and treatments provided daily, weekly, monthly, or yearly, and the amount of income they produce. The analysis shows how income is derived; whether from cash, personal checks, insurance payments, or government-related programs. It also shows adjustments and

<table>
<tr><td colspan="4" align="center">BANK DEPOSIT   08/18/—</td></tr>
<tr><td colspan="4" align="center">BANK: First National</td></tr>
<tr><td colspan="4" align="center">TOTAL DEPOSIT: $ 571.63</td></tr>
</table>

#	BANK/CHECK #	DESCRIPTION	AMOUNT
1	RD Initial	KEELER 2120424	9.75
2	IVF	KEELER 2120424	18.03
3	payment;	HUNT 1060612	14.83
4	AARP;	ABRAMEK 1110117	14.83
5	AARP;	EMERSON 1121515	9.58
6	AARP;	DAVENPORT 1122716	6.36
7	AARP;	OFNER 1060913	9.58
8	AARP;	THRAN 1012414	6.36
9	BANKERS LI;	HEDRICK 1082613	83.98
10	BANKERS LI;	BASANKO 2032324	6.36
11	IC;	DEHART 2051513	83.98
12	IC;	SWARTZ 1061916	9.58
13	IC;	CAMPBELL 2051021	6.36
14	IC;	CAMPBELL 2051021	10.04
15	IC;	CAMPBELL 2051021	6.36
16	IC;	SWARTZ 1081213	14.83
17	IC;	GENTERT 1031009	260.82

FIGURE 13-10 Check register

payments. A medical assistant may be asked to provide regular practice analyses for an employer.

By reviewing the practice analysis, a physician can make important management decisions that will increase income. The first block of data shown in the Daily Report for Sydney Carrington in Figure 13-11 on the firm's practice analysis lists the daily transactions and dollar volume of each physician. Period-to-date and year-to-date totals are shown in the second and third blocks of data.

Cross-Posting Report

A computer system can track the application of fees for group practices when the physicians provide service for one another's patients. Fees can be reported on a daily, weekly, or monthly basis by means of a cross-posting report as shown in Figure 13-12.

IN YOUR OPINION

1. How can a background in pegboard accounting help you with computerized accounting?
2. Will the introduction of computerized accounting in medical offices result in the addition or loss of jobs for medical assistants who are no longer needed for pegboard accounting? Explain your answer.
3. What steps can be taken to make the transition from a pegboard system to a computerized system easier for staff members?

REFERENCES

Gartee, Richard, and Doris D. Humphrey. *The Medical Manager.* Cincinnati, Ohio: South-Western Publishing Co., 1995.*

Taylor, Dorothy, A., and Lewis B. Keeling. *Medical Pegboard Procedures.* Cincinnati, Ohio: South-Western Publishing Co., 1987.*

*Currently published by Delmar Publishers.

TOTALS FOR 04/03—

Doctor	Charges	Receipts	Adjustments	Net A/R	Total A/R	# Proc.	Serv Chg	Tax Chg
1. James Monroe, M.D.	0.00	−24.00	0.00	24.00	46.00	0	0.00	0.00
3. Sydney Carrington, M.D.	0.00	−266.00	0.00	266.00	969.20	0	0.00	0.00
TOTAL	0.00	−290.00	0.00	290.00	1,015.20	0	0.00	0.00

PERIOD-TO-DATE TOTALS FOR 01/01/— – 04/03—

Doctor	Charges	Receipts	Adjustments	Net A/R	Total A/R	# Proc.	Serv Chg	Tax Chg
1. James Monroe, M.D.	202.00	144.00	12.00	46.00	46.00	7	. . . .	. . . .
2. Frances Simpson, M.D.	206.00	0.00	40.00	166.00	166.00	5	. . . .	. . . .
3. Sydney Carrington, M.D.	1,401.00	422.80	9.00	969.20	969.20	27	. . . .	. . . .
TOTAL	1,809.00	566.80	61.00	1,181.20	1,181.20	39	. . . .	. . . .

YEAR-TO-DATE TOTALS FOR 01/01/— – 04/03/—

Doctor	Charges	Receipts	Adjustments	Net A/R	Total A/R	# Proc.	Serv Chg	Tax Chg
1. James Monroe, M.D.	202.00	144.00	12.00	46.00	46.00	7	. . . .	. . . .
2. Frances Simpson, M.D.	206.00	0.00	40.00	166.00	166.00	5	. . . .	. . . .
3. Sydney Carrington, M.D	1,401.00	422.80	9.00	969.20	969.20	27	. . . .	. . . .
TOTAL	1,809.00	566.80	61.00	1,181.20	1,181.20	39	. . . .	. . . .

FIGURE 13-11 Daily practice analysis (Adapted from Gartee and Humphrey, *The Medical Manager, Student Edition, Version 5.3,* copyright 1995, Delmar Publishers)

Cross-Posting Totals for: 08/10/—

Primary Physician: Sydney Carrington

Repeating Physician	Charges	Adjustments	Payments
James Monroe, M.D.	187.50	35.00	132.50
Frances Simpson, M.D.	200.00		100.00

FIGURE 13-12 Cross-posting report

Chapter Activities

PERFORMANCE BASED ACTIVITIES

1. Set up a summary for a daily log. In the columns "Office Visit," "Laboratory," "Injections," and "Emergencies," list the medical fees given here. Then analyze the summary to determine the types of service performed most often. Based on the summary, which staff members do you think are busiest?

Brook Raines	Level IV Office Visit, New Patient, $125; Urinalysis, $16; Complete Blood Check, $15
Martin Omar	Level III Office Visit, Established Patient, $58; Allergy Injection, $35
Majik Bonak	Level IV Office Visit, Established Patient $87; DPT shot, $35
Michelle Chung	Emergency Visit, $150
Charles Victor	Level III Office Visit, Established Patient, $58; Throat Culture, $26
Susan Ankar	Emergency Hospital Visit, $60
Barbara Ross	Allergy Injection, $30
Ashley Wilson	Level III Office Visit, New Patient, $83
Lawrence Rawley	Emergency Visit, $120
Santigo Mendez	Level III Office Visit, Established Patient, $58

(DACUM 8.1, 8.4, 8.6)

	Patient Identification	Office Visit	Laboratory	Injections	Emergencies
1.	_____	_____	_____	_____	_____
2.	_____	_____	_____	_____	_____
3.	_____	_____	_____	_____	_____
4.	_____	_____	_____	_____	_____
5.	_____	_____	_____	_____	_____
6.	_____	_____	_____	_____	_____
7.	_____	_____	_____	_____	_____
8.	_____	_____	_____	_____	_____
9.	_____	_____	_____	_____	_____
10.	_____	_____	_____	_____	_____

2. Following the procedures outlined in this chapter, determine the current balance for each of these patients (use the form on the following page):

	Old Balance	Today's Charges	Today's Payment
David Sebert	0	$60, 22, 16	$85
Rawley Ashburn-Myers	$16	$48, 38, 16	$75
Nancy O'Grady	$323	$46, 75, 18	$125
Tishee Bryant	$86	$46, 34, 22	$135
Carmen Sanchez	0	$70, 36, 20, 18	$120
Roulff Berquest	$122	$85, 25, 18	$175

Old Balance + Today's Charges – Today's Payment = New Balance

Patient	Old Balance	Today's Charges	Today's Payment	New Balance
1. _____	_____	_____	_____	_____
2. _____	_____	_____	_____	_____
3. _____	_____	_____	_____	_____
4. _____	_____	_____	_____	_____
5. _____	_____	_____	_____	_____
6. _____	_____	_____	_____	_____

(DACUM 8.1, 8.4, 8.6)

3. Complete the following chart by filling in the correct responses.

Situation	Action/Answer
An established patient has arrived at the medical office. Trace the path of his computerized superbill from creation to end of visit.	
On days the computerized monthly billing is prepared, the computer is tied up so frequently that patients must wait for their superbills. Develop a correction for this problem.	
Some medical assistants in your office continue to use a typewriter for keying letters even though the computer is available. Make suggestions for involving all medical assistants in computing.	
Your employer, who was out of town for several days, asked another physician to treat her patients. Now your employer wants to know the dollar amount of fees that were applied to other physicians. Explain how you will develop this information.	

(DACUM 3.4, 8.1, 8.4, 8.6)

EXPANDING YOUR THINKING

1. Compare the steps for entering information for a new patient's account in (1) the computer system used at your mentoring practice, and (2) the system used at school. Summarize the similarities and differences.

Process to Enter a New Patient's Account

Steps *Medical Practice System*   *School System*

1. _____   _____

2. _____   _____

3. _____   _____

4. _____   _____

5. _____   _____

6. _____   _____

7. _____   _____

8. _____   _____

9. _____   _____

10. _____   _____

Additional Steps

_____   _____

_____   _____

_____   _____

_____   _____

_____   _____

_____   _____

_____   _____

_____   _____

_____   _____

_____   _____

_____   _____

_____   _____

Chapter 14

Health Insurance and Alternative Financing Plans

CHILOQUIN, OREGON

Health care is such an involved issue. I understand why people are confused. As I process health insurance forms to be sent to a variety of public and private insurance companies, I see how expensive health care really is. Some people think the government should pay the health care costs for people who can't pay for their own care. These government programs are not free, of course. Your taxes and mine pay for them.

Oregon was one of the first states to put some limits on its Medicaid program, and it caused quite an uproar in the state and across the country. Our legislature made a list of 709 ailments and their treatments and ranked them according to the cost of treatment and the likely success of treatment. For example, pneumonia was No. 1 because it is inexpensive to treat and is usually curable. Procedures such as neonatal care for newborns weighing less than 1½ pounds, coronary bypass operations for patients over 80, and bone marrow transplants for advanced breast cancer patients were near the bottom; they are very expensive and not often successful in prolonging life. These patients might be covered by other types of insurance, of course, but Oregon's legislature said that there's no such thing as a free health care program, and we have to draw the line somewhere.

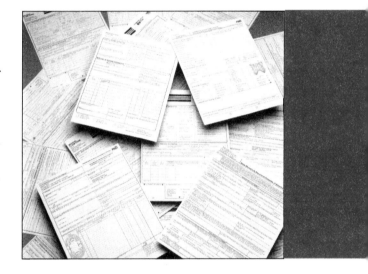

When I first heard about government guaranteed health care for all people, I thought it was a good idea. I still think these programs are necessary, but I, along with a lot of other people, have a lot of questions. You could classify them under the heading of personal responsibility, I guess. It bothers me when a heart attack patient continues to smoke cigarettes after being removed from an oxygen tent, and I wonder how long the state can pay for the health care needs of women who have no source of income but continue to have babies. I wonder how many people think as I do?

Christen Johannsen
Medical Assistant/Claims Examiner

PERFORMANCE BASED COMPETENCIES

After completing this chapter, you should be able to:

1. Use current procedural terminology and ICD-9 coding. (DACUM 8.2)
2. Analyze and use current third-party guidelines for reimbursement. (DACUM 8.3)
3. Place a patient in a diagnosis-related group (DRG). (DACUM 8.2)
4. Complete an HFCA-1500 form. (DACUM 8.3)
5. Set up an audit trail for health insurance claims. (DACUM 8.3)

HEALTHSPEAK

Basic insurance Insurance benefits that cover physicians' fees, hospital expenses, and surgical fees as determined by the plan contract, usually after payment of a deductible by the patient.

Blue Cross and Blue Shield Nonprofit insurers organized under the laws of individual states; generally, Blue Shield pays for physicians' services and Blue Cross covers hospital costs.

Commercial insurance For-profit companies offering individual or group health insurance.

Comprehensive insurance Combination of basic and major medical insurance.

Copayment Percent of medical expenses for which the patient is responsible beyond the deductible.

Deductible Amount paid by a patient prior to initiation of insurance benefits.

Diagnosis-related group (DRG) Method of classifying patients into categories based on the primary diagnosis.

Group insurance Coverage of a group of people based on a common characteristic, such as employment at a company.

Major medical insurance Insurance designed to offset potentially catastrophic expenses from a lengthy illness or accident.

Medicaid Government health insurance program that protects the poor.

Medicare Government health insurance program that protects the elderly.

Prospective payment Term describing a method of flat fee pricing.

Workers' compensation insurance Employer-paid insurance that provides health care and income to employees and their dependents when employees suffer work-related injuries or illness.

From 1965 to 1991, spending on health care in the United States soared from 5.9 to 13.2 percent of all spending in the economy. National health care costs are expected to continue to soar, as shown in Figure 14-1, from *Newsweek,* October 4, 1993. Sixteen percent of all government expenditures are on health care, up from 2.6 percent in 1965. No country in the world has experienced the same rapid growth in health care costs relative to other expenditures, such as food, housing, and education. Each additional dollar required for health care is one less dollar in the consumer's pocket for food and clothing, in the employer's pocket for wages and investment, or in the government's pocket for schools and roads.

Someone has to pay for this level of care. Because few families can afford to pay the expenses of a catastrophic illness or even the routine medical expenses of a family, most Americans purchase insurance protection individually or through an organization. The federal government's Medicare and the states' Medicaid programs cover health care for the elderly and the poor. Again, according to *Newsweek,* October 4, 1993, 78 percent of all medical bills are paid by insurance or government.

Health insurance enables people to prepare financially for the high cost of an unexpected illness or injury by purchasing protection for an annual premium. Over the last two decades, escalating health care costs have generated sev-

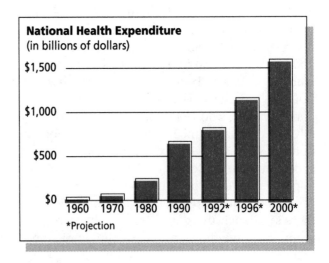

FIGURE 14-1 The soaring cost of health care (Courtesy of *Newsweek,* October 4, 1993, Source: Congressional Budget Office)

eral alternative financing plans besides the traditional private office, fee-for-service physician arrangement.

As a medical assistant, you will learn the differences among the plans under which patients are covered. Frequently, you will interpret benefits for patients in order to collect the practice's fees properly. Although patients are ultimately responsible for paying their accounts, they usually pay only a small portion of the costs of illnesses or accidents themselves, and some form of insurance pays for the remainder. Because the livelihoods of the physician and staff of a medical facility depend on income from insurance sources, managing insurance payments will be a fundamental part of your duties as a medical assistant.

Types of Health Insurance Coverage

In general, health insurance can be categorized in three ways: basic coverage, major medical coverage, and comprehensive coverage. The amount of premium a subscriber or purchaser pays determines the degree of protection a policy offers.

BASIC INSURANCE

Although insurance policies vary widely, certain general benefits are available in most basic policies. The physician's fee, hospital expenses up to a maximum amount, and surgical fees as determined in the contract are generally covered by basic insurance. Payment may be based on a "usual and customary fee," or the content may specify a stated amount. Many policies require a deductible or copayment from the patient with the patient typically paying the first $100, $200, or more of annual medical costs in addition to 20 percent of the remaining charges. For example, the patient whose medical expenses amount to $500 during one year might be required to pay a $200 deductible and an additional $60 ($500 − $200 × 20 percent). The insurance company would reimburse the patient for $240.

Hospital benefits for basic insurance may pay a certain dollar amount for a specified number of days, or they may pay full charges for a specific type of room, usually semi-private (two patients per room), for a specified number of days. Inpatient services such as laboratory tests, x-rays, operating room, anesthesia, surgical dressings, and some outpatient services, though not all, are usually included (Figure 14-2). Some plans cover extended care at a skilled nursing facility after a patient's release from a hospital. A basic policy usually covers all or a portion of maternity care.

MAJOR MEDICAL INSURANCE

Major medical, or catastrophic, insurance takes up where basic insurance leaves off and is designed to help offset huge medical expenses that would result from a lengthy illness or serious accident. Most major medical policies include a deductible amount as well as a coinsurance provision that calls for an additional percentage, usually 20 percent, to be paid by the patient. Benefits, which usually range from $10,000 to unlimited coverage, determine the amount of premium. They cover health services and supplies beyond those available in basic policies, including the services of special nurses, rental of medical equipment, prosthetic devices, and related items (Figure 14-3).

COMPREHENSIVE MAJOR MEDICAL INSURANCE

Comprehensive major medical insurance combines the benefits of basic medical and major medical protection. Coverage usually includes a small deductible and provides broad medical treatment under one contract.

Health Care Financing Plans

Americans have a choice of several major types of health care financing plans. They are Blue Cross and Blue Shield, commercial insurance companies, health maintenance organizations, preferred provider organizations, Medicare and Medicaid, and other government programs.

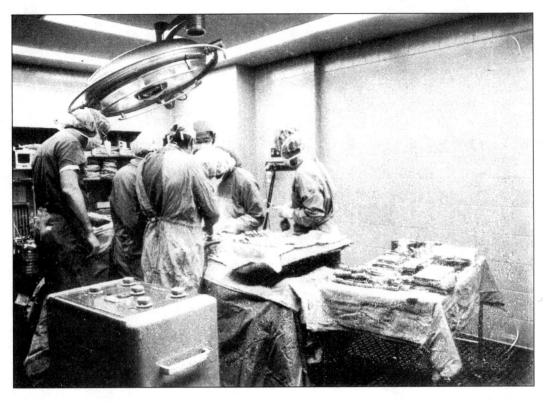

FIGURE 14-2 Operating room services are among the in-patient services that are usually covered by basic insurance.

BLUE CROSS AND BLUE SHIELD

Blue Cross and Blue Shield are nonprofit insurers organized under the laws of the individual states and regulated by boards of directors made up of public representatives, physicians, and other health care providers. Generally, Blue Shield plans pay for the services of physicians and other providers, and Blue Cross plans pay for hospital services. A patient may subscribe to either plan or to a combined plan. Each Blue Cross/Blue Shield plan develops and administers its own benefits package, although both plans usually cover groups of people with a common characteristic; for example, all the employees of a single company.

Commercial Insurance Companies

Aetna Life and Casualty, Prudential Insurance, Equitable Life Assurance Society, The Travelers Companies, and other similar companies are for-profit organizations that offer individual or group basic health and major medical insurance for an annual premium. In addition to health coverage, most sell other forms of insurance such as fire, theft, life, and casualty insurance.

HEALTH MAINTENANCE ORGANIZATIONS

About 50 million people belong to health maintenance organizations (HMOs). For a monthly pay-in-advance membership or annual prepayment, each insured person is guaranteed physician and hospital services for little or no additional charge. Patients are attracted to HMOs because they guarantee no unexpected medical costs.

Health maintenance organizations sometimes operate their own clinics with a salaried staff of physicians, or they may contract with groups of private physicians to provide service to members. In general, HMO members receive full medical services only if they use the physician groups and hospitals who participate in the plan, although under some plans emergency care will be covered outside the service area. When members are ill, they go to HMO clinics

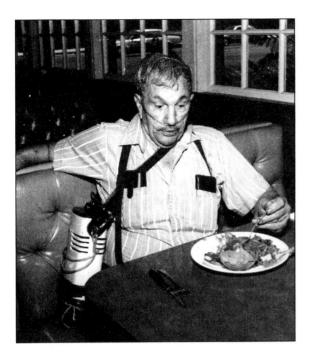

FIGURE 14-3 Major medical insurance benefits cover services and supplies beyond those available in basic policies, including the rental of medical equipment. (Courtesy of Huber and Spatz, *Homemaker/Home Health Aide,* 4th ed., copyright 1994, Delmar Publishers)

paperwork activity, the HMO requires fewer employees. According to *Newsweek* of October 4, 1993, there are 1300 different claims forms from insurers in this country. One consulting firm estimates that the United States could save $50 billion per year in administration costs if its health care were structured similarly to the Canadian plan, in which government pays most bills.

With no profit incentive for ordering additional tests and procedures, HMO physicians are less likely to duplicate laboratory procedures or ask for secondary tests. Studies have shown that fee-for-service physicians order 50 percent more chest x-rays and EKGs than do HMO physicians.

Health maintenance organizations have been the center of controversy between managers of health financing groups and the medical community. While HMOs appear to limit expenses, physicians and hospitals argue that they may also limit care. When an extra x-ray reads negative for the average patient, it becomes an unnecessary expense; however, a second x-ray that finds a formerly undetected carcinoma may save a patient's life.

to see physicians who are salaried employees; if they need hospitalization, they are admitted to HMO-approved hospitals. The bill is sent to the HMO, and the members spend little or no money beyond the monthly or annual membership fee. In essence, a patient's choice of care is limited in exchange for a prepaid, preset price.

Health maintenance organizations differ in the services they provide, with some offering options such as prescriptions, nursing home care, and related expenses. An HMO may cover the entire cost of a medical or hospital service or may require a small charge for each visit or services. Since HMOs operate within a fixed budget based on prepayment, the HMO has a financial incentive to reduce the use of hospital facilities and emergency care, thus emphasizing "wellness" and "wellness checks" as a method of reducing expenses.

Two factors contribute to an HMO's ability to afford the promise to guarantee no unexpected costs. First, paperwork expenses are less for HMOs because there are no insurance forms to fill out. By eliminating time-consuming

PREFERRED PROVIDER ORGANIZATIONS

Preferred provider organizations (PPOs) offer another alternative to traditional health care financing through contracts between groups of physicians, hospitals, and a health insurer. The PPO provides medical services to the insurer at preset, usually lower, fees in return for a large number of referrals. In a PPO, a large buyer of group insurance such as a major corporation or a union agrees to send all members of the group, usually employees of the company, to physicians or hospitals affiliated with the PPO in return for volume discounts. Patients get 80 to 100 percent reimbursement for treatment costs. Unlike some HMO physicians, PPO physicians are not employees of the organization; therefore, they can continue to provide service under the traditional fee-for-service arrangement. Because major corporations, with approximately 130 million employees and dependents, are the largest buyers of health care coverage in the United States, PPOs are attractive both to physicians and corporations.

In an effort to fill beds during a time when out-patient service is growing, hospitals often organize PPOs and sign up their staff physicians to ensure that patients will be admitted to their facility. The PPO is then marketed to major employers who agree to refer all their employees to participating physicians and the hospital. Under the typical PPO arrangement, the insurer pays the entire bill, or all but a small deductible, as long as the patient uses only the preferred providers. Patients may use other providers as long as they are willing to pay the difference in cost. A related organization, called an exclusive provider organization (EPO), attempts to prevent patients from using providers who are not affiliated by eliminating all reimbursement when a provider outside the EPO is used. Yet another alternative related to both HMOs and PPOs resembles an HMO run from scattered private offices rather than a central clinic. The physicians are self-employed and get a standard fee per member patient per year.

Preferred Provider Organizations offer advantages and disadvantages for participating physicians, patients, and insurers. Physicians often decide to participate in a PPO because they can continue a traditional fee-for-service, office-based practice while at the same time affiliating with an organization that broadens the patient referral base. Also, PPOs frequently promise rapid turnaround on payment of claims, thereby improving the practice's cash flow and reducing collection expenses.

In exchange for this broader base, the doctor must be willing to give up some control over the practice. For example, PPOs rely heavily on utilization reviews, requiring physicians to submit their practices and procedures to the scrutiny of a third party. Under some PPO arrangements, the organization must grant prior approval before a physician can treat a patient. A further disadvantage of a physician's participating in a PPO is the 15 to 20 percent reduction of fees to which the provider must agree. For the arrangement to be financially satisfactory, the physician needs a large number of new patients or referrals. Individual physicians may join more than one PPO or HMO and at the same time continue to treat patients with traditional health plans.

For the patient, many PPOs provide "first dollar coverage," meaning that no deductible or copayment is required. However, the patient who seeks care from a non-PPO provider must personally pay a large portion of the fee. As a medical assistant, you should be knowledgeable about the PPOs your employer accepts and advise patients if the physician drops out after participating in a PPO for some time.

In theory, corporations, unions, and other insurers pay lower premiums because of two factors: (1) the PPO maintains tight control over the type and frequency of service each physician can provide; and (2) the PPO is able to negotiate reduced fees from some physicians and hospitals. Because PPOs are a relatively new phenomenon, research is still being conducted on actual cost savings.

MEDICARE, MEDICAID, AND OTHER GOVERNMENT PROGRAMS

The fastest growing segment of the U.S. population is the group over 100 years old, according to *The Futurist* magazine, August, 1990. The second fastest growing population group is 85 to 100 years old. Life span is also increasing, from a life expectancy of 68 years in 1950 to 76 years in 1993.

As might be expected and research confirms, the elderly are the biggest users of health care services in this country. Although people over age 65 comprised 13 percent of the U.S. population in 1993, they consumed one third of total health care services. The largest expenditures occurred during the last year of life.

As older people usually do not work and may depend on Social Security benefits, they cannot afford expensive health care. To address this problem, the U.S. government developed Medicare in 1965 to protect older citizens from the costs of illnesses (Figure 14-4). Medicaid, a similar program, was created to provide health services for the poor.

An aging population means continued increase in the rate of growth for Medicare spending. From 1993 to 2030, new entrants into the labor force will increase by 20 percent while the number of people over the age of 65 will double, or increase by 100 percent, according to a

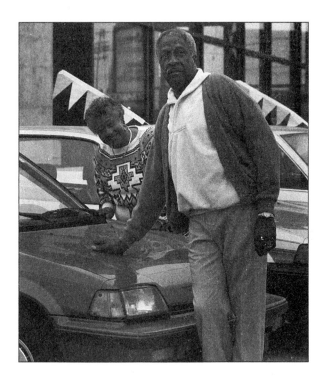

FIGURE 14-4 Americans aged 65 and over are protected by Medicare.

Sixty Minutes report of December 3, 1993. In 1965, the government became the largest purchaser of health care in this country, according to the January 26, 1987 issue of *Newsweek*. In 1960, patients and their insurance companies paid 56 percent of all health costs with government paying only 44 percent. By 1991, the government was paying 78 percent of all health care, with patients and their insurance companies paying only 22 percent of costs.

Medicare

Medicare protects Americans 65 and over and disabled citizens under 65. The coverage consists of two parts: A, hospital insurance; and B, medical insurance. Medicare hospital insurance pays for most but not all of a patient's hospital treatment and related expenses, and Medicare medical insurance pays 80 percent of reasonable physician's fees and related medical charges minus a deductible amount. In each state, an administering agency, often a large insurance company such as Equitable Life Assurance Society or Nationwide Insurance, is named to process Medicare claims. Since claims may be

handled in a slightly different manner by the administering agency in each state, each state should be contacted for specific instructions. The local Medicare office in each area can provide the name of the administrator. Also, Parts A and B may be administered by two different contractors.

Medicare recipients are issued cards showing whether they have hospital benefits or a combination of hospital and medical benefits. The card also shows the Medicare identification number, which is needed for reporting Medicare claims. When a new Medicare patient registers with the medical office, the medical assistant should photocopy the Medicare card and store the photocopy in the patient's medical record.

Medicaid

Medicaid is a financial assistance program developed jointly by the federal government and the states to provide health care for the poor. Benefits offered are similar to other insurance programs, although they differ in amount from state to state. Medicaid generally pays the deductible amount charged under Medicare and the 20 percent not covered by Medicare medical insurance. Again, the local Medicaid office should be called to determine what Medicaid benefits are paid in a specific state.

Medicaid claim forms are filed with the state administering agency, which determines whether the claim will be paid. Time limits for filing claims vary from state to state, and late claims may be rejected by the administrator. Individuals should contact their local agencies for information regarding filing deadlines and procedures. A Medicaid patient is issued an identifying card and number. The medical assistant should photocopy the card when a Medicaid patient registers and place the copy in the patient's medical record.

Other Government Programs

Military personnel and civilian employees of the federal government are covered under special insurance programs. Because the number of patients covered under one of these plans in the average medical office is small, only a brief overview is provided here. When a patient enrolled in one of the programs comes under the care of the physician, the medical assistant should ask the patient for a brochure or other documentation that explains the benefits before making an insurance claim. Some restrictions exist for use of medical services off-base; therefore, this documentation should be carefully reviewed.

CHAMPUS CHAMPUS refers to the Civilian Health and Medical Program of the Uniformed Services (Army, Navy, Air Force, Marines, and Coast Guard). This program covers medical care not directly related to military service (for example, viral infection) for uniformed service personnel and their families. Although most uniformed services families obtain their medical care from government facilities, they are paid CHAMPUS benefits if they are referred to a private physician. The provider must be authorized by CHAMPUS (Figure 14-5).

Military dependents who prefer to be treated by a civilian medical facility can receive treatment by providing the office with a non-availability statement or authorization issued by the commander of the military hospital. This statement should be attached to the CHAMPUS claim reporting form.

CHAMPVA CHAMPVA refers to the Civilian Health and Medical Program of the Veterans Administration and is similar to CHAMPUS. Those covered are (1) dependents of totally disabled veterans whose disabilities are service related, and (2) surviving dependents of veterans who have died from service-related disabilities.

FEHB Active and retired civilian employees of the federal government and their dependents may enroll in the Federal Employees' Health Benefits Program, which is administered by the Civil Service Commission through private insurers. The program is voluntary and offers similar benefits to the basic coverage and major medical coverage of other programs.

WORKERS' COMPENSATION INSURANCE

Workers' compensation insurance laws in each state require employers to purchase insurance that provides health care and income to employees and their dependents when the employee suffers or dies from a work-related injury or illness (Figure 14-6). The employer pays all premiums for workers' compensation

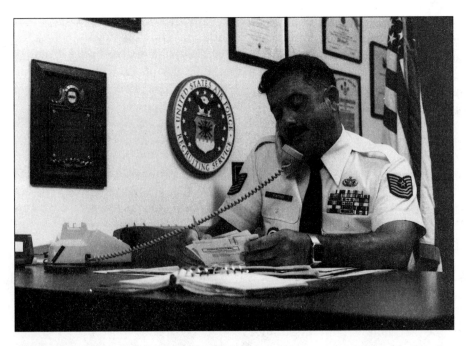

FIGURE 14-5 The CHAMPUS program covers medical care that is not directly related to the military for uniformed service personnel and their families.

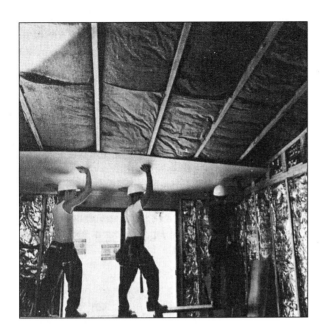

FIGURE 14-6 Workers' compensation insurance provides health care and income when an employee suffers a work-related injury, illness, or death. (Courtesy of Lewis, *Carpentry*, copyright 1995, Delmar Publishers)

insurance to a private carrier in return for protection from financial liability. Excluded from the workers' compensation laws in some states are domestic workers, farmers, and employees of small companies. Federal workers' compensation laws have been enacted to provide benefits for people employed by the federal government.

The purpose of workers' compensation insurance is to return the employee to work. This includes providing medical treatment, hospital care, surgery, and therapy from the time of injury or diagnosis of an illness until recovery. In the case of total or partial disability, income benefits are paid to the injured or ill worker. If an employee is killed on the job or dies from a job-related disease or disability, a moderate funeral expense and living expenses are provided for the dependents. Benefits vary from state to state, so the Bureau of Workers' Compensation in each state must be contacted for an explanation of that state's law.

Claims for workers' compensation insurance are made with the Bureau of Workers' Compensation in each state. Because the claim forms for the states differ, the medical assistant should

contact the patient's employer for a copy of the proper form. The attending physician is required to make a report before an employee may collect benefits under a claim. A workers' compensation insurance form from one state is shown in Figure 14-7.

Prospective Payment System

Diagnosis-related group is a term that describes a method of prospective pricing in which a hospital is paid a flat fee for medical service for Medicare patients based on an average cost of service, not on the actual cost per patient. The prospective pricing, or prospective payment, system was enacted in 1983 for hospitalized Medicare patients in an effort to reduce the cost of hospital care for the elderly.

As originally set up in 1965, Medicare payments were "passed along"; that is, hospitals assigned whatever cost they wished for medical care and passed the bill along to the government. Physicians, too, who treated Medicare patients could decide what fees were "customary" and pass along their bills to Medicare, which paid, usually without question. There was virtually no control over fee setting for either physicians or hospitals, and health care costs for the elderly skyrocketed. Predictably, those in control of financing government programs began to look for ways to contain expenses.

DIAGNOSIS-RELATED GROUPS

The Health Care Financing Administration (HCFA), which manages Medicare and Medicaid, in an effort to set a standard for hospital costs for Medicare patients, adopted a plan developed at Yale University in the late 1960s. With minor changes, the plan, called diagnosis-related groups, was written into law in the Social Security Amendments Act in 1983. A diagnosis-related group (DRG) is a method of classifying patients into categories based on the primary diagnosis. There are 467 DRGs, or categories, and every hospitalized Medicare patient must be placed in one of them. The categories

1. Type answers to All questions and file original with the Workers' Compensation Commission within 72 hours after first treatment.
2. DO NOT FAIL to forward to the Workers' Compensation Commission PROGRESS REPORTS and FINAL REPORT upon discharge of patient.

DO NOT WRITE IN THIS SPACE

WORKERS' COMPENSATION COMMISSION

WCC CLAIM #

EMPLOYER'S REPORT Yes ☐ No ☐

This is First Report ☐   Progress Report ☐   Final Report ☐

EVERY QUESTION MUST BE ANSWERED AND FORM SIGNED

1. Name of Injured Person:
Maureen A. Santega
Soc. Sec. No. 610-98-7432
D.O.B. 7/19/69
Sex M ☐ F ☑

2. Address: (No. and Street)
905 Raymond Lane
(City or Town) Atlanta
(State) GA
(Zip Code) 30385-8893

3. Name and Address of Employer:
Majors Concrete Company, 238 Leaf Lane, Atlanta, GA 30342-3329

4. Date of Accident or Onset of Disease:
4/9/—
Hour: A.M. ☑ P.M. ☐

5. Date Disability Began:
4/9/—

6. Patient's Description of Accident or Cause of Disease:
Concrete truck struck and backed over patient's foot while she was pouring concrete at job site

7. Medical description of Injury or Disease:
massive bruising to left foot, no broken bones, great deal of pain associated with bruises

8. Will Injury result in:
(a) Permanent defect?   Yes ☐   No ☑   If so, what?   (b) Disfigurement   Yes ☐   No ☑

9. Causes, other than injury, contributing to patients condition:
None

10. Is patient suffering from any disease of the heart, lungs, brain, kidneys, blood, vascular system or any other disabling condition not due to this accident?
Give particulars: No

11. Is there any history or evidence present of previous accident or disease? Give particulars:
No

12. Has normal recovery been delayed for any reason? Give particulars:
No

13. Date of first treatment:
4/10/—
Who engaged your services?
patient

14. Describe treatment given by you:
Darvon, 100 mg q4h prn for pain

15. Were X-Rays taken?
Yes ☑ No ☐
By whom? — (Name and Address)
Edwin Gordon, M.D. 802 Manor Lane, Atlanta 30303
Date 4/10/—

16. X-Ray Diagnosis:
No broken bones

17. Was patient treated by anyone else?
Yes ☐ No ☑
By whom? — (Name and Address)   Date

18. Was patient hospitalized?
Yes ☐ No ☑
Name and Address of Hospital   Date of Admission: Date of Discharge:

19. Is further treatment needed?
Yes ☐ No ☑
For how long?
20. Patient was ☑ will be ☐ able to resume regular work on: 4/14
Patient was ☐ will be ☐ able to resume light work on:

21. If death ensued give date: 22. Remarks: (Give any information of value not included above)

23. I am a qualified specialist in:
orthopedics
I am a duly licensed Physician in the State of:
Maryland
I was graduated from Medical School (Name)
Johns Hopkins
Year 1967

Date of this report: 6/21/—   (Signed) *John N. Sparks, M.D.*

Address: 8504 Capricorn Drive Atlanta GA 30312
(This report must be signed PERSONALLY by Physician)
Phone: (404) 544-0078

FIGURE 14-7 Sample workers' compensation claim form

are derived from all of the possible diagnoses identified in *International Classification of Diseases,* 9th Edition, *Clinical Modification* (ICD-9-CM). Diseases are classified into twenty-three major diagnostic categories based on organ systems; they are broken down further into 467 distinct groups. All patients in the same DRG can be expected to respond in a clinically similar manner, which, if averaged statistically, will result in about equal use of the hospital's facilities and resources, according to *DRGs and the Prospective Payment System.*

Five pieces of information are needed to place a patient in a DRG:

1. The patient's principal diagnosis and up to four complications
2. The treatment procedures performed
3. The patient's age
4. The patient's sex, and
5. The patient's status at discharge

The DRG program works in the following manner. After a patient is diagnosed, the hospital sends diagnostic information to the administering agency and receives a fixed fee based on the average cost of treating the patient's condition. If the patient's condition is corrected at less than average cost, the hospital makes money. However, if the patient's problem is more severe than average and takes more hospital days, physician time, and hospital resources than average, the hospital loses money. As an example, a Medicare patient diagnosed by a physician as suffering heart failure and shock would be classified in DRG 157, and the hospital would be reimbursed the amount allowed for that particular classification. In severe cases where expenses become catastrophic, an additional sum called an "outlier" is paid to offset the hospital's huge losses. The DRG system rewards efficiency in providing care, and a hospital that treats patients for less than the DRG payment receives a built-in bonus.

SIGNIFICANCE OF DRGs

Diagnosis-related groups caused a dramatic change in the way hospitals treat Medicare patients, and both hospitals and physicians argue that patients may not receive the treatment they need because of cost-cutting measures to stay within DRG limits. However, proponents of the system point out that physicians should not order duplicate procedures and services.

In an effort to maintain financial stability, hospitals have formed boards of physicians and other providers to set standards for what tests, procedures, and services are necessary to treat patients assigned to each DRG. Since physicians are responsible for diagnosing the condition that places a patient in a DRG, hospitals exert great pressure on them to make realistic diagnoses and to treat within the DRG payment system. Extra tests, procedures, and services are not allowed except in unusual cases.

The concept of DRGs and prospective payment is highly controversial because, based on Medicare's success in reducing costs, private insurance companies are now drawing plans for establishing their own standards. The time when hospitals and physicians can establish costs without outside review has passed.

IN YOUR OPINION

1. From the medical assistant's viewpoint, what are the advantages and disadvantages of the variety of health care financing plans available to patients?
2. What procedures should a medical assistant follow when presented with CHAMPUS, CHAMPVA, or other coverage when questions arise?
3. Since DRGs were developed to standardize hospital charges only, why are they important to private practice medical assistants?

Filing an Insurance Claim

Payments by insurance companies, or third-party carriers, represent a large portion of a medical practice's income. Therefore, as a medical assistant, it is extremely important that you understand the claims process if you file insurance claims or help patients file their own claims.

FOLLOWING THE ROUTE OF A CLAIM

Patients with insurance coverage must file claims with their carriers explaining the services received and the costs accrued. Although patients are responsible for filing their own claims, some medical offices have found that their collection rate is better if they complete the forms for the patients. Patients often are uncertain about how the form should be filled in, or they delay mailing the form, which delays the physician's payment. Physicians have reduced this problem somewhat by requiring patients to pay at the time of their visit and collect reimbursement from their insurance carriers. Computers have also contributed to more efficient claim filing, since many software systems used in medical offices automatically print an insurance claim form at the end of each patient's visit. Some medical offices use modems for quick electronic filing of a claim with an insurance company.

Once a claim form has been properly completed and signed by the physician and patient, it is mailed to the carrier's claim department or, in the case of a government agency, to the agency's administrator. The claims examiner evaluates the form and determines whether the patient's benefits cover the services provided. If the claim form is improperly filled out, incomplete, unsigned by either the patient or the physician, or in any way questionable, the form will be returned and the claim will not be paid. The form can be resubmitted; however, because payment takes from one to six weeks from the time a form is received in the claims department, resubmissions reduce a practice's cash flow and should be avoided whenever possible. When the insurance examiner is satisfied that all conditions of coverage have been satisfactorily met, the claims department mails a check for the covered services, minus the deductible or co-payment, to the patient or the physician.

ASSIGNMENT OF PAYMENT

A physician may elect to accept assignment of the patient's benefits under Medicare and other government insurance programs. This means that the physician agrees to accept an amount predetermined by the third-party carrier instead of charging usual and customary fees, which may be more or less. Many physicians will not accept assignment of benefits. This is a matter about which a medical assistant should be clear before completing a claim form.

INSURANCE CODING SYSTEMS

Two types of codes are used to standardize information for insurance claim forms. They are CPT-4 for identifying procedures, treatments, and services, and ICD-9-CM for identifying diagnoses.

CPT-4

CPT-4 codes, developed by the American Medical Association (AMA), are listed in the book, *Current Procedural Terminology,* Fourth Edition, which identifies individual medical procedures, treatments, and services for all specialties by a five-digit code. The book lists all the procedures, treatments, and service for each specialty and identifies each with its own code. Most insurance companies require the use of CPT-4 codes on claim forms; as a medical assistant, you will refer to the book frequently when completing claim forms.

Selecting a code to represent the level of service for a patient visit depends on seven components: history, examination, medical decision making, nature of the problem, counseling, coordination of care, and time required. A medical assistant may take a course in CPT-4 coding for in-depth understanding.

Physicians mark on the superbill the service they performed, so the medical assistant will not be called upon to make all the decisions regarding how service should be coded. A medical assistant who has a question about the level or type of service performed should check with the physician before filing a claim form. A comprehensive superbill that lists most of the treatments, procedures, and services performed by specialty practice and matches them with a CPT code is an excellent time saver. This enables the physician to identify clearly the CPT designation simply by marking the service.

Successful coding depends on proper documentation. Each code must be supported by evidence of treatment, procedures, or service, or the practice will not be reimbursed for the amounts submitted. Inaccurate or incomplete documentation of claims can put a practice at legal risk.

Several sample procedures and treatments and their codes are listed below, on the superbill in Figure 14-8 and on the HCFA-1500 and dental forms in Figures 14-9a and 14-9b. A hypothetical fee is listed for each service. Refer to Figure 14-8 and analyze the manner in which the CPT codes, ICD codes, and fees are used to document services.

1. Look at the section of the superbill called Office Visits. This established patient was charged $46 for an Intermediate Office Visit during which the physician performed an examination to help arrive at a diagnosis. The CPT code range for established patients is 99211 to 99215, depending on the duration and complexity of the visit. The range for new patients, is 99201 to 99205. All doctors do not list all levels on the superbill. The level of service is determined by the length of time the physician spends with the patient and the complexity of the problem. When assigning levels of service, the physician takes into consideration three key components:

   - The amount of history taking necessary to clearly understand the problem
   - The level of physical examination necessary to adequately evaluate the patient
   - The complexity of the problem and the amount of medical decision-making necessary to determine an adequate treatment plan

   When assigning higher levels of service, the physician also determines the mortality risk associated with the patient's condition.

2. Look at the section of the superbill called Laboratory Services. These laboratory services, which are identified with a CPT code, were performed to help the physician arrive at a diagnosis.

Chest x-ray	CPT code 71010	Fee $50.00
EKG	CPT code 93000	Fee $58.00
Electrolytes	CPT code 80003	Fee $35.00

   Several CPT codes are shown in the following list.

99213	Level III Office Visit, Established Patient	52.00
99214	Level IV Office Visit, Established Patient	79.00
99215	Level V Visit, Established Patient	130.00
99222	Level II Initial Hospital Care	145.00
99231	Subsequent Hospital Care	67.00
99238	Hospital Discharge	83.00
85007	Complete Blood Count	15.00
87060	Throat Culture	25.00
87086	Urine Culture	27.00
81000	Urinalysis	17.00

3. Look at the Diagnosis section of the superbill immediately under the words Attending Physician's Statement. The diagnosis code 402.00 for hypertension with heart involvement is marked. In addition, the physician diagnosed angina, ICD-9 413.9, and spontaneous hypoglycemia ICD-9 251.2. The hypoglycemia was added in the Other Diagnosis line. These diagnoses were reached through a combination of the physician's examination and the laboratory results.

ICD-9-CM

Standard nomenclature for diagnoses is contained in the *International Classification of Diseases, 9th Edition, Clinical Modification,* which is available from the AMA. Only Medicare, Blue Cross/Blue Shield plans, and some private insurance companies require diagnosis codes on their claim forms. However, it is wise to use these codes to speed the processing of a claim even if a carrier does not require them. Diagnosis codes are made up of three digits that are followed by a decimal point and one or two additional digits. Claims submitted with a three- or four-digit code where a four- or five-level code is available will be returned for proper coding. The first three numbers identify the primary diagnosis and the extra digits differentiate within the diagnosis area. Several diagnosis codes are shown in the following list and on the HCFA-1500 form in Figure 14-8 on page 296.

244	Acquired hypothyroidism
250.9	Diabetes
251.2	Spontaneous hypoglycemia
401.0	Hypertension
402.00	Hypertension with heart involvement (Fifth digit must be included)
413.9	Angina
414.0	Unstable arteriosclerotic heart disease
490	Bronchitis
493.9	Asthma

PLEASE DO NOT STAPLE IN THIS AREA

CARRIER

PICA

HEALTH INSURANCE CLAIM FORM

PICA

| 1. MEDICARE (Medicare #) | MEDICAID (Medicaid #) | CHAMPUS (Sponsor's SSN) | CHAMPVA (VA File #) | GROUP HEALTH PLAN (SSN or ID) | FECA BLK LUNG (SSN) | OTHER ☒ (ID) | 1a. INSURED'S I.D. NUMBER 238-58-6871 | (FOR PROGRAM IN ITEM 1) |

2. PATIENT'S NAME (Last Name, First Name, Middle Initial)
Hammond, John, S.

3. PATIENT'S BIRTH DATE MM 08 DD 15 YY — SEX M ☒ F

4. INSURED'S NAME (Last Name, First Name, Middle Initial)
Hammond, John, S.

5. PATIENT'S ADDRESS (No., Street)
5168 Oak Grove Terrace

6. PATIENT RELATIONSHIP TO INSURED Self ☒ Spouse ☐ Child ☐ Other ☐

7. INSURED'S ADDRESS (No., Street)
5168 Oak Grove Terrace

CITY Atlanta   STATE GA

8. PATIENT STATUS Single ☐ Married ☒ Other ☐

CITY Atlanta   STATE GA

ZIP CODE 30304-5475   TELEPHONE (Include Area Code) (404) 628-9109

Employed ☒ Full-Time Student ☐ Part-Time Student ☐

ZIP CODE 30304-5475   TELEPHONE (INCLUDE AREA CODE) (555) 628-9109

9. OTHER INSURED'S NAME (Last Name, First Name, Middle Initial)

10. IS PATIENT'S CONDITION RELATED TO:

11. INSURED'S POLICY GROUP OR FECA NUMBER
TN 75281

a. OTHER INSURED'S POLICY OR GROUP NUMBER

a. EMPLOYMENT? (CURRENT OR PREVIOUS) YES ☐ ☒ NO

a. INSURED'S DATE OF BIRTH MM 08 DD 15 YY — SEX M ☒ F ☐

b. OTHER INSURED'S DATE OF BIRTH MM DD YY SEX M ☐ F ☐

b. AUTO ACCIDENT? PLACE (State) YES ☐ ☒ NO

b. EMPLOYER'S NAME OR SCHOOL NAME
Acme Computers

c. EMPLOYER'S NAME OR SCHOOL NAME

c. OTHER ACCIDENT? YES ☐ ☒ NO

c. INSURANCE PLAN NAME OR PROGRAM NAME
Acme Computers

d. INSURANCE PLAN NAME OR PROGRAM NAME

10d. RESERVED FOR LOCAL USE

d. IS THERE ANOTHER HEALTH BENEFIT PLAN? YES ☐ ☒ NO If yes, return to and complete item 9 a-d.

READ BACK OF FORM BEFORE COMPLETING & SIGNING THIS FORM.
12. PATIENT'S OR AUTHORIZED PERSON'S SIGNATURE I authorize the release of any medical or other information necessary to process this claim. I also request payment of government benefits either to myself or to the party who accepts assignment below.

SIGNED *John S. Hammond*   DATE 4/14/—

13. INSURED'S OR AUTHORIZED PERSON'S SIGNATURE I authorize payment of medical benefits to the undersigned physician or supplier for services described below.

SIGNED

PATIENT AND INSURED INFORMATION

DATE	DESCRIPTION	CHARGE	CREDIT PAYMENT	ADJUSTMENT	CURRENT BALANCE	PREVIOUS BALANCE	NAME	ACCT. NUMBER
4/14/-	O.V., Lab, Xray	189.00			189.00		John S. Hammond	839

This is your RECEIPT for this amount ⇧

⇧ This is a STATEMENT of your account to date

ATTENDING PHYSICIAN'S STATEMENT
Patient *John Hammond*   Date of Service *4/14/—*

DIAGNOSES ARE ICD-9-CM CODED

☐ 401.0	Hypertension	☐ 227.3	Pituitary Neoplasm	☐ 242.2	Hyperthyroidism
☒ 402.00	Hypertension with heart involvement	☐ 193.0	Thyroid Neoplasm	☐ 244	Hypothyroidism
☐ 786.50	Chest pain	☐ 490	Bronchitis	☐ 240.9	Goiter
☒ 413.9	Angina	☐ 324.0	Emphysema	☐ 242.3	Thyroid Nodule
☐ 428.0	C H F	☐ 493.9	Asthma	☐ 245.9	Thyroiditis
☐ 425	Cardiomyopathy	☐ 079.9	Viral Syndrome	☐ 250.9	Diabetes
☐ 427.9	Cardiac Arrhythmia	☐ 558.9	Gastroenteritis		

OTHER DIAGNOSIS *Spontaneous Hypoglycemia (251.2)*

AMA CURRENT PROCEDURAL TERMINOLOGY - 4TH EDITION

1. OFFICE VISITS

	New	Established	FEE
Limited Visit	☐ 99201	☐ 99211	
Intermediate Visit	☐ 99202	☒ 99212	46.00
Extended Visit	☐ 99203	☐ 99213	
Comprehensive Visit	☐ 99204	☐ 99214	

2. HOSPITAL SERVICES
Hospital: ☐ Metro ☐ _____
Admission/Hist. & Phy. ☐ 99222
Admit Date: _____ 19 ____
ICU Visits ☐ 90270
____ visits @ ____ ea.
Hospital Visits ☐ 99231
____ visits @ ____ ea.
Hospital Visits Limited ☐ 90250
____ visits @ ____ ea.
(All Service Dates Below)
Date of Discharge _____ 19 ___

3. EMERGENCY ROOM
Brief Service ☐ 90505 ☐ 90540
Extended Service ☐ 90517 ☐ 90570

4. HOSPITAL CONSULTATIONS
Limited ☐ 90600
Intermediate ☐ 90605
Extended ☐ 90610
Complex ☐ 90620
Referring Physician _____

5. IMMUNIZATIONS - INJECTIONS
☐ TET ☐ Flu ☐ Pneumovax ☐ 90720
☐ Testosterone
☐ T-B Tine Test
☐

6. LABORATORY SERVICES

	CPT	FEE
☒ Chest Xray (PA)	71010	50.00
☒ EKG	93000	58.00
☐ CBC	85007	
☐ Urinalysis	81000	
☐ SMAC-20	80019	
☐ T-4	83440	
☐ Pap Smear	88100	
☐ Sed Rate	85650	
☐ Occult Blood Stool	82770	
☐ Glucose	84340	
☐ Cholesterol	82465	
☐ Protime	85610	
☐ Potassium	84132	
☐ WBC	84048	
☐ Hemoglobin	85018	
☒ Electrolytes	80003	35.00
☐ Electrolytes, BUN, CR	80005	
☐ Thyroid Profile (T-7)	82756	
☐ TSH	84443	
☐ T3 RIA	84480	
☐ Thyroid Antimicro. Antibodies	85694	
☐ Prolactin	84146	
☐ Testosterone	84401	
☐ Glycohemoglobin	83020	
☐ SMAC - 20/T4	80019	
☐ Calcium	82310	
☐ Triglycerides	84478	
☐ Culture (Urine)	87086	
☐ Sensitivity (Urine)	87086	
☐ Culture (Throat Strep)	87060	
☐ Lateral Skull Film	70240	
☐ Blood Handling	99000	

7. OTHER SERVICES FEE

TODAY'S FEES $ 189.00

AUTHORIZATION TO PAY PHYSICIAN DIRECT

I hereby authorize payments directly to the undersigned Physician of the Medical Benefits, if any, otherwise payable to me for his services described above. I understand that I am responsible for the charges not covered by this authorization. I hereby authorize the undersigned Physician to release any medical information necessary to process this form.

Sign. _____ Date _____

PATIENTS—Insurance claims handling procedures are explained on the reverse of the Pink Copy. KEEP THIS RECORD FOR INCOME TAX AND INSURANCE CLAIM FILING.

Return: ____ Days ____ Weeks ____ Mo.
Your Next Appointment _____
Day   Month   Date   Time   AM PM

John H. Sparks, M.D.

FIGURE 14-8 Superbill used with HCFA-1500 claim form

HEALTH INSURANCE CLAIM FORM

APPROVED OMB-0938-0008

PICA

1. MEDICARE (Medicare #) MEDICAID (Medicaid #) CHAMPUS (Sponsor's SSN) CHAMPVA (VA File #) GROUP HEALTH PLAN (SSN or ID) FECA BLK LUNG (SSN) OTHER ☒ (ID)

1a. INSURED'S I.D. NUMBER (FOR PROGRAM IN ITEM 1)
283-58-6871

2. PATIENT'S NAME (Last Name, First Name, Middle Initial)
Shields, Nancy V.

3. PATIENT'S BIRTH DATE: 08 15 41 SEX M ☐ F ☒

4. INSURED'S NAME (Last Name, First Name, Middle Initial)
SAME

5. PATIENT'S ADDRESS (No., Street)
5168 Oak Terrace

6. PATIENT RELATIONSHIP TO INSURED
Self ☒ Spouse ☐ Child ☐ Other ☐

7. INSURED'S ADDRESS (No., Street)
5168 Oak Terrace

CITY: Decatur   STATE: GA

8. PATIENT STATUS
Single ☐ Married ☒ Other ☐
Employed ☒ Full-Time Student ☐ Part-Time Student ☐

CITY: Decatur   STATE: GA

ZIP CODE: 30033-8823   TELEPHONE (Include Area Code): (404) 721-9001

ZIP CODE: 30033-8823   TELEPHONE (INCLUDE AREA CODE): (555) 721-9001

9. OTHER INSURED'S NAME (Last Name, First Name, Middle Initial)
Shields, John H.

10. IS PATIENT'S CONDITION RELATED TO:

11. INSURED'S POLICY GROUP OR FECA NUMBER
TN 75281

a. OTHER INSURED'S POLICY OR GROUP NUMBER
US 8123976

a. EMPLOYMENT? (CURRENT OR PREVIOUS) ☐ YES ☒ NO

a. INSURED'S DATE OF BIRTH: 08 15 41 SEX M ☐ F ☒

b. OTHER INSURED'S DATE OF BIRTH: 02 10 40 SEX M ☒ F ☐

b. AUTO ACCIDENT? PLACE (State) ☐ YES ☒ NO

b. EMPLOYER'S NAME OR SCHOOL NAME
Marshall Industries

c. EMPLOYER'S NAME OR SCHOOL NAME
United Surgical

c. OTHER ACCIDENT? ☐ YES ☒ NO

c. INSURANCE PLAN NAME OR PROGRAM NAME
MarshInd Plan

d. INSURANCE PLAN NAME OR PROGRAM NAME
United Surgical Plan

10d. RESERVED FOR LOCAL USE

d. IS THERE ANOTHER HEALTH BENEFIT PLAN?
☒ YES ☐ NO *If yes*, return to and complete item 9 a-d.

READ BACK OF FORM BEFORE COMPLETING & SIGNING THIS FORM.
12. PATIENT'S OR AUTHORIZED PERSON'S SIGNATURE I authorize the release of any medical or other information necessary to process this claim. I also request payment of government benefits either to myself or to the party who accepts assignment below.

SIGNED *Nancy Shields*   DATE 4/20/—

13. INSURED'S OR AUTHORIZED PERSON'S SIGNATURE I authorize payment of medical benefits to the undersigned physician or supplier for services described below.

SIGNED *Nancy Shields*

14. DATE OF CURRENT: ILLNESS (First symptom) OR INJURY (Accident) OR PREGNANCY(LMP)   02 25 —

15. IF PATIENT HAS HAD SAME OR SIMILAR ILLNESS. GIVE FIRST DATE MM DD YY

16. DATES PATIENT UNABLE TO WORK IN CURRENT OCCUPATION
FROM   TO

17. NAME OF REFERRING PHYSICIAN OR OTHER SOURCE
Dr. Frances Morgan

17a. I.D. NUMBER OF REFERRING PHYSICIAN
8439-71-10

18. HOSPITALIZATION DATES RELATED TO CURRENT SERVICES
FROM   TO

19. RESERVED FOR LOCAL USE

20. OUTSIDE LAB? $ CHARGES
☐ YES ☒ NO

21. DIAGNOSIS OR NATURE OF ILLNESS OR INJURY. (RELATE ITEMS 1,2,3 OR 4 TO ITEM 24E BY LINE)

1. 402.00 Hypertension with heart involvement
2. 413.9 Angina
3.
4.

22. MEDICAID RESUBMISSION CODE   ORIGINAL REF. NO.

23. PRIOR AUTHORIZATION NUMBER

24. A DATE(S) OF SERVICE From To		B Place of Service	C Type of Service	D PROCEDURES, SERVICES, OR SUPPLIES (Explain Unusual Circumstances) CPT/HCPCS MODIFIER	E DIAGNOSIS CODE	F $ CHARGES	G DAYS OR UNITS	H EPSDT Family Plan	I EMG	J COB	K RESERVED FOR LOCAL USE
04 14 —		3		99214	1 and 2	79 00	1				
04 14 —		3		71010	1 and 2	50 00	1				
04 14 —		3		93000	1 and 2	50 00	1				
04 14 —		3		80003	1 and 2	35 00	2				

25. FEDERAL TAX I.D. NUMBER   SSN ☐ EIN ☐

26. PATIENT'S ACCOUNT NO.
839

27. ACCEPT ASSIGNMENT? (For govt. claims, see back)
☐ YES ☒ NO

28. TOTAL CHARGE $ 214 00

29. AMOUNT PAID $ 0

30. BALANCE DUE $ 214 00

31. SIGNATURE OF PHYSICIAN OR SUPPLIER INCLUDING DEGREES OR CREDENTIALS (I certify that the statements on the reverse apply to this bill and are made a part thereof.)

Signature on file

SIGNED   DATE

32. NAME AND ADDRESS OF FACILITY WHERE SERVICES WERE RENDERED (If other than home or office)

33. PHYSICIAN'S, SUPPLIER'S BILLING NAME, ADDRESS, ZIP CODE & PHONE #
John H. Sparks, M.D.
8504 Capricorn Drive
Atlanta GA 30033-7775
(404) 555-6078
PIN#   GRP#

(APPROVED BY AMA COUNCIL ON MEDICAL SERVICE 8/88)   **PLEASE PRINT OR TYPE**

FORM HCFA-1500 (U2) (12-90)
FORM OWCP-1500   FORM RRB-1500

FIGURE 14-9a   Completed HCFA-1500 claim form

Please Type or Print

TO BE COMPLETED BY EMPLOYEE

1. PATIENT NAME: JAMIE ARSTON
2. RELATIONSHIP TO EMPLOYEE: SELF / SPOUSE / CHILD ✓ / OTHER
3. SEX: M / F ✓
4. PATIENT BIRTHDATE: MO. 11 / DAY 30 / YEAR 74
5. IF FULL TIME STUDENT — SCHOOL: Colton High School — CITY: Darby, PA

6. EMPLOYEE NAME — FIRST: Joseph / MIDDLE / LAST: Arston
EMPLOYEE'S BIRTHDATE: MO. 7 / DAY 10 / YEAR 40
7. EMPLOYEE SOCIAL SECURITY NO.: 711-76-8194
8. MARITAL STATUS: ☐ Single / Divorced ☐ / ☑ Married / Separated ☐
SPOUSE'S BIRTHDATE: MO. 3 / DAY 10 / YEAR 42

9. EMPLOYEE MAILING ADDRESS: 7002 Lansdown Ave.
CITY, STATE: DARBY, PA — ZIP: 19010
10. EMPLOYER (COMPANY) NAME AND ADDRESS: ABC Company, 321 Chestnut St, Darby, PA 19010

11. GROUP NUMBER
12. BRANCH
13. ARE OTHER FAMILY MEMBERS EMPLOYED? NO ☑ YES ☐ — EMPLOYEE NAME — SOC. SEC. NO.
14. NAME AND ADDRESS OF EMPLOYER IN ITEM 13.

15. IS PATIENT COVERED BY ANOTHER DENTAL PLAN? NO ☑ YES ☐ If yes, please give: DENTAL PLAN NAME — NAME AND ADDRESS OF CARRIER
15a. IF PATIENT IS A DEPENDENT CHILD, ARE THE LEGAL PARENTS DIVORCED OR SEPARATED FROM EACH OTHER? NO ☑ YES ☐

15b. I HAVE REVIEWED THE FOLLOWING TREATMENT PLAN. I AUTHORIZE RELEASE OF ANY INFORMATION RELATING TO THIS CLAIM.
SIGNED (PATIENT, OR PARENT IF MINOR): Joseph Arston — DATE: 2/21/—
15c. I HEREBY CERTIFY THAT THE ABOVE INFORMATION IS CORRECT.
EMPLOYEE SIGNATURE: Joseph Arston — DATE: 2/22/—

TO BE COMPLETED BY DENTIST

16. DENTIST NAME — FIRST: Gary / MIDDLE: L. / LAST: Brother D.D.S.
17. MAILING ADDRESS: 230-B Rachel Avenue
CITY, STATE: Darby, PA — ZIP: 19010
18. DENTIST SOC. SEC. OR T.I.N.: 210-10-9870
19. DENTIST LICENSE NO.: 16-024
20. DENTIST PHONE NO.: 608-237-4102

24. IS TREATMENT RESULT OF OCCUPATIONAL ILLNESS OR INJURY? NO ✓ YES — IF YES, ENTER BRIEF DESCRIPTION AND DATES
25. IS TREATMENT RESULT OF AUTO ACCIDENT? NO ✓
26. OTHER ACCIDENT?
27. ARE ANY SERVICES COVERED BY ANOTHER PLAN? ✓
28. IF PROSTHESIS, CROWN OR INLAY, IS THIS INITIAL PLACEMENT? ✓ — (IF NO. REASON FOR REPLACEMENT) — 29. DATE OF PRIOR PLACEMENT

21. FIRST VISIT DATE CURRENT SERIES
22. PLACE OF TREATMENT: OFFICE X / HOSP. / ECF / OTHER
23. RADIOGRAPHS OR MODELS ENCLOSED? NO / YES ✓ / HOW MANY?
30. IS TREATMENT FOR ORTHODONTICS? ✓ — IF SERVICES ALREADY COMMENCED, ENTER — DATE APPLIANCES PLACED — MOS. TREATMENT REMAINING

DENTIST - CHECK ONE:
☐ PRETREATMENT ESTIMATE
☑ STATEMENT OF ACTUAL SERVICES

IDENTIFY MISSING TEETH WITH "X"

31. EXAMINATION AND TREATMENT PLAN - LIST IN ORDER FROM TOOTH NO. 1 THROUGH TOOTH NO. 32 — USE CHARTING SYSTEM SHOWN

ADMINISTRATIVE USE ONLY

Tooth No. or Ltr.	Surface	DESCRIPTION OF SERVICES (Including X-Rays, Prophylaxis, Materials Used, etc.)	Date Service Performed Mo.	Day	Yr.	Procedure Number	FEE	
		Examination	2	21	--	00120	20 00	
		Prophylaxis	2	21	--	0110	45 00	
14	M	Amalgam - 1 surface	2	21	--	02140	55 00	

32. REMARKS FOR UNUSUAL SERVICES

TOTAL FEE CHARGED: 120 00

Administrative Use Only
Patient's Eligible Date: Mo.____ Day____ Yr.____
Patient's Effective Date: Mo.____ Day____ Yr.____
Patient's Termination Date: Mo.____ Day____ Yr.____
Verified by____
Date Verified Mo.____ Day____ Yr.____

TO BE COMPLETED BY DENTIST
I HEREBY CERTIFY THAT THE PROCEDURES AS INDICATED BY DATE HAVE BEEN COMPLETED AND THAT THE FEES SUBMITTED ARE THE ACTUAL FEES I HAVE CHARGED *THIS PATIENT* AND INTEND TO ACCEPT FOR THESE PROCEDURES.
DENTIST'S SIGNATURE: Gary L. Brother — DATE: 2/22/—

DIRECTION TO PAY BENEFITS TO DENTIST
I HEREBY DIRECT BENEFITS PAYABLE TO THE ATTENDING DENTIST.
EMPLOYEE'S SIGNATURE: Joseph Arston — DATE: 2/21/—

IMPORTANT — to insure the proper processing of this claim, please check the accuracy of the following:
Employee Questions — 1 through 15a, b, & c
Dentist Questions — 16 through 32, dates of services, & procedure numbers
If initial prosthesis, list date(s) of extraction(s) for teeth being replaced.

Batch # _____

FIGURE 14-9b Completed dental claim form

ICD-9 coding is a complex issue and many times, physician's office personnel code conditions incorrectly. Incorrect codes often appear on superbills because a single code cannot represent all aspects of one condition. A good example is hypertension, which is coded differently depending upon associated problems. Because a general code for hypertension often appears on the superbill, this condition can be easily miscoded. Several hypertension related ICD-9 codes are shown below.

401.0	Malignant hypertension
401.1	Benign hypertension
402.00	Hypertension with heart involvement
403.00	Hypertension with renal involvement
405.09	Hypertension due to brain tumor

SUPERBILL AS DOCUMENTATION

Most superbills provide a complete list of procedures and treatments and their accompanying codes; many also list diagnoses and diagnosis codes. Space is given for writing the charge for each service and for the physician to write a diagnosis. Formerly, a superbill could be submitted in place of a completed HCFA-1500 form. At present, the trend is away from this practice. Medicare and many other insurers will no longer accept the superbill. This practice varies by insurance carrier because many companies are using computer scanners on the claims.

Completing a Universal Health Insurance Claim Form

A Universal Health Insurance Claim Form (HCFA-1500), developed by the AMA, has been adopted for use by most group and individual insurance claim organizations, HMOs, PPOs, and government health programs. Some carriers, however, require their own special form for reporting claims.

The HCFA-1500 form is divided into two sections: Patient and Insured Information Section and Physician or Supplier Information Section. The Patient and Insured Section contains eleven spaces for information and two

spaces for signatures; the Physician or Supplier Information Section consists of nineteen spaces for information, and one space for the physician's signature. A description of each space on the HCFA-1500 form and its relevance to Medicare, Medicaid, and private insurance carriers is given below. For Blue Shield claims, refer to the local plan. Completed medical and dental forms are shown in Figures 14-9a and 14-9b.

BASIC PROCEDURES FOR COMPLETING THE HCFA-1500 FORM

The numbered items below correspond to the numbered spaces on the HCFA-1500 form.

1. and 1a. Mark the patient's type of insurance. Indicate the patient's insurance identification number, Medicare number, or Medicaid number, including any letters that are a part of the identification. To ensure accuracy, you should ask the patient for an insurance identification card that shows the complete number. For Medicare, use the number on the beneficiary's red, white, and blue health insurance card. The Medicaid identification number is assigned by the local administering agency. For Blue Shield, use the number on the subscriber's identification card, which is usually referred to as the "identification" or "certification" or "contract" number.

2. Type the patient's last name followed by the first name and middle initial.

3. Type the patient's birth date in numerals using six digits; for example, June 3, 1943 should be typed 06/03/43. For Medicare, type "DNA" (Does Not Apply). Mark whether the patient is male or female.

4. Type the insured's name (the name of the person to whom the policy was issued). If the insured and the patient are the same, you may type "Same." For Medicare, type "DNA."

5. Type the patient's full address and phone number. Place the street address on the first line of section five, the city and state on the second line, and the ZIP code and complete phone number, including area code, on the third line of section five.

6. Mark the correct box indicating the patient's relationship to the insured.

7. Type the insured's full address and phone number.

8. Mark the correct box(es) to indicate the patient's marital and employment status. **Note:** In items 9, a, b, c, d and 11, a, b, c, d, the HCFA-1500 form asks for information about insurance under which the patient is covered. These two sections can be confusing, as item 11 continues with information that began in line 7, essentially skipping over items 9 and 10. To make this part of the form simpler, you should skip to instruction 11 below, then return to items 9 and 10.

9. Complete items 9, a, b, c, d. If the file indicates the patient is covered by any other health insurance, type the name of the other policyholder, the other insured's policy or group number, the other policyholder's birth date and sex, the other policyholder's employer or school name, and the name of the additional insurance plan or program. If the file shows no record of any other health insurance coverage, type "DNA."

10. Complete items 10, a, b, c. Mark the proper boxes indicating whether the cause of the patient's condition was related to employment, auto accident, or other accident.

11. Complete items 11, a, b, c, d. Type the identification number of the insured's group, if this is a group claim, or FECA number. If the patient is not covered by group insurance, type "DNA." Type the insured's birth date and mark the box indicating the patient's sex. Type the insured employer's name or school name, and the name of the insurance or program. Check the correct box to indicate another health benefit plan.

12. and 13. Secure the patient's signature or the signature of the patient's parent or guardian. The signature in box 12 gives the patient's permission for the physician to release medical information to the insurance carrier. Patient signatures may be kept on file, which gives the doctor's office authority to file the claim without a personal signature. A signature in box 13 gives the patient's permission for the insurance company to pay the physician directly. When an illiterate or physically handicapped enrollee signs by marking an "x," a witness must sign next to the mark and enter an address.

Complete the following items only if a comprehensive superbill will not be attached to the claim forms.

14. Type the date of the first symptoms of the illness or the date of the injury. If the reason for the visit is a suspected pregnancy, write the date of the last menstrual period (LMP).

15. If the patient has had the same or similar illness, type the date the symptoms first appeared.

16. Some patients may be unable to work in their current occupation because of the current illness or condition. If this has occurred, type the dates the patient did not work.

17. and 17a. Type the name and identification number of the referring physician or agency.

18. If the patient was previously hospitalized due to the current illness, insert the correct dates.

19. Leave this space blank.

20. If the patient received services from an outside laboratory, check the appropriate box and insert the charge for the service.

21. Look at the medical record on the superbill to determine the diagnosis(es). Type the diagnosis and diagnosis codes.

22. In some cases, the patient may have previously submitted a claim for the same illness. If so, the Medicaid resubmission code must be inserted in this section, along with the original reference number.

23. Prior authorization is required for certain services that Medicaid will not reimburse without prior approval. A special number is issued for prior authorization, and it must be entered on the form before payment will be made for the services in question.

24. To complete section 24, type across the page. Complete each column of line 1 before going to line 2.
    A. List the date(s) of service shown in the medical record or on the superbill. Continue to Column B.
    B. and C. Place of Service and Type of Service codes are specific for each insurance carrier and may differ among carriers and Medicare or Medicaid. You must refer to each carrier's service codes to complete this information. For Nancy Shields the number "3" is used. For the MarshInd Plan "3" indicates "office" was the place

of service. Typical codes are shown in Figure 14-10. Continue to Column D.

D. The information for this section is given on the superbill and in the medical record. Identify the procedures code being used, commonly CPT-4, by inserting the name of the code in the heading of 24D. Fill in the code for the first procedure. This is likely to be an office visit. The CPT-4 code for established patient office visits range from 99211 to 99215. Explain any unusual circumstances to help in processing the claim.

E. Refer to section 21 of the claim form. Use the number 1, 2, 3, 4 or the ICD-9-CM code shown in section 21 to relate the date of service and the procedure to the appropriate diagnosis.

F. From the physician's fee schedule, determine the fee for each procedure. Type the amount in the "Charges" column. Proceed to line 2 of box 24.

G. For Medicare: If "From" and "To" are entered in Column A indicating a series of identical services, give the number of services here.

H. For Medicare, leave this blank. For Medicaid, the blocks for EPSDT (Early and Periodic Screening for Diagnosis and Treatment of Children) and Family Planning are used to indicate whether these services are involved and should be checked if appropriate. If marked, funds especially designated for these purposes will be used for reimbursement.

I. and J. These boxes are rarely used. These have to do with Emergencies and Coordination of Benefits. Ignore these sections.

K. Leave blank.

Go to line 2. Continue across the page and complete each column in the same manner as line 1. Repeat as necessary. Complete the following items.

25. Fill in the physician's social security number or federal tax identification number. A federal tax identification number is generally

---

Place of Service Codes:

1	(IH)	Inpatient Hospital
2	(OH)	Outpatient Hospital
3	(O)	Doctor's Office
4	(H)	Patient's Home
5		Day Care Facility (PSY)
6		Night Care Facility (PSY)
7	(NH)	Nursing Home
8	(SNF)	Skilled Nursing Facility
9		Ambulance
0	(OL)	Other Locations
A	(IL)	Independent Laboratory
B	(ASC)	Ambulatory Surgical Center
C	(RTC)	Residential Treatment Center
D	(STF)	Specialized Treatment Facility
E	(COR)	Comprehensive Outpatient Rehabilitation Facility
F	(KDC)	Independent Kidney Disease Treatment Center

Type of Service Codes:

1	Medical Care
2	Surgery
3	Consultation
4	Diagnostic X-Ray
5	Diagnostic Laboratory
6	Radiation Therapy
7	Anesthesia
8	Assistance at Surgery
9	Other Medical Service
0	Blood or Packed Red Cells
A	Used DME
F	Ambulatory Surgical Center
H	Hospice
L	Renal Supplies in the Home
M	Alternate Payment for Maintenance Dialysis
N	Kidney Donor
V	Pneumococcal Vaccine
Y	Second Opinion on Elective Surgery
Z	Third Opinion Elective Surgery

FIGURE 14-10 Typical place of service and type of service codes

used when the physician or supplier provides services in a group practice or is employed by a hospital or other institution. Check the appropriate box.

26. Key the patient's account number. If none, type "DNA."

27. Mark the correct box to indicate whether the physician accepts assignment of benefits under a government-funded program. This does not include FEHB and does not refer to Medicaid.

28. Fill in the amount of the total charge.

29. Fill in any amount that was paid by another source, for example, another insurance carrier. If none was paid by another source, type "0."

30. Fill in the balance due.

31. The physician or a person designated by the physician must sign and date the form. This block must be completed although the doctor's stamp is acceptable.

32. If services were rendered outside the physician's office or the patient's home, key the name and address of the person or facility providing the service. If not, type "DNA."

33. Fill in the physician's full address and telephone number. This information may be preprinted or rubber stamped.

Copy the form for the medical office files. Mail the original to the insurance carrier.

SUPPLEMENTAL PROCEDURES FOR COMPLETING AN HCFA-1500 FORM

1. Provide complete information about procedures, treatments, and diagnoses.

2. Give procedure and treatment codes and diagnosis codes.

3. List DRGs for hospital patients.

4. List all dates accurately.

5. Obtain all necessary signatures.

6. Check for agreement of diagnoses and treatments.

7. List all charges. Do not summarize.

8. Provide accurate totals.

9. Double check the insurance policy number.

10. Submit forms to the proper administering agency. Call the local carrier's office for an address, if you do not know it.

11. Submit forms to all carriers that provide coverage to the patient.

12. Provide a detailed report of nonstandard treatments.

13. List each service separately for each visit.

14. Combine office and hospital visits if the fee is the same for each visit.

15. Itemize laboratory work separately from office visits.

16. Itemize injections separately.

17. Itemize x-rays separately.

18. Provide detailed information regarding excision of tumors. List the type, number, category, size, weight, and location of tumors.

19. Provide detailed information regarding lacerations. List the length, location, and type of repair.

20. Itemize special materials.

21. List federal identification numbers and provider identification numbers.

22. Submit claims to the insurance carrier promptly.

23. File a copy of the claim form in the patient's medical record.

24. Retrieve the patient's ledger card and place a check mark in the date column.

25. Establish an audit trail for the claim (see below).

ESTABLISHING AN AUDIT TRAIL

An audit trail should be established to determine the status of all insurance claims at all times. This is especially important for medical offices that file a large number of insurance claims for patients. When a carrier fails to make a timely reimbursement, the medical assistant must call or write the company, determine the problem, and assist in rectifying the situation. An alert medical assistant should be able to give an up-to-date status report on a claim at any time if the physician or patient inquires. Two simple methods of tracing claims are discussed in the next section.

Claims Register

A claims register is a continuing log that lists the following information about each claim submitted to an insurance carrier: (1) the claim number, (2) the patient's name, (3) the carrier,

(4) the date the claim was submitted, (5) the amount of the claim, (6) dates of follow-up requests, and (7) final disposition of the claim, including (a) the date the claim was made, (b) the amount paid, and (c) any difference between the amount of the claims and the amount paid.

For greatest efficiency, complete the claims register when an insurance claim form is mailed to the carrier, or keep all claims in a stack to be registered at the end of each day. Depending on the number of forms submitted, one sheet from the claims register can be used for several days. When the sheet is full, continue listing claims on a new page.

The follow-up date refers to a future date when an inquiry should be made if the carrier has not responded. Since most claims require two to six weeks for processing, a date six weeks away is realistic. People who work with the various carriers learn how long a claim takes for processing, and can adjust the follow-up dates accordingly. A claims register is shown in Figure 14-11.

Tickler File

A tickler file is a dated file that holds a copy of each claim form until it is paid. In a tickler file, primary dividers are labeled with the name of each month, and two sets of folders list the numbers 1–31. One set of folders is placed behind the divider for the current month, and the second set is placed behind the divider for the upcoming month. Follow the procedures below for using a tickler file (Figure 14-12).

1. When the claim form is submitted to the insurance carrier, place a copy of the form in the proper folder behind a date approximately six weeks in advance. (For example, for a claim submitted on June 1, file the copy of the claim form in the folder for July 15.)

2. When a claim is paid, record the payment on the patient's ledger card, then remove the copy of the claim form from the tickler file. (Destroy this copy, since another copy should already be filed in the patient's medical record.)

3. At the end of each billing period, review all claim forms in the tickler file to determine which claims are more than six weeks old. Begin the follow-up procedure described in the next section.

Follow-up Procedure

When payment has not been received from a carrier at the end of six weeks (or the next billing period after six weeks), write a follow-up letter asking for payment and enclose a copy of the claim form. Enter the date of the letter in the claim register and record a new follow-up date two to six weeks away. Or, attach a copy of the letter to the file copy of the claim form in the tickler file and return it to the tickler file in a folder dated before the next billing period. Con-

INSURANCE CLAIMS REGISTER

Claim No.	Patient	Carrier	Claim Submitted Date	Claim Submitted Amount	Follow-up Date	Claim Paid Date	Claim Paid Amount	Difference (Submitted - Paid)	
1 601	Clara Vinings	Liberty Mutual	5/17	62.00	6/30	6/2	54.00	8.00	1
2 602	Jason Martin	Blue Shield	5/17	26.00	6/30	6/15	20.00	6.00	2
3 603	Anthony Garcia	Nationwide	5/18	78.00	6/30				3
4 604	Barbara Cosby	Aetna Life Casualty	5/18	26.00	6/30	6/4	26.00	—	4
5 605	Gerard Jackson	Blue Shield	5/23	84.00	7/7				5
6									6
7									7
8									8
9									9
10									10
11									11
12									12
13									13
14									14
15									15

FIGURE 14-11 Claims Register

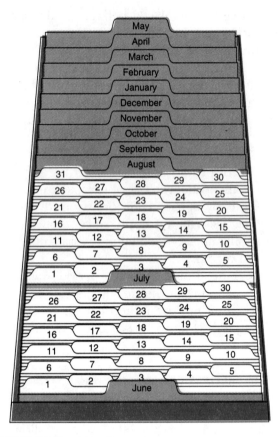

FIGURE 14-12 Tickler file

tinue with the collection process discussed in Chapter 15 until the claim is paid.

Computerizing the Claims Process

Computers have revolutionized the processing of claims. With a few simple commands, the medical assistant can instruct the computer to print insurance forms daily, weekly, or monthly. The computer can also track the forms on a standard schedule, thus providing an up-to-date analysis of each form's location in the insurance cycle.

Most medical software is capable of automatically printing the HCFA-1500 form, and the instruction to bill the insurance company for patient charges is coded when the information is entered on the patient's first visit. When the medical assistant instructs the program to print an insurance form, it searches through the transactions previously posted to the account from the superbill and prints complete details about each office visit, procedure, or service.

Most computer systems can print individually or in bulk on a daily, weekly, or monthly basis at the rate of two to four forms a minute, depending on the printer. The computer will even print two forms automatically if the patient has two insurance policies. In medical offices that do not prepare insurance forms for patients, the program can generate a detailed superbill for the patient to attach to the insurance form.

Look at the computer-completed HCFA-1500 form in Figure 14-13. A computer program enters the correct information for each patient onto the form as it is fed into the computer, providing a detailed description of the services provided. This form provides the insurer with all the information needed to quickly process the insurance claim. The computer program eliminates the tedious task of handwriting the information onto the form and greatly reduces errors.

Some government agencies do not accept the HCFA-1500 form. It is possible to program most computer systems to accept various other formats for claims forms. An example is the Workers' Compensation First Report of Injury form shown in Figure 14-7. The computer can also be programmed to produce the Attending Physician's Report and other relevant forms.

IN YOUR OPINION

1. Should the medical assistant complete claims forms for patients? Explain your thinking.
2. Would you prefer to work with a claims register or a tickler file? Explain your answer.
3. What should you do if you find yourself often using a typewriter because one of the insurance forms is not built into your software?

REFERENCES

"Ask the Doctor," *Ladies Home Journal*, February, 1995, p. 114.

Beck, Melinda. "The Gray Nineties," *Newsweek*, October 14, 1993.

DRGs and the Prospective Payment System: A Guide for Physicians. Chicago: American Medical Association, 1986.

PLEASE DO NOT STAPLE IN THIS AREA

Epsilon Life & Casualty
P.O. Box 189
Macon, GA 31298

APPROVED OMB-0938-0008

CARRIER

| | PICA | | **HEALTH INSURANCE CLAIM FORM** | PICA | |

1. MEDICARE ☐ (Medicare #) MEDICAID ☐ (Medicaid #) CHAMPUS ☐ (Sponsor's SSN) CHAMPVA ☐ (VA File #) GROUP HEALTH PLAN ☐ (SSN or ID) FECA BLK LUNG ☐ (SSN) OTHER ☒ (ID)

1a. INSURED'S I.D. NUMBER (FOR PROGRAM IN ITEM 1)
756575675

2. PATIENT'S NAME (Last Name, First Name, Middle Initial)
Evans   Patricia

3. PATIENT'S BIRTH DATE MM DD YY
12 13 40   M ☐ SEX F ☒

4. INSURED'S NAME (Last Name, First Name, Middle Initial)
Evans   Patricia G

5. PATIENT'S ADDRESS (No., Street)
8907 Harbor Drive

6. PATIENT RELATIONSHIP TO INSURED
Self ☒ Spouse ☐ Child ☐ Other ☐

7. INSURED'S ADDRESS (No., Street)
8907 Harbor Drive

CITY
Madison   STATE C A

8. PATIENT STATUS
Single ☐ Married ☐ Other ☐

CITY
Madison   STATE C A

ZIP CODE
95653   TELEPHONE (Include Area Code) ( )

Employed ☐ Full-Time Student ☐ Part-Time Student ☐

ZIP CODE
95653   TELEPHONE (INCLUDE AREA CODE) ( )

9. OTHER INSURED'S NAME (Last Name, First Name, Middle Initial)

10. IS PATIENT'S CONDITION RELATED TO:

11. INSURED'S POLICY GROUP OR FECA NUMBER

a. OTHER INSURED'S POLICY OR GROUP NUMBER

a. EMPLOYMENT? (CURRENT OR PREVIOUS)
YES ☐ NO ☒

a. INSURED'S DATE OF BIRTH MM DD YY   SEX M ☐ F ☐

b. OTHER INSURED'S DATE OF BIRTH MM DD YY   SEX M ☐ F ☐

b. AUTO ACCIDENT?   PLACE (State)
YES ☐ NO ☐

b. EMPLOYER'S NAME OR SCHOOL NAME

c. EMPLOYER'S NAME OR SCHOOL NAME

c. OTHER ACCIDENT?
YES ☐ NO ☐

c. INSURANCE PLAN NAME OR PROGRAM NAME

d. INSURANCE PLAN NAME OR PROGRAM NAME

10d. RESERVED FOR LOCAL USE

d. IS THERE ANOTHER HEALTH BENEFIT PLAN?
YES ☐ NO ☐ If yes, return to and complete item 9 a-d.

READ BACK OF FORM BEFORE COMPLETING & SIGNING THIS FORM.

12. PATIENT'S OR AUTHORIZED PERSON'S SIGNATURE I authorize the release of any medical or other information necessary to process this claim. I also request payment of government benefits either to myself or to the party who accepts assignment below.

SIGNED Signature on File   DATE 02/03/—

13. INSURED'S OR AUTHORIZED PERSON'S SIGNATURE I authorize payment of medical benefits to the undersigned physician or supplier for services described below.

SIGNED Signature on File

14. DATE OF CURRENT: MM DD YY 12 30 ◄ ILLNESS (First symptom) OR INJURY (Accident) OR PREGNANCY(LMP)

15. IF PATIENT HAS HAD SAME OR SIMILAR ILLNESS. GIVE FIRST DATE MM DD YY 01 10 —

16. DATES PATIENT UNABLE TO WORK IN CURRENT OCCUPATION
FROM MM DD YY   TO MM DD YY

17. NAME OF REFERRING PHYSICIAN OR OTHER SOURCE
Leland W Groves, M.D.

17a. I.D. NUMBER OF REFERRING PHYSICIAN

18. HOSPITALIZATION DATES RELATED TO CURRENT SERVICES
FROM 01 26 —   TO 01 31 —

19. RESERVED FOR LOCAL USE

20. OUTSIDE LAB? $ CHARGES
YES ☐ NO ☐

21. DIAGNOSIS OR NATURE OF ILLNESS OR INJURY. (RELATE ITEMS 1,2,3 OR 4 TO ITEM 24E BY LINE)
1. 174.9
2. ___.___
3. ___.___
4. ___.___

22. MEDICAID RESUBMISSION CODE   ORIGINAL REF. NO.

23. PRIOR AUTHORIZATION NUMBER

24.
A DATE(S) OF SERVICE From MM DD YY — To MM DD YY	B Place of Service	C Type of Service	D PROCEDURES, SERVICES, OR SUPPLIES (Explain Unusual Circumstances) CPT/HCPCS | MODIFIER	E DIAGNOSIS CODE	F $ CHARGES	G DAYS OR UNITS	H EPSDT Family Plan	I EMG	J COB	K RESERVED FOR LOCAL USE
01 10 —	3		99214	174.9	50 00	1				
01 10 —	3		76088	174.9	125 00	1				
01 10 —	3		71020	174.9	58 00	1				
01 26 —	3		99223	174.9	180 00	1				
01 31 —	3		99238	174.9	38 00	1				
01 27 — 01 31 —	3		99232	174.9	208 00	1				

25. FEDERAL TAX I.D. NUMBER   SSN ☐ EIN ☐

26. PATIENT'S ACCOUNT NO.

27. ACCEPT ASSIGNMENT? (For govt. claims, see back)
YES ☒ NO ☐

28. TOTAL CHARGE $ 659 00

29. AMOUNT PAID $ 00

30. BALANCE DUE $ 659 00

31. SIGNATURE OF PHYSICIAN OR SUPPLIER INCLUDING DEGREES OR CREDENTIALS (I certify that the statements on the reverse apply to this bill and are made a part thereof.)
Signature on File

SIGNED   DATE

32. NAME AND ADDRESS OF FACILITY WHERE SERVICES WERE RENDERED (If other than home or office)

33. PHYSICIAN'S, SUPPLIER'S BILLING NAME, ADDRESS, ZIP CODE & PHONE #
9169876543
Sydney Carrington & Assoc.
34 Sycamore St. Suite 300
Madison, CA 94303
PIN#   GRP#

790-0115(12/90) (OCR) 1 pt.

(APPROVED BY AMA COUNCIL ON MEDICAL SERVICE 8/88)   **PLEASE PRINT OR TYPE**

FORM HCFA-1500 (U2) (12-90)
FORM OWCP-1500   FORM RRB-1500

PATIENT AND INSURED INFORMATION   PHYSICIAN OR SUPPLIER INFORMATION

FIGURE 14-13 Computerized insurance form (Adapted from Gartee and Humphrey, *The Medical Manager, Student Edition, Version 5.3,* copyright 1995, Delmar Publishers)

Esterbrook, Greg. "The Revolution in Medicine," *Newsweek,* January 26, 1987.

Gartee, Richard, and Doris D. Humphrey. *The Medical Manager.* Cincinnati, Ohio: South-Western Publishing Co., 1995.*

Humphrey, Doris, and Kathie Sigler. *The Modern Medical Office: A Reference Manual.* Cincinnati, Ohio: South-Western Publishing Company, 1990.*

Kotoski, Gabrielle M. *CPT Coding Made Easy.* Gaithersburg, Maryland: Aspen Publishers, Inc., 1993.

Medical Collection Study Course. Chicago: American Medical Association, 1986.

Medicare Special Bulletin, March 6, 1992. U.S. Government Printing Office.

Physician Reimbursement Under DRGs: Problems and Prospects. Chicago: American Medical Association, 1984.

"Population Trends," *The Futurist,* August, 1990, p. 40.

Samuelson, Robert J. "Healthcare: How We Got into This Mess," *Newsweek,* October 4, 1993, p.31.

"Sixty Minutes," December 3, 1993.

*Currently published by Delmar Publishers.

Chapter Activities

PERFORMANCE BASED ACTIVITIES

1. Contact the administrative office of an HMO and a PPO in your area. Ask for the information shown in the chart. Compare the two types of plans.
   a. What benefits do the plans offer?
   b. What are the provisions of the physician's contract?
   c. Who pays for the plan and when is it paid?
   d. What are the advantages for the insured person and the physician?

Comparison of HMO and PPO Plans

	HMO Plan	PPO Plan
Covered Benefits	_____	_____
Physician's Contract Provisions	_____	_____
Who Pays the Plan	_____	_____
When Is the Plan Paid	_____	_____
Advantages for the Patient	_____	_____
Advantages for the Physician	_____	_____

(DACUM 8.3)

2. Review the procedures and codes on pages 295 and 299 and the superbill on page 296. List the correct CPT-4 codes, ICD-9 codes, and fees for patients with the services and diagnoses listed below:

BARBARA GONZALES	CPT CODE	ICD CODE	FEE
SERVICE			
Level III			
Established Patient	_____		_____
CBC	_____		_____
Urinalysis	_____		_____
DIAGNOSIS			
Goiter		_____	
Hyperthyroidism		_____	

FRED CHEN	CPT CODE	ICD CODE	FEE
SERVICE			
Intermediate Visit			
Established Patient	_____		_____
Throat Culture	_____		_____
CBC	_____		_____
DIAGNOSIS			
Bronchitis		_____	

JUANITA DAVIS	CPT CODE	ICD CODE	FEE
SERVICE			
Level IV			
Established Patient	_____		_____
Chest X-ray	_____		_____
EKG	_____		_____
CBC	_____		_____
Urinalysis	_____		_____
Electrolytes	_____		_____
DIAGNOSIS			
Cardiac Arrhythmia		_____	

(DACUM 8.2)

3. What is the medical assistant's responsibility at each step in the health insurance claim process? Fill out the chart below.

Step	Medical Assistant's Responsibility
1. Completing Form	
2. Form Signatures	
3. Form Mailing	
4. Claim Examination	
5. Form Return (if incomplete)	
6. Form Resubmission (if original was incomplete)	
7. Check Sent to Patient or Physician	
8. Account Credited	

(DACUM 8.3)

EXPANDING YOUR THINKING

1. Call or visit the business office of a local hospital and inquire about the effect of DRGs on the hospital, physicians, and patients. Based on your research, write a short analysis of the value of DRGs.

DRGs Analysis

Effect on Hospital

_____

_____

_____

Effect on Physicians

_____

_____

_____

Effect on Patients

_____

_____

_____

2. Contact the claims department of two major insurers and inquire about the types of problems the department encounters when processing patients' health claims. Make a list of the problems and suggest how the medical assistant can help correct the problem. What conclusions can you draw from the information? (You may call Blue Cross/Blue Shield, The Travelers, Aetna, or other health insurance companies.)

	Problems with Claim Forms	*How Medical Assistant Can Assist in Correction*
Insurer 1	_____	_____
	_____	_____
	_____	_____
	_____	_____
	_____	_____
Insurer 2	_____	_____
	_____	_____
	_____	_____
	_____	_____
	_____	_____

Conclusions Drawn:

_____

_____

_____

_____

_____

_____

3. Visit your local library or a physician's office and review a copy of the CPT-4 and ICD-9-CM manuals. Make a list of ten procedures or treatments you recognize and ten diagnoses you have heard about.

Medical Diagnoses   *Diagnosis Code*

_____   _____

_____   _____

_____   _____

_____   _____

_____   _____

_____   _____

_____   _____

_____   _____

_____   _____

_____   _____

Chapter 15

Billing and Collection

MORRISTOWN, NEW JERSEY

My brother works for a large computer company in the Direct Marketing Division. They sell computer components to consumers via phone, fax, and mail orders. He told me a story about their overdue accounts which I've been able to apply to our sports medicine and rehabilitation clinic here in New Jersey.

Eric said that at one point his division had one of the highest percentages of unpaid bills in the company. Management assembled a task force to look into causes of the problem. The task force began by assuming that people who hadn't paid their bills were "deadbeats" or unwilling or unable to pay their bills. The task force conducted a survey and discovered that almost every overdue invoice had some sort of problem that originated in the company's own order entry department!

That's when I started thinking of our patients who had not paid their bills as "people with a problem" instead of "deadbeats." Maybe, I thought, they just don't understand the billing codes and charges. I am constantly wrestling with codes and revisions to codes and regulations; and, sometimes, even I don't understand. No wonder our patients are sometimes baffled by our billing.

When I started investigating the bills, I found a lot of errors in our patient files. If pa-

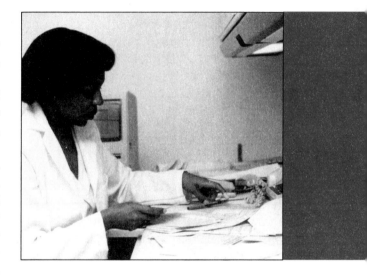

tients receive bills with the wrong spelling, birth date, address, or initials, they may think the bill was meant for someone else and sent to them by mistake. These days, we have patients audit their own information sheets for up-to-date data every six months. We've changed our invoice format so that it's self-explanatory and we include a pamphlet on how to read the invoice. Our receivable figure, I'm happy to say, has steadily decreased since we've put more work into the process at the beginning.

Rebecca Greyling
Accounts Receivable Supervisor

PERFORMANCE BASED COMPETENCIES

After completing this chapter, you should be able to:
1. Compare the advantages of internal billing and external billing. (DACUM 8.4)
2. Evaluate different methods of internal billing. (DACUM 8.1)
3. Manage the collection process. (DACUM 8.4)

HEALTHSPEAK

Account aging Method for reporting how long an account has been due.

Collection Process for expediting overdue accounts.

Cycle billing Method for spreading billing over the whole month instead of sending all bills at the same time.

Invoice Statement of services.

Payables Amount of money owed by a practice to those from whom it purchases goods and services.

Receivables Amount of money owed to a practice by those who purchase its services.

Patient billing may take many forms, from the simple to the complex. Whatever method is used, it must be managed efficiently and expeditiously if a medical practice is to succeed. If patients do not pay their bills, the practice will not be able to pay its bills, including the salaries of the physicians and the staff. An organized, standard billing system based on a schedule that fits the practice, combined with accurate, complete records, makes billing a relatively simple task.

A routine statement of services mailed during the regular billing cycle usually suffices to collect patient accounts; however, when patients fail to pay their bills, the practice must attempt to collect. Collection can take many forms, from a series of letters, to personal telephone calls, to the services of a collection agency. If all of these efforts fail, the medical office can take a patient to court for nonpayment. Collection by means of a lawsuit is a costly procedure, however, and should be avoided when possible. Often this expensive process can be forestalled by simply calling the person responsible for the bill and asking if she or he understood it, if the bill is accurate, and if there are any problems with the bill.

When a pegboard accounting system is used to maintain financial records, billing and collection activities are completed by hand. If the office uses a computer system, the computer produces billing statements, aging reports, and collection notices.

Billing Patients

Billing may be handled internally by a medical assistant who devotes some portion of the day or perhaps even the entire day to accounts control. Or, it may be contracted through an external service that manages billing for several different clients for a monthly or annual fee. In either case, the medical assistant must be knowledgeable about the process to manage the office's billing and collection records accurately and efficiently. If you, as a medical assistant, are asked to handle the billing for the practice, you will be required to concentrate, to work for large blocks of uninterrupted time, and to have a clear understanding of the account aging process. Since you will usually work alone at this task without much supervision, organizational skills and maturity are important assets.

INTERNAL BILLING

Internal billing takes a variety of forms, depending on the size of the practice. Billing can be as simple as requiring payment at the time of service or as complex as cycle billing that spans several days each month. The best billing system is one that meets the needs of the individual practice, and the simpler the system, the better. Although some practices require complex billing systems, complexity itself does not always guarantee better payment results. Several methods of billings from simple to complex are discussed in the next section. The individual practice must determine which method is best suited for its size, financial objectives, and patient load.

Superbill as Statement at Time of Service

The best opportunity for collection of an account is at the time of service, and it is becoming increasingly common for practices to require payment at that time. The superbill, which is given to each patient at the end of a visit, serves as the first statement and eliminates the time and expense of preparing and mailing a statement. Another advantage is that the practice receives the income immediately and can earn interest if the money is deposited in an interest-bearing account. To encourage payment, some medical offices accept major credit cards, as well as cash and checks, making it possible for almost everyone to pay immediately.

Even in practices that do not require payment at the time of service, patients should be encouraged to pay when they are given the superbill. Old balances can often be collected at the same time with a bit of subtlety and tact. While handing the superbill to the patient, a medical assistant might make one of the following comments:

- "Here is your superbill, Mrs. Mara. The charge is $46."
- "Mr. Silvano, do you want to write a check or pay cash for today's visit?"
- "If it's helpful, Ms. Riegert, we take VISA and MasterCard as well as cash or a check."
- "Mr. Itani, today's charge is $46, and you have a balance of $28 from the last visit. Would you like to pay the entire account today?"

Billing Statement

The practice that mails a billing statement has two options: (1) mailing a copy of the ledger card as a statement, which is faster, or (2) sending a special statement form, which is time-consuming but looks more professional (Figure 15-1). In either case, a self-addressed return envelope may be enclosed to make payment simple.

Ledger Card as Statement

If a practice uses the ledger card as a statement, the medical assistant should copy all the ledger cards with outstanding balances once during each billing cycle, enclose each in a window envelope, and mail it to the person responsible for the account. Since the ledger card shows the history of all the account's charges, credits, and adjustments, in addition to the patient's name and address, minimal time will be spent on billing. To eliminate the need to check each card individually, all ledger cards showing outstanding balances can be coded with colored strips doubled over the top of the cards so the color is visible. When an account is paid in full, the colored strip is removed.

Another method to identify accounts with outstanding balances is to store the past due ledger cards in a special "Unpaid" or "Balance

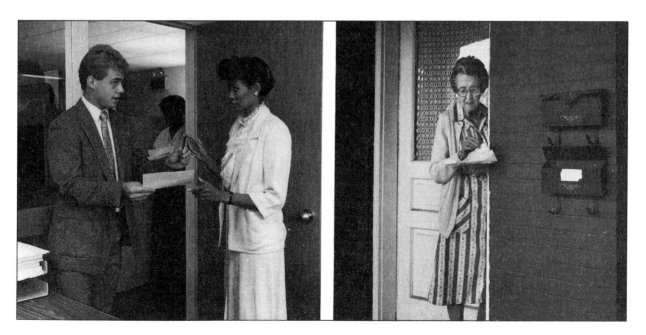

FIGURE 15-1 Some medical offices require payment at the time of service; other practices mail a billing statement to the patient.

Due" section of the file. See Figures 15-2 and 15-3 for illustrations of the two methods. There is, however, one disadvantage to using ledger cards as statements. Because the information on the ledger card is handwritten and transfers through carbon when the superbill is completed, the copied ledger card is not an attractive method of billing.

Special Statement Form

A special statement form, typed or printed and mailed in a window envelope, looks more professional and attractive. The statement lists most of the same information shown on a ledger card; however, only the services performed since the last statement, along with any previous balance, are shown. This method is less efficient

LEDGER SHEET
JOHN H. SPARKS, M.D.

Romero Sanchez 407
253-A Lost Creek Circle
Atlanta, GA 30033-2289

| DATE | DESCRIPTION | CHARGE | CREDITS | | CURRENT BALANCE |
			PAYMENT	ADJUSTMENT	
4/17/--	O.V., Xray	55.00	30.00		25.00
6/14/--	O.V., Lab	40.00	30.00		35.00

FIGURE 15-2 Ledger card color-coded for outstanding balance

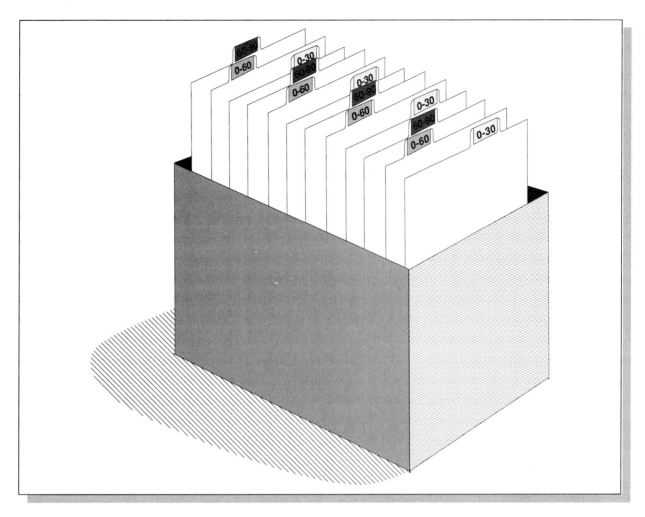

FIGURE 15-3 Ledger card stored in special filing section

than mailing a copy of the ledger card, but it makes a better impression for the practice. A special statement form is shown in Figure 15-4.

Computerized Statement

The most sophisticated billing method is accomplished with a computer. If the office is computerized, during each billing cycle the medical assistant will direct the program to search the patient database and print statements for patients with outstanding balances (Figure 15-5). The program automatically ages accounts at the same time. For overdue accounts, the computer can also print a series of pre-written collection letters to remind patients of their balances.

The medical assistant can process the billings while attending to other duties simply by entering the beginning and ending account numbers and instructing the computer to print. Look at the computerized sample monthly statement in Figure 15-6. The top of the form is perforated, so the patient can tear it off and return it to the medical office. Since the top shows the account name and number, the amount currently due, and the statement date, all the necessary posting information will be received when the patient returns the top with the payment.

The bottom portion of the statement, which the patient keeps, shows the old balance, the date of service, the family member treated, each procedure and charge, any payments, and the current amount due.

After all statements are printed, they can be inserted in window envelopes and mailed to the responsible parties.

STATEMENT

Telephone
(615) 555-8726

Alyson Malik, M.D.
423 West Main Street
Lebanon, TN 37087-0000

Mr. Amrit Singh
2203 Van Loan Drive
Lebanon, TN 37087-0000

| DATE | FAMILY MEMBER | PROFESSIONAL SERVICE | CHARGE | CREDITS | | BALANCE |
				PAYMTS	ADJ.	
			BALANCE FORWARD			
3/27	Michael	EV, S, HV				192 —
We have received payment from your insurance company. Please pay the remaining amount.						
WE NOW ACCEPT VISA/MASTERCARD FOR YOUR CONVENIENCE						
LAST BILL BEFORE COLLECTIONS						
		PAY LAST AMOUNT IN THIS COLUMN				

FIGURE 15-4 Special statement form

MONTHLY BILLING AND CYCLE BILLING

The size of a practice usually determines the billing schedule. In a single-physician or small group practice, monthly billing may be the most efficient method. However, in a large practice, the flexibility of cycle billing offers certain advantages.

Monthly Billing

In a monthly billing system, all accounts are billed at the same time, usually near the end of the month. This means that the medical assistant will devote one or two days to the billing task and mail all statements at the same time. Monthly billing offers the advantage of continu-

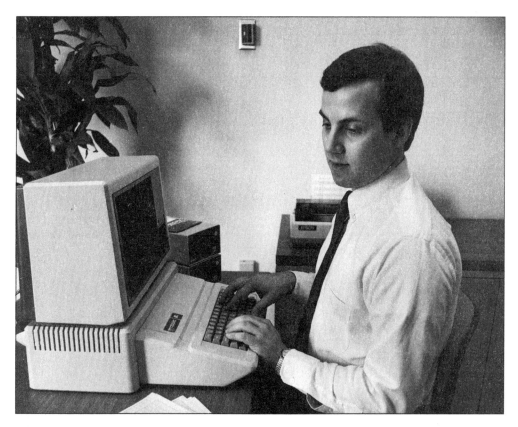

FIGURE 15-5 Computerized statements are the most sophisticated method of billing patients.

ity, allowing the assistant to plan other responsibilities around the billing schedule.

The disadvantage of monthly billing is that a medical assistant may neglect other activities during this billing time, or become overworked and harassed. To avoid these problems, the medical assistant may prepare billing statements intermittently over a one- or two-week period and store them until the mailing date. However, if several days pass between the time statements are prepared and mailed, a message to "Disregard if payment has already been made" should be printed on the form. Patients become annoyed and the practice appears disorganized if a statement arrives several days after payment has been made.

Cycle Billing

Cycle billing offers a feasible alternative for practices that cannot devote the full services of a medical assistant to billing for one or more days each month. With this system, the alphabet is divided into sections and patients are billed according to where the first letter of their last names fall in the alphabet. Each month statements are prepared on the same schedule. Then they can be mailed as they are completed, or held and mailed at one time. A typical cycle billing schedule is shown here. The system can be varied as needed by the individual practice:

1. Divide the alphabet into four sections: A–F, G–L, M–R, S–Z.
2. Prepare statements for patients whose last names begin with A through F on Monday and mail them on Tuesday of Week 1.
3. Prepare statements for patients whose last names begin with G through L on Monday and mail them on Tuesday of Week 2.
4. Prepare statements for patients whose last names begin with M through R on Monday and mail them on Tuesday of Week 3.
5. Prepare statements for patients whose last names begin with S through Z on Monday and mail them on Tuesday of Week 4.

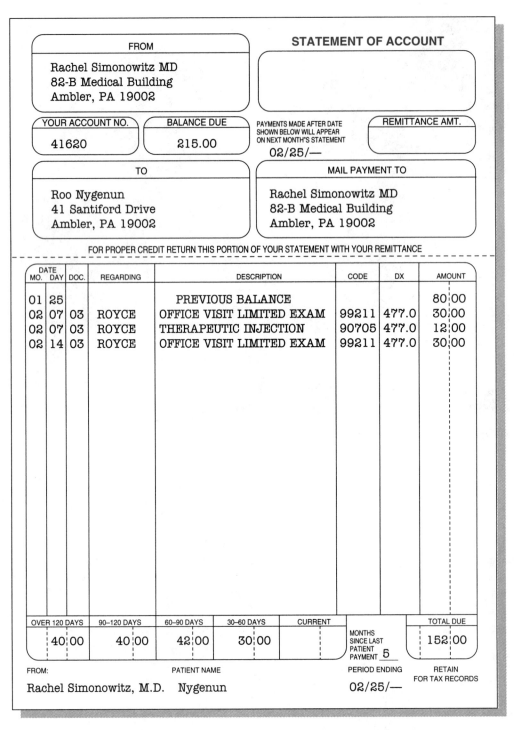

FIGURE 15-6 Computerized statement

Billing is a time-consuming yet necessary activity if a practice is to remain financially viable. To relieve the stress of unbroken paperwork, schedule routine breaks. It is important, however, not to become too involved in another activity that delays the billing and results in a last-minute rush to get statements mailed.

EXTERNAL BILLING SERVICE

An outside billing service can be hired to manage patient accounts. The service maintains all ledger cards; posting debits and credits from copies of superbills provided by the medical office. It prepares monthly statements, usually by computer, and mails them with a request that payment be returned to the billing service. In addition, it makes deposits directly to the practice's bank account and prepares a report outlining all transactions. External billing services are valuable for practices that employ only a small clerical staff or that have a large number of patients. By placing the billing function with an outside agency, the office eliminates a time-consuming clerical task. When an office uses such a service, the medical assistant acts as liaison between the service and the office, and is responsible for coordinating activities between the two.

IN YOUR OPINION

1. Consider the advantages and disadvantages of using the superbill as a statement, mailing a copy of the ledger card as a statement, or preparing a monthly statement. Which procedure is best?
2. Why is it important to age accounts on a regular basis?
3. In addition to time savings, what advantages does computer billing offer over billing accomplished by pegboard accounting?

The Collection Process

According to the American Medical Association's *Medical Collection Study Course,* 90 to 95 percent of patients pay their medical bills on time; 5 to 10 percent are slow to pay; and about 2 percent have no intention of paying. The collection process is geared to the 5 to 10 percent who are slow to pay. Other measures, such as taking the patient to court, are used for the 2 percent who do not intend to pay. Once a collection agency becomes involved with a patient's account, the medical assistant refers all patient calls regarding the account to the agency.

The purposes of the collection process are (1) to determine if there are errors on the bills, (2) to remind patients of their overdue balances, (3) to encourage them to pay their bills, and (4) to help them find a way to pay their bills if they have financial difficulties. As a medical assistant who handles billing, you may also manage collections, or the practice can contract to have collections made by a private service. Since using an agency is expensive, only large, long-overdue accounts should be given to a collection agency. Usually, accounts of more than $100 that are six months or more overdue are turned over to an agency, while the medical assistant manages routine collections. Filing a lawsuit for nonpayment is the ultimate collection procedure.

Typically, however, collection is attempted by letter or telephone or by a combination of the two methods. The initial contact comes through letters, and telephone collections are instituted only after an account ages and the patient has made no response to letters.

AGING ACCOUNTS

A process called account aging identifies how long an account is overdue. This means that past due accounts are coded according to the length of time they have been unpaid. In a pegboard accounting system, color-coded strips are attached to the ledger cards to show the age of an account, or the cards can be stored behind a color-coded divider in an "Unpaid" file. For example, a red code might be used for accounts one month overdue, a blue code for accounts two months overdue, and other colors for additional months overdue. A written code such as "OD2/6/18—" should be written on the ledger card to indicate when the overdue notice was mailed, meaning "Overdue notice No. 2 mailed on June 18."

Computer account aging is very simple. By giving the appropriate commands, the medical assistant can have the computer system automatically age the accounts at the end of each month before printing billing statements. The program may age accounts according to several criteria; for example, by past due balance, zero balance, or credit balance accounts. Accounts can also be aged by government agency category or by insurance carrier. Therefore, all Medicare or Medicaid accounts would be aged separately from other accounts.

The practice may also wish to have an accounts receivable report printed showing each overdue account, the balance overdue, and a breakdown of the length of time the account is overdue. This breakdown is usually divided into accounts 0–30 days overdue, 31–60 days overdue, 61–90 days overdue, and 90 days or more overdue. The computer may also generate other reports from the accounts receivable report. For example, the medical assistant may wish to reprint a report showing accounts that have been delinquent for more than 90 days or accounts that are delinquent by more than a certain dollar amount.

The top portion of an accounts receivable report is shown in Figure 15-7. Notice the regular accounts that are past due—seven by 31–60 days, four by 61–90 days, and four over 90 days. One Medicaid account is past due by 61–90 days. Figure 15-7 also shows a delinquent accounts report. Notice that this is a listing of four regular accounts overdue by $100 for which no payment has been made since May 30, 19—. The addresses and telephone numbers of the responsible parties are listed, so you may contact the person to begin the collection process.

Aging systems differ according to the type of patient served. For example, a private patient's account is aged differently from a Medicare patient's account. This occurs because federal reimbursement takes time, and the patient may be unprepared to pay without the reimbursement. In a computerized billing system, the accounts are automatically aged, and the aging code is shown on the computerized ledger card. A typical aging code for a private patient follows.

- **S:** Superbill given to patient at time of visit.
- **1:** Itemized statement mailed when account is past due one month.
- **2:** Itemized statement with overdue notice mailed when account is past due two months.
- **3:** Letter stating, "We have not received payment for your account," when account is past due three months.
- **4:** Letter stating, "Your account is overdue" when account is past due four months; or
- **4T:** Telephone call reminding patient of overdue account and offering to help arrange a payment schedule.
- **5** or **5T:** Letter or telephone call stating, "Your account will be turned over to a collector," when account is past due five months.

- **6:** Certified letter stating, "Your account was turned over to a collection agency," when account is past due six months. No further telephone calls are necessary, as they might antagonize the patient and leave the medical assistant open to verbal abuse.
- **7:** Collection agency attempts to collect.
- **8:** Lawsuit filed.

COLLECTION LETTERS SERIES

Medical offices send collection letters to encourage patients and third-party carriers to pay overdue balances. The series of letters to the patient begins after two statements are mailed and the superbill has brought no response. Because the claims process is lengthy for third-party carriers, a collection letter to carriers is not considered valuable until after sixty days have passed.

Collection Letters to Patients

Lack of payment is not considered serious until after sixty days. When the patient has not responded to the superbill, to the statement, or to the statement with an "Overdue" remark at the end of sixty days, a series of collection letters begins. A typical collection letter series is shown in Figures 15-8 through 15-11.

Collection Letters to Third-Party Carriers

Patients are not the only source of late payment. Often private and government insurance groups also need to be reminded of overdue balances. Because the claims units of most insurance companies and government agencies are very large, with many employees of varying levels of experience, the delay can be caused by an overburdened claims department, by a form that has been lost in transit, by a misfiled form, by an inexperienced employee, or by several other reasons. The claims units are concerned with hundreds or thousands of claims, and one misfiled form from a private practice is of little consequence. As a medical assistant, if you maintain a current claims register or tickler and take firm control of the practice's collection procedures, you can make a difference in the promptness with which a claim is paid.

Many patients have private medical plans or qualify for government insurance; therefore, the

```
REGULAR                  ACCOUNTS RECEIVABLE REPORT              07/06/--

ACCOUNT  NAME        BALANCE   CURRENT    0-30    31-60    61-90   OVER 90

   1     Mason        325.00    50.00   118.00    70.00    12.00    75.00
   2     Tiebot        68.00     0.00     0.00    44.00    24.00     0.00
   3     Rohn         483.00     0.00     0.00   435.00     0.00    48.00
   4     Rosa          53.00     0.00     0.00    53.00     0.00     0.00
   5     Bradshaw     358.00    40.00     0.00    34.00    24.00   260.00
   6     South        273.00     0.00   200.00    73.00     0.00     0.00
   8     Capowitz     350.00   138.00     0.00   212.00     0.00     0.00
   9     Adam         282.00     0.00    35.00     0.00   227.00    20.00

   8 Accounts       2,192.00   228.00   353.00   921.00   287.00   403.00

Medicaid               Accounts Receivable Report               07/06/--

ACCOUNT  NAME        BALANCE   CURRENT    0-30    31-60    61-90   OVER 90

   7     Myers-Brooke   12.00     0.00     0.00     0.00    12.00     0.00

   1 Account           12.00     0.00     0.00     0.00    12.00     0.00

   9 Accounts       2,204.00   228.00   353.00   921.00   299.00   403.00

------------------------------------------------------------------------

REGULAR     DELINQUENT ACCOUNTS MORE THAN $200.00    NO PAYMENT SINCE 05/30/--

ACCOUNT NAME AND ADDRESS     DATE    AMOUNT   BALANCE   31-60    60-90   OVER 90

  3 Ms. Suzanne Rohn        00/00/--    0.00   483.00   435.00     0.00    48.00
    P.O. Box 360            none
    Cincinnati, OH 45249

  5 Mr. Matthew Bradshaw    04/14/--   40.00   358.00    34.00    24.00   260.00
    1914 Galen Drive        Cash
    Blue Ash, OH 45236      555-3083

  8 Ms. Patricia Capowitz   04/14/--   60.00   350.00   212.00     0.00     0.00
    890 Tower Place         Personal Check
    Cincinnati, OH 45242    555-4581

  9 Mr. Arthur Adam         02/21/--   65.00   282.00     0.00   227.00    20.00
    601 Springfield Terr.   Insurance Payment
    Montgomery, OH 45249    555-8412

  4 Accounts                Totals           1,473.00   681.00   251.00   318.00
```

FIGURE 15-7 Computerized accounts receivable report

Rachel Simonowitz, M.D.
82-B Medical Building
Ambler, PA 19002

June 14, 19—

Mr. Roo Nygenun
41 Santiford Drive
Ambler, PA 19002

Dear Mr. Nygenun:

Your account with our office is
three months past due, and you
have not responded to our
previous requests for payment.
Please pay your balance of $152
at this time, or contact us with an
explanation of why you
cannot pay.

Please call me at 555-7823 if you
have a question about your
account. Otherwise, we expect
your payment immediately.

Sincerely,

Casey Husted
Accounts Manager

FIGURE 15-8 First collection letter to patient

Rachel Simonowitz, M.D.
82-B Medical Building
Ambler, PA 19002

July 15, 19—

Mr. Roo Nygenun
41 Santiford Drive
Ambler, PA 19002

Dear Mr. Nygenun:

Your son, Royce, was seriously ill
in March when he came to
Dr. Simonowitz for treatment.
Dr. Simonowitz was pleased to use
her experience and education to
treat Royce, and it was in this
same spirit of cooperation that we
expected you to pay your account
within a reasonable amount of
time.

Four months have passed and you
have still not remitted the $152
outstanding balance on your
account. We cannot continue to
keep your unpaid account on our
books. If you are experiencing
financial difficulties, please call
the office so we can arrange a
payment schedule that is
agreeable to both of us.

Sincerely,

Casey Husted
Accounts Manager

FIGURE 15-9 Second collection letter to patient

Rachel Simonowitz, M.D.
82-B Medical Building
Ambler, PA 19002

August 14, 19—

Mr. Roo Nygenun
41 Santiford Drive
Ambler, PA 19002

Dear Mr. Nygenun:

You have not replied to our previous notices regarding your unpaid balance of $152. Unless we hear from you personally within 14 days, your account will be given to the Ambler Medical Collection Service.

Do not wait any longer to contact me at 555-7823 if you wish to maintain your previous good credit record with Dr. Simonowitz. As previously suggested, we will cooperate in arranging a suitable payment schedule if needed.

Sincerely,

Casey Husted
Accounts Manager

FIGURE 15-10 Third collection letter to patient

Rachel Simonowitz, M.D.
82-B Medical Building
Ambler, PA 19002

September 17, 19—

CERTIFIED MAIL

Mr. Roo Nygenun
41 Santiford Drive
Ambler, PA 19002

Dear Mr. Nygenun:

This is our final attempt to collect your account of $152, which is six months past due. You have ignored all our previous letters [or letters and phone calls], so we have no alternative but to turn over your account to a collection company.

Your account is being assigned to Ambler Medical Collection Service, which will pursue whatever legal means is necessary to collect this debt. If you contact me at 555-7823 within seven days, we will retrieve your account from the collection service to protect your credit rating.

Sincerely,

Casey Husted
Accounts Manager

FIGURE 15-11 Fourth collection letter to patient

medical assistant may need to write these carriers. In offices where the medical assistant files claims for patients, a follow-up collection policy is important to maintain strong cash flow. When agencies do not pay in full or question or deny a claim, the assistant will have to determine the nature of the problem and notify the patients. Figures 15-12 through 15-17 illustrate several kinds of correspondence relating to insurance claims.

TELEPHONE COLLECTIONS

Patients who do not respond to collection letters cannot ignore a ringing telephone. Therefore, when a practice has received no payment after mailing several collection letters, a telephone call is in order to inquire about the past due balance. In medical offices where collections are handled internally, you as a medical assistant will assume the responsibility for telephone collections (Figure 15-18).

Telephone inquiries about unpaid bills are awkward, and you must use your best human relations skills to put the patient at ease while at the same time establishing control of the conversation. The purpose of a telephone inquiry is fourfold: (1) to inquire if there is a problem, error, or misunderstanding about the bill; (2) to remind the patient of the bill; (3) to stimulate the person to pay; and (4) to help find a way for the person to pay.

Telephone collection calls can be made at the end of the collection series or at any point during the collection process. Several Dos and Don'ts for telephone collection are listed in Figure 15-19. Refer to Chapter 6 for a review of general telephoning techniques.

Telephone collection is an effective method when handled properly; on the other hand, this task can become unpleasant if it is perceived negatively. Remember, each person who charges a product or service is morally, ethically, and legally bound to pay. Although some people are slow to pay, they should not be allowed to overlook the account. Although the medical assistant's patience may be tested at times, telephone collections are valuable in reaching people who ignore letters. Think of telephone collection as a method for the practice and the patient mutually to figure out a way for the bill to be paid.

Truth-In-Lending

Health insurance does not always cover the cost of a physician's service, and not all patients are covered by health insurance. Therefore, physicians occasionally find it necessary to extend credit, or "carry" an account over a period of time, allowing the patient to make several small, scheduled payments. For the privilege of receiving credit, patients must pay finance charges on the unpaid balance, just like an interest charge on a credit card. This substitutes for interest the practice could earn if fees were paid at the time of service and placed in an interest-bearing account. In other words, when a practice is willing to offer payment alternatives, it should not lose money doing so.

The Consumer Credit Protection Act of 1968, commonly called the Truth-in-Lending Act, requires providers of installment credit to state the charges in writing clearly and to express the interest as an annual rate. This law applies to medical practices as well as to other lenders; therefore, each time an account is to be paid "on time" a truth-in-lending letter should be written to the responsible person outlining the terms of the credit and the annual rate of interest. A cover letter and a truth-in-lending disclosure are shown in Figures 15-20 and 15-21.

IN YOUR OPINION

1. Why is it important for accounts to be aged? What results might occur from improperly aging accounts?
2. As a medical assistant, what could you do to make collection calls easier for both the patient and yourself?
3. What protections do truth-in-lending letters offer to both the patient and the practice?

REFERENCES

"Consumerism." *World Book Encyclopedia.*
Gartee, Richard, and Doris D. Humphrey. *The Medical Manager.* Cincinnati, Ohio: South-Western Publishing Co., 1995.*
Humphrey, Doris, and Kathie Sigler. *The Modern Medical Office: A Reference Manual.* Cincinnati, Ohio: South-Western Publishing Co., 1990.*
Medical Collection Study Course. Chicago: American Medical Association, 1986.
*Currently published by Delmar Publishers.

Rachel Simonowitz, M.D.
82-B Medical Building
Ambler, PA 19002

June 15, 19—

Mrs. Sarika Javis
7823 Midland Circle
Paoli, PA 19301

Dear Mrs. Javis:

Medicaid has notified us that no payment will be made on your account with Dr. Simonowitz since you no longer qualify for the program. When a government agency does not pay, the patient is responsible for the account.

Please pay your outstanding balance of $286 within the next thirty days or, if you prefer, call me at 555-7823, so we can arrange a payment plan that will be satisfactory for both you and Dr. Simonowitz.

Sincerely,

Casey Husted
Accounts Manager

FIGURE 15-12 Letter to patient regarding Medicaid's refusal to pay

Rachel Simonowitz, M.D.
82-B Medical Building
Ambler, PA 19002

June 15, 19—

Miss Lisa Izzo
982-B Chesterbrook Boulevard
Wayne, PA 19087

Dear Miss Izzo:

Your personal record in our office is incomplete and does not provide the information necessary for us to file a claim with your insurance company. If you will answer the questions below that apply to you and return the letter to this office within ten days, we will be happy to submit the necessary paperwork to collect payment.

1. Medicare number
2. Medicaid number
3. Blue Cross/Blue Shield Group Number
4. Blue Cross/Blue Shield Contract Number
5. Name of Blue Cross/Blue Shield Subscriber
6. Other Insurance, HMO, or PPO Name and Address
7. Other Insurance, HMO, or PPO policy or identification number

Thank you for your cooperation. We will contact you as soon as we hear from your carrier.

Sincerely,

Casey Husted
Accounts Manager

FIGURE 15-13 Letter to patient asking for insurance information

Rachel Simonowitz, M.D.
82-B Medical Building
Ambler, PA 19002

June 17, 19—

Mr. Todd Ingram
78 Lenape Drive
Berwyn, PA 19312

Dear Mr. Ingram:

Metropolitan Insurance has informed us that the annual deductible on your health insurance policy has not been met, and they will not pay for Dr. Simonowitz's services on May 2. Since payment of an account is the patient's responsibility, we would appreciate your sending us a check for the outstanding balance of $98.

Please contact your insurance carrier directly if you have a question about their denial of payment. If I can be of further help, please call me at 555-7823.

Sincerely,

Casey Husted
Accounts Manager

FIGURE 15-14 Letter informing patient of carrier's refusal to pay

Rachel Simonowitz, M.D.
82-B Medical Building
Ambler, PA 19002

June 17, 19—

The Travelers
90 Merrick Avenue
East Meadow, NY 11554

Ladies and Gentlemen:

Patient Name: Holly Sparkman
Insured Name: John Sparkman
Contract No.: GA 87600J
I.D. No.: 415-89-3765
Date of Service: April 28, 19—
Date Claim Submitted: May 1, 19—

A claim for the above patient was submitted on May 1, 19—, and we have not yet received payment. Will you please determine the status of the claim and let me know immediately whether there is a problem and, if not, when payment will be mailed.

A copy of the original claim form is enclosed. We will appreciate your prompt response to this inquiry.

Sincerely,

Casey Husted
Accounts Manager

FIGURE 15-15 Inquiry letter to insurance company

Rachel Simonowitz, M.D.
82-B Medical Building
Ambler, PA 19002

June 20, 19—

Medicare
Pennsylvania Blue Shield
Box 65, Blue Shield Building
Camp Hill, PA 17011

Ladies and Gentlemen:

Patient Name: Mary Ann
                    Thomasini
Patient Address: 678 Penn Pike
                    Malvern, PA 19832
Medicare No.: 483-2878-32a

A claim form documenting
Dr. Rachel Simonowitz's treatment
of Mrs. Elise Jaeger on April 3,
19— was filed with your office on
April 6, 19—, and we have no
response to the claim.

A copy of the original claim is
enclosed. Please check your files
and notify us on the status of this
claim as soon as possible.

Sincerely,

Casey Husted
Accounts Manager

FIGURE 15-16 Inquiry to Medicare administrator regarding patient's claim

---

Rachel Simonowitz, M.D.
82-B Medical Building
Ambler, PA 19002

June 20, 19—

Ms. Barbara Hopewell
Personnel Supervisor
Markson Services
86 Hudson Lane
Ambler, PA 19002

Dear Ms. Woodson:

Employee: Randall Palmer
Date of Service: May 2, 19—

The claim submitted on behalf of
Mr. Randall Palmer to Aetna Life
and Casualty has not been paid.
Please contact the carrier and
inquire about the status of this
claim; then inform us immediately
of your findings.

When insurance companies fail to
make payment for a medical claim
within eight weeks, the policy of
this office is to bill the patient. If
you have a question, please call
me at 555-7823.

Sincerely,

Casey Husted
Accounts Manager

FIGURE 15-17 Letter to employer regarding workers' compensation claim

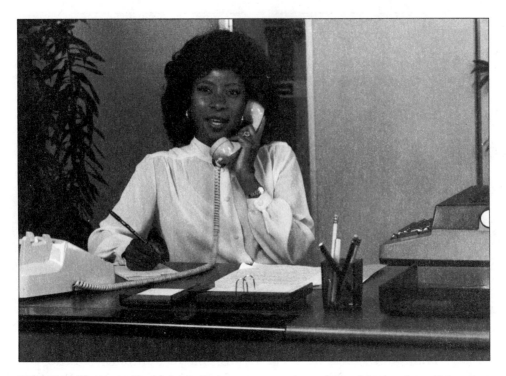

FIGURE 15-18 When collection letters receive no response, the medical assistant needs to call the patient to inquire about the past due balance.

Do

- Organize your thoughts before calling.
- Identify the person to whom you are speaking. Ask for the person responsible for the account.
- Display a cooperative attitude.
- Speak on patient's level.
- Listen respectfully to the person.
- Help the person think of multiple ways of solving the payment problem.
- Review the patient's past payment history.
- Ask for a specific payment date.
- Ask for partial payment when full payment cannot be paid.
- Refer the person to the physician if treatment is questioned.
- Prompt answers by asking questions about the payment problem.
- Wait for the patient to answer.
- Record results of the call in the patient's file.
- Tabulate results of all such calls to create an overdue account profile for the practice.

Don't

- Speak to anyone unfamiliar with the account.
- Act harsh, belligerent, or threatening.
- Use insurance "legalese" language.
- Interrupt patients in an unkind or tactless manner.
- Threaten or argue.
- Dive right into a conversation without thinking.
- Put the patient in the position of correcting your information.
- Leave the payment date unclear.
- Make an impossible ultimatum.
- Discuss the value of medical treatment the patient received.
- Allow the individual to flounder for excuses.
- Help the patient with excuses about why payment has not been made.
- Try to remember everything the patient said.

FIGURE 15-19 Dos and don'ts for telephone collection

Rachel Simonowitz, M.D.
82-B Medical Building
Ambler, PA 19002

June 15, 19—

Mr. Chamois Reilly
42 Jennings Drive
Ambler, PA 19002

Dear Mr. Reilly:

As you and Dr. Simonowitz agreed in the office last week, your balance of $736 will be paid on an installment plan over the next six months. Two copies of a truth-in-lending disclosure statement showing the amount of money financed and the annual finance charge are enclosed. Please read the statement carefully, sign on the line called "Guarantor's Signature," and return one copy of the form to me.

If you have any questions, Mr. Reilly, please call me at 555-7823. Your first payment is due August 1, 19—.

Sincerely,

Casey Husted
Accounts Manager

FIGURE 15-20 Cover letter for truth-in-lending statement

Rachel Simonowitz, M.D.
82-B Medical Building
Ambler, PA 19002

Truth-In-Lending

This Truth-in-Lending Disclosure is made in compliance with the Consumer Credit Protection Act.

<u>Chamois Reilly</u>	<u>Chamois Reilly</u>
Patient's Name	Guarantor's Name

<u>605</u>	<u>42 Jennings Drive</u> <u>Ambler, PA 19002</u>
Patient Number	Address

1. Cash Price Medical Fee $886
2. Less Cash Down
   Payment   150
3. Unpaid Balance of
   Cash Service   736
4. Amount Financed   736
5. Finance Charge   73.60
6. Total of Payment
   (4 plus 5)   809.60
7. Deferred Payment Price   809.60
8. Annual Percentage Rate   10%

The total of $809.60 is payable to Dr. Rachel Simonowitz at the address shown above in six (6) installments of $134.70 beginning August 1, 19— and due on the first day of each month thereafter through January 1, 19—.

_____   _____
Date   Guarantor's Signature

FIGURE 15-21 Truth-in-lending disclosure statement

Chapter Activities

PERFORMANCE BASED ACTIVITIES

1. Assume that you have been hired to handle collections at a private practice with three physicians. Collections have not been made since the last collection manager left six months ago. Most of the patients are covered by private or group insurance and a few patients are covered by Medicare. Write your recommendations for starting the collections process again, giving your reasons for each recommendation.

   Recommended Steps for Collection

Type of Account	Steps	Why
1. Private Insurance	1. _____	1. _____
	2. _____	2. _____
	3. _____	3. _____
	4. _____	4. _____
	5. _____	5. _____
2. Group Insurance	1. _____	1. _____
	2. _____	2. _____
	3. _____	3. _____
	4. _____	4. _____
	5. _____	5. _____
3. Medicare	1. _____	1. _____
	2. _____	2. _____
	3. _____	3. _____
	4. _____	4. _____
	5. _____	5. _____
4. Other	1. _____	1. _____
	2. _____	2. _____
	3. _____	3. _____
	4. _____	4. _____
	5. _____	5. _____

   (DACUM 2.7, 3.1, 8.1, 8.4)

2. Write a series of four form collection letters to mail to private insurers who do not pay claims promptly. Use the heading provided. (DACUM 2.11, 8.4)

   > ### *Garibaldi Medical Center*
   > 314 Walnut Street
   > San Francisco, CA 94122
   > (415) 555-1213

3. Write the dialogue for three conversations you would have with a patient who refuses to pay her account. Assume you call the first time when the account is three months overdue, the second time when the account is four months overdue, and the third time when the account is five months overdue. List in the chart below the key points to make and the patient's likely questions and objections. Role play your situations with a member of your class.

Key Points   *Patient Questions*   *Patient Objections*

Conversation 1.

Conversation 2.

Conversation 3.

(DACUM 1.1, 1.2, 1.6, 2.3, 8.4)

EXPANDING YOUR THINKING

1. Compare the advantages and disadvantages of internal and external collection. Come to a conclusion about which method you would prefer.

Internal Collection

Advantages and Benefits   *Disadvantages*

1.

2.

3.

4.

5.

6.

7.

8.

External Collection

Advantages and Benefits   *Disadvantages*

1.

2.

3.

4.

5.

6.

7.

8.

2. With a team of three other classmates, consider the following situation. Suppose you wish to improve the cash flow in your office, especially concerning patients who do not pay in a timely manner. First, brainstorm suggestions you and your teammates have for correcting this situation. As a team, use the forms below to analyze the advantages and disadvantages of each suggestion.

   a. Brainstorm: First, take five minutes for each person to make an individual list of suggestions. Then, go around the group and collect one suggestion from each person until you have collected all of the suggestions below. Do not discuss the suggestions yet—just list them.

Individual List

Group List

b. Analysis: List the advantages and disadvantages of each suggestion.

Suggestion   *Advantages*   *Disadvantages*

3. Add your personal suggestions on the form below to the list of Dos and Don'ts for telephone collection given on page 328.

Tone of Voice

Words to Use or Avoid

Helpful Questions

Making Sure You Gain Commitment to Pay the Bill

Portfolio Assessment

 Choose one of the following two exercises depending on whether you are using the medical management software or the pegboard system of accounting. If you are using a computer, advance knowledge and skill in using the specific software for your equipment is necessary, as software instructions are not given in this text. The computer exercises are designed specifically for *The Medical Manager,* but other practice management software can be used successfully. If you are using *The Medical Manager,* follow the directions in the student textbook for entering, manipulating, and printing data. If you are using other practice management software, follow directions in the software manual in order to complete the exercises.

Warning! Use *The Medical Manager* software only if you have completed *The Medical Manager* tutorial. *Do not* merge the following problem with *The Medical Manager* if you are still working the tutorial. If you do so, you will confuse the system and incorrect answers will occur in the tutorial for the remainder of the course.

(DACUM 3.1, 3.3, 3.4, 8.2, 8.4, 8.6)

Exercise I

1. Establish new accounts for the five patients whose patient registration forms are given in Portfolio Figures IV-1, IV-2, IV-3, IV-4, and IV-5. Include all insurance information. Follow the directions provided in *The Medical Manager* or other software.
2. Post accounts for the five patients based on information given in Portfolio Figures IV-6, IV-7, IV-8, IV-9, and IV-10.
3. Prepare a daily report for Dr. Carrington for February 17, 19—.
4. Print insurance forms for each patient in Portfolio Figures IV-6 through IV-10.

(DACUM 8.1, 8.2, 8.4, 8.6)

Exercise II

If you do not use a computerized medical billing package for recording patient transactions, follow the directions below:

1. Post in the daily log (in Portfolio Figure IV-11) for 2/17/19— the accounts of the five new patients in Portfolio Figures IV-6 through IV-10.
2. Calculate the total for the today's charge column of the daily log.
3. Key and print insurance forms for each of the new patients based on the information found in Portfolio Figures IV-1 through IV-10 by copying the insurance form produced in Portfolio Figure IV-12 for each of the five patients.

Doctor: Carrington, #3
Bill Type: 11
Extended Info: Yes

Patient Registration Form

Sydney Carrington and Associates - 34 Sycamore Street - Madison, CA 95653

TODAY'S DATE: **2/17/—**

Swazar	Monique	S.	(916) 555-4032	(916) 555-6960
RESPONSIBLE PARTY LAST NAME	FIRST NAME	MI	(AREA CODE) HOME PHONE	(AREA CODE) WORK PHONE

5168 Oak Grove Terrace
MAILING ADDRESS

345-91-4023	F	10/8/47
SOCIAL SECURITY NUMBER	SEX M/F	DATE OF BIRTH

STREET ADDRESS (IF DIFFERENT)

Random Action Toys
EMPLOYER NAME

Madison	CA	95653
CITY	STATE	ZIP CODE

2022 Arden Lane
EMPLOYER ADDRESS

Dr. Matthews
REFERRED BY:

Madison CA 95653	(916) 249-3062
EMPLOYER (CITY, STATE, & ZIP)	PHONE

IF YOU HAVE DEPENDENTS WHO ARE ALSO BEING SEEN AS PATIENTS, PLEASE FILL IN:

Angela Swazar
FIRST DEPENDENT'S NAME

SECOND DEPENDENT'S NAME

6/10/74	F	Daughter	415-62-9109
DATE OF BIRTH	SEX	RELATIONSHIP	SOC. SECURITY #

DATE OF BIRTH	SEX	RELATIONSHIP	SOC. SECURITY #

Madison High School	(916) 436-1032
EMPLOYER OR SCHOOL	PHONE

EMPLOYER OR SCHOOL	PHONE

610 Lansbury Lane Madison CA 95651
ADDRESS OF EMPLOYER OR SCHOOL

ADDRESS OF EMPLOYER OR SCHOOL

INSURANCE INFORMATION: (YOU DO NOT NEED TO FILL IN ADDRESS IF YOUR INSURANCE IS MEDICARE, MEDICAID, CHAMPUS, OR BC/BS)

Pan American Health Ins	2236-082345	Random Action Toys
NAME OF PRIMARY INSURANCE COMPANY	IDENTIFICATION #	GROUP NAME AND/OR #

4567 Newberry Rd	Los Angeles	CA	98706	(213) 456-7654
ADDRESS	CITY	STATE	ZIP	PHONE

INSURED PERSON'S NAME (IF DIFFERENT FROM THE RESPONSIBLE PARTY)	ADDRESS (IF DIFFERENT)	CITY	STATE	ZIP

SOCIAL SECURITY # PHONE	WHAT IS THE RESPONSIBLE PARTY'S RELATIONSHIP TO THE INSURED?

SECONDARY INSURANCE:

NAME OF SECONDARY INSURANCE COMPANY	IDENTIFICATION #	GROUP NAME AND/OR #

ADDRESS	CITY	STATE	ZIP	PHONE

INSURED PERSON'S NAME (IF DIFFERENT FROM THE RESPONSIBLE PARTY)	ADDRESS (IF DIFFERENT)	CITY	STATE	ZIP

SOCIAL SECURITY # PHONE	WHAT IS THE RELATIONSHIP TO THE INSURED?

PORTFOLIO FIGURE IV-1

To the student: Assign a Patient No. → *Patient No:*

Doctor: Carrington, #3
Bill Type: 11
Extended Info: No

Patient Registration Form

Sydney Carrington and Associates - 34 Sycamore Street - Madison, CA 95653   TODAY'S DATE: *2/17/—*

Bonaker	*Arash*	*S.*	*(408) 230-6019*	*None*
RESPONSIBLE PARTY LAST NAME	FIRST NAME	MI	(AREA CODE) HOME PHONE	(AREA CODE) WORK PHONE

82-B Rolling Lane		*328-41-6891*	*M*	*2/10/21*
MAILING ADDRESS		SOCIAL SECURITY NUMBER	SEX M/F	DATE OF BIRTH

STREET ADDRESS (IF DIFFERENT)   EMPLOYER NAME

Morgan Hill	*CA*	*98076*	
CITY	STATE	ZIP CODE	EMPLOYER ADDRESS

Daughter — Mandy Braun		
REFERRED BY:	EMPLOYER (CITY, STATE, & ZIP)	PHONE

IF YOU HAVE DEPENDENTS WHO ARE ALSO BEING SEEN AS PATIENTS, PLEASE FILL IN:

FIRST DEPENDENT'S NAME   SECOND DEPENDENT'S NAME

DATE OF BIRTH	SEX	RELATIONSHIP	SOC. SECURITY #		DATE OF BIRTH	SEX	RELATIONSHIP	SOC. SECURITY #

EMPLOYER OR SCHOOL   PHONE   EMPLOYER OR SCHOOL   PHONE

ADDRESS OF EMPLOYER OR SCHOOL   ADDRESS OF EMPLOYER OR SCHOOL

INSURANCE INFORMATION: (YOU DO NOT NEED TO FILL IN ADDRESS IF YOUR INSURANCE IS MEDICARE, MEDICAID, CHAMPUS, OR BC/BS)

Medicare	*7212462 342*	
NAME OF PRIMARY INSURANCE COMPANY	IDENTIFICATION #	GROUP NAME AND/OR #

ADDRESS	CITY	STATE	ZIP	PHONE

INSURED PERSON'S NAME (IF DIFFERENT FROM THE RESPONSIBLE PARTY)	ADDRESS (IF DIFFERENT)	CITY	STATE	ZIP

SOCIAL SECURITY #	PHONE	WHAT IS THE RESPONSIBLE PARTY'S RELATIONSHIP TO THE INSURED?

SECONDARY INSURANCE:

Medicare Plus	*231038743188*	
NAME OF SECONDARY INSURANCE COMPANY	IDENTIFICATION #	GROUP NAME AND/OR #

34567 Arbor Ave	*Madison*	*CA*	*95653*	*(800) 675-4354*
ADDRESS	CITY	STATE	ZIP	PHONE

INSURED PERSON'S NAME (IF DIFFERENT FROM THE RESPONSIBLE PARTY)	ADDRESS (IF DIFFERENT)	CITY	STATE	ZIP

SOCIAL SECURITY #	PHONE	WHAT IS THE RELATIONSHIP TO THE INSURED?

PORTFOLIO FIGURE IV-2

To the student: Assign a Patient No. → Patient No: | Doctor: Carrington, #3
Bill Type: 11
Extended Info: Yes

Patient Registration Form

Sydney Carrington and Associates - 34 Sycamore Street - Madison, CA 95653   TODAY'S DATE: **2/17/—**

Hight	**Mark**	**W**	**(916) 328-6203**	**(916) 426-0295**
RESPONSIBLE PARTY LAST NAME	FIRST NAME	MI	(AREA CODE) HOME PHONE	(AREA CODE) WORK PHONE

1203 Northern Avenue
MAILING ADDRESS

602-31-4304   **M**   **10/2/60**
SOCIAL SECURITY NUMBER   SEX M/F   DATE OF BIRTH

STREET ADDRESS (IF DIFFERENT)

Rathbone Marble Works
EMPLOYER NAME

Madison   **CA**   **95653**
CITY   STATE   ZIP CODE

2020 Netherland Road
EMPLOYER ADDRESS

None
REFERRED BY:

Madison CA 95042   **(916) 430-3001**
EMPLOYER (CITY, STATE, & ZIP)   PHONE

IF YOU HAVE DEPENDENTS WHO ARE ALSO BEING SEEN AS PATIENTS, PLEASE FILL IN:

Sandra B. Hight
FIRST DEPENDENT'S NAME

SECOND DEPENDENT'S NAME

7/3/64   **F**   **Wife**   **203-91-1110**
DATE OF BIRTH SEX RELATIONSHIP SOC. SECURITY #

DATE OF BIRTH   SEX   RELATIONSHIP   SOC. SECURITY #

Mosaics For You   **(916) 203-6010**
EMPLOYER OR SCHOOL   PHONE

EMPLOYER OR SCHOOL   PHONE

2019 Lawrence Ave.   Madison   CA   95642
ADDRESS OF EMPLOYER OR SCHOOL

ADDRESS OF EMPLOYER OR SCHOOL

INSURANCE INFORMATION: (YOU DO NOT NEED TO FILL IN ADDRESS IF YOUR INSURANCE IS MEDICARE, MEDICAID, CHAMPUS, OR BC/BS)

Pan American Health Ins   **2064394**   **Rathbone Marble Works**
NAME OF PRIMARY INSURANCE COMPANY   IDENTIFICATION #   GROUP NAME AND/OR #

4567 Newberry Rd   **Los Angeles**   **CA**   **98706**   **(213) 456-7654**
ADDRESS   CITY   STATE   ZIP   PHONE

Mark
INSURED PERSON'S NAME (IF DIFFERENT FROM THE RESPONSIBLE PARTY)   ADDRESS (IF DIFFERENT)   CITY   STATE   ZIP

self

SOCIAL SECURITY #   PHONE   WHAT IS THE RESPONSIBLE PARTY'S RELATIONSHIP TO THE INSURED?

SECONDARY INSURANCE:

NAME OF SECONDARY INSURANCE COMPANY   IDENTIFICATION #   GROUP NAME AND/OR #

ADDRESS   CITY   STATE   ZIP   PHONE

INSURED PERSON'S NAME (IF DIFFERENT FROM THE RESPONSIBLE PARTY)   ADDRESS (IF DIFFERENT)   CITY   STATE   ZIP

SOCIAL SECURITY #   PHONE   WHAT IS THE RELATIONSHIP TO THE INSURED?

PORTFOLIO FIGURE IV-3

Doctor: Carrington, #3
Bill Type: 11
Extended Info: Yes

Patient Registration Form

Sydney Carrington and Associates - 34 Sycamore Street - Madison, CA 95653   TODAY'S DATE: **2/17/—**

Rambo	James	H	(916) 823-4304	(916) 826-3341
RESPONSIBLE PARTY LAST NAME	FIRST NAME	MI	(AREA CODE) HOME PHONE	(AREA CODE) WORK PHONE

203 Lebanon Rd		931-40-9016	M	2/10/45
MAILING ADDRESS		SOCIAL SECURITY NUMBER	SEX M/F	DATE OF BIRTH

Leaf Control Industries

STREET ADDRESS (IF DIFFERENT)		EMPLOYER NAME

Wallace	CA	95039	1291 North Flushing Way
CITY	STATE	ZIP CODE	EMPLOYER ADDRESS

Alice Arons, M.D.	Palo Alto CA 94033	(916) 236-4019
REFERRED BY:	EMPLOYER (CITY, STATE, & ZIP)	PHONE

IF YOU HAVE DEPENDENTS WHO ARE ALSO BEING SEEN AS PATIENTS, PLEASE FILL IN:

Cynthia Rambo	Lucas Snider
FIRST DEPENDENT'S NAME	SECOND DEPENDENT'S NAME

5/14/90	F	Daughter	921-60-3019	2/14/92	M	Son	203-91-6011
DATE OF BIRTH	SEX	RELATIONSHIP	SOC. SECURITY #	DATE OF BIRTH	SEX	RELATIONSHIP	SOC. SECURITY #

Palo Alto Grade School	(916) 202-3041	Palo Alto Preschool	
EMPLOYER OR SCHOOL	PHONE	EMPLOYER OR SCHOOL	PHONE

Palo Alto CA 95039	Palo Alto CA 95039
ADDRESS OF EMPLOYER OR SCHOOL	ADDRESS OF EMPLOYER OR SCHOOL

INSURANCE INFORMATION: (YOU DO NOT NEED TO FILL IN ADDRESS IF YOUR INSURANCE IS MEDICARE, MEDICAID, CHAMPUS, OR BC/BS)

Epsilon Life Insurance	2360481	Rawley Towers
NAME OF PRIMARY INSURANCE COMPANY	IDENTIFICATION #	GROUP NAME AND/OR #

P.O. Box 189	Macon	GA	31298	(800) 908-7654
ADDRESS	CITY	STATE	ZIP	PHONE

same				
INSURED PERSON'S NAME (IF DIFFERENT FROM THE RESPONSIBLE PARTY)	ADDRESS (IF DIFFERENT)	CITY	STATE	ZIP

SOCIAL SECURITY #	PHONE	WHAT IS THE RESPONSIBLE PARTY'S RELATIONSHIP TO THE INSURED?

SECONDARY INSURANCE:

Fringe Benefit Center	835 204906	
NAME OF SECONDARY INSURANCE COMPANY	IDENTIFICATION #	GROUP NAME AND/OR #

123 Mission Corners	San Mateo	TX	78723	(800) 678-9565
ADDRESS	CITY	STATE	ZIP	PHONE

Marsha Rambo	P.O. Box 356	Madison	CA	95653
INSURED PERSON'S NAME (IF DIFFERENT FROM THE RESPONSIBLE PARTY)	ADDRESS (IF DIFFERENT)	CITY	STATE	ZIP

415-72-6903	(916) 875-3256	wife
SOCIAL SECURITY #	PHONE	WHAT IS THE RELATIONSHIP TO THE INSURED?

PORTFOLIO FIGURE IV-4

Doctor: Carrington, #3
Bill Type: 11
Extended Info: Yes

Patient Registration Form

Sydney Carrington and Associates - 34 Sycamore Street - Madison, CA 95653

TODAY'S DATE: **2/17/—**

Stryker	Margaret	S.	(408) 231-6013	(408) 234-9060
RESPONSIBLE PARTY LAST NAME	FIRST NAME	MI	(AREA CODE) HOME PHONE	(AREA CODE) WORK PHONE

Rt. 6, Road 43
MAILING ADDRESS

230-91-7063	F	3/4/53
SOCIAL SECURITY NUMBER	SEX M/F	DATE OF BIRTH

STREET ADDRESS (IF DIFFERENT)

Honeybee Industries, Inc.
EMPLOYER NAME

Woodside	CA	98075
CITY	STATE	ZIP CODE

2001 Wanabee Drive
EMPLOYER ADDRESS

Anna Rosenberg, M.D.
REFERRED BY:

Woodside CA 98075	(408) 632-8210
EMPLOYER (CITY, STATE, & ZIP)	PHONE

IF YOU HAVE DEPENDENTS WHO ARE ALSO BEING SEEN AS PATIENTS, PLEASE FILL IN:

FIRST DEPENDENT'S NAME

SECOND DEPENDENT'S NAME

DATE OF BIRTH	SEX	RELATIONSHIP	SOC. SECURITY #

DATE OF BIRTH	SEX	RELATIONSHIP	SOC. SECURITY #

EMPLOYER OR SCHOOL   PHONE

EMPLOYER OR SCHOOL   PHONE

ADDRESS OF EMPLOYER OR SCHOOL

ADDRESS OF EMPLOYER OR SCHOOL

INSURANCE INFORMATION: (YOU DO NOT NEED TO FILL IN ADDRESS IF YOUR INSURANCE IS MEDICARE, MEDICAID, CHAMPUS, OR BC/BS)

Cross and Shield	2732619002	Honeybee Industries, Inc.
NAME OF PRIMARY INSURANCE COMPANY	IDENTIFICATION #	GROUP NAME AND/OR #

435 Embarcadero	Madison	CA	95653	(415) 623-5093
ADDRESS	CITY	STATE	ZIP	PHONE

INSURED PERSON'S NAME (IF DIFFERENT FROM THE RESPONSIBLE PARTY)	ADDRESS (IF DIFFERENT)	CITY	STATE	ZIP

SOCIAL SECURITY #	PHONE	self WHAT IS THE RESPONSIBLE PARTY'S RELATIONSHIP TO THE INSURED?

SECONDARY INSURANCE:

NAME OF SECONDARY INSURANCE COMPANY	IDENTIFICATION #	GROUP NAME AND/OR #

ADDRESS	CITY	STATE	ZIP	PHONE

INSURED PERSON'S NAME (IF DIFFERENT FROM THE RESPONSIBLE PARTY)	ADDRESS (IF DIFFERENT)	CITY	STATE	ZIP

SOCIAL SECURITY #	PHONE	WHAT IS THE RELATIONSHIP TO THE INSURED?

PORTFOLIO FIGURE IV-5

To the student:
This should be the next
number in your system
↓

Sydney Carrington & Associates P.A.
34 Sycamore Street Suite 300
Madison, CA 95653

Date: 2/17/—

Time: 10:00

Patient: Angela Swazar

Guarantor: Monique Swazar

Voucher No.:

Patient No:

Doctor: 3 - S. Carrington, M.D.

	CPT	DESCRIPTION	FEE		CPT	DESCRIPTION	FEE		CPT	DESCRIPTION	FEE
☐	99211	Office Visit Minimal		☐	72110	X-Ray Lumbrosacral Complete		☐	99070	Supplies and Materials	
☐	99212	Office Visit Focused		☐	73030	X-Ray Shoulder, Complete (3)		☐	99070.1	Sling	
☒	99213	Office Visit Expanded	40.00	☐	73070	X-Ray Elbow Ap & Lat Views		☐	99070.2	Catheterization Supplier	
☐	99214	Office Visit Detailed		☐	73560	X-Ray Knee Ap & Lat		☐	68900	Cast Application - Lower Leg	
☐	99215	Exam Comprehensive Hist/Phys		☐	76088	Mammary Ductogram Complete		☐	68902	Cast Application - Upper Leg	
☐	90086	Exam Complex Hist Phys		☐	76140	X-Ray Interpret & Consult		☒	29075	Cast Application - Lower Arm	48.00
☐	90606	Exam & Evaluate Intermediate		☐	76300	Thermography		☐	68906	Cast Application - Up Arm/Shld	
☐	90610	Exam & Evaluate Extended		☐	76499	X-Ray Entire Spine, (4) Views		☐	68915	Cast Application - Wrist-Ankle	
☐	90620	Exam Compre. W/Hist & Phys		☐	81000	Urinalysis		☐	68920	Body Cast	
☐	90642	Exam Follow-up Intermediate		☐	82951	Glucose Tolerance Test		☐	69050	Cast Charge	
☐	90643	Exam Follow-up Extended		☐	84550	Uric Acid: Blood Chemistry		☐	29700	Cast Removal W/Exam	
☐	92002	Exam Intermediate (New Pat)		☐	85014	Hematocrit		☐	30930	Fract Nasal Turbinate Therap	
☐	95860	Electromyography 1 Extremity		☐	85022	CBC		☐	35001	Repair of Aneurysm	
☐	95869	Electromyography: Ltd. Spec M		☐	85031	Hemogram, Comp Blood Work		☐	42826	Tonsillectomy - Age 12 or Over	
☐	99032	Counseling - 50 Minutes		☐	86287	Hepatitis B Surface Antigen		☐	66830	Removal of 2nd Mem Cataract	
☐	99033	Counseling - 25 Minutes		☐	86289	Hepatitis B Antibody Core		☐	97010	Treatment - Hot	
☐	90110	Home Care Service (New Pat)		☐	86291	Hepatitis B Antibody		☐	97110	Exercise Therapeutic	
☐	90150	Home Care Service (Estab Pat)		☐	86296	Hepatitis A Antibody		☐	97124	Massage	
☐	90215	Admiss Hist/Phys Intermediate		☐	87070	Culture		☐	97128	Ultrasound	
☐	99223	Admiss Hist/Phys Comprehen		☐	87210	Wet Mount		☐	97720	Extremity testing for strength	
☐	99232	Hospital Visit Expanded		☐	88150	Pap Smear		☐	97752	Muscle Testing, Torque Curves	
☐	90260	Hospital Visit Intermediate		☐	93000	Electrocardiogram		☐	53670	Catheterization Incl Supplies	
☐	90270	Hospital Visit Extended		☐	99000	Lab Special Handling		☐	77263	Treatment Planning - Complex	
☐	99238	Hospital Visit Discharge Exam		☐	-583	Hepatitis Profile # 1		☐	77290	Simulation - Complex	
☐	90510	Emergency Room Care Limited		☐	femlab	Female Lab Series		☐	77300	Central Axis Dose	
☐	90515	Emerg Room Care Intermediate		☐	-gtt-3	Glucose Tolerance Test - 3 hour		☐	77305	Simple Isodose Plan	
☐	90941	Homodialysis		☐	-gtt-5	Glucose Tolerance Test - 5 hour		☐	77333	Shielding Block - Regular	
☐	71020	X-Ray Chest Pa B Lat		☐	pre-op	Pre-operative Routine Labs		☐	77336	Continuing Physics/Week	
☐	71010	Radiological Exam Entire Spine		☐	90701	Immunization		☐	77415	Port Film Verification	
				☐	90749	Injection		☐	77420	3-B MEV, Daily, Complex	

	ICDA CODE DIAGNOSIS			ICDA CODE DIAGNOSIS			ICDA CODE DIAGNOSIS	
☐	783.1	Abnormal Weight Gain	☐	921.1	Contusions of Eyelids/Periocular	☐	575.2	Obstruction of Gallbladder
☐	783.2	Abnormal Weight Loss	☐	780.3	Convulsions	☐	742.2	Pain: Lower back
☐	461.9	Acute Sinusitis	☐	352.9	Cranial Neuralgia	☐	481.0	Pneumococcal Pneumonia
☐	346.2	Allergic Headache	☐	300.4	Depression	☐	V22.2	Pregnancy
☐	006.3	Amebic Liver Abscess	☐	311	Depression	☐	722.0	Prolapse/Protrusion Cervical IVD
☐	285.9	Anemia	☐	830.6	Dislocated Hip	☐	593.9	Renal Insufficiency
☐	783.0	Anorexia	☐	830.9	Dislocated Shoulder	☐	727.6	Rupture Achilles Tendon
☐	440.0	Atherosclerosis	☐	487.0	Flu	☐	727.8	Rupture Flexor Tendon Hand/Wrist
☐	353.0	Brachial Plexus Irritation	☐	802.0	Fracture - Nasal Closed	☐	355.0	Sciatic Nerve Root Lesion
☐	174.9	Breast Cancer	☐	892.0	Fractured Fibula	☐	564.1	Spastic Colon
☐	185.0	Cancer of the Prostate	☐	891.2	Fractured Tibia	☐	842.5	Sprained Ankle
☐	442.81	Carotid Artery	☐	780.1	Hallucinations	☒	841.2	Sprained Wrist
☐	354.0	Carpal Tunnel Syndrome	☐	477.9	Hay Fever	☐	538.8	Stomach Pain
☐	366.9	Cataract	☐	573.3	Hepatitis	☐	918.1	Superficial Injury to Eye (Comea)
☐	353.3	Cervical Dorsal Outlet Syndrome	☐	553.3	Hiatal Hernia	☐	524.6	Temporo-Mand Joint Syndrome
☐	721.0	Cervical Osteo/Spondyloarthritis	☐	009.0	Ill-defined Intestinal Infections	☐	353.3	Thoratic Nerve Root Compression
☐	571.4	Chronic Hepatitis	☐	919.5	Insect Bite, Nonvenom, Infected	☐	721.2	Thoratic Spondylo/Osteoarthritis
☐	473.9	Chronic Sinusitis	☐	721.3	Lumbar Osteo/Spondyloarthritis	☐	474.0	Tonsillitis
☐	571.5	Cirrhosis of the Liver	☐	353.1	Lumbosacral Plexus Lesion	☐	386.0	Vertigo
☐	892.5	Combo Fibula/Tibia Fracture	☐	346.9	Migraine Headache	☐	480.0	Viral Pneumonia
☐	460.0	Common Cold	☐	721.1	Neuro-Vascular Compression	☐	V20.2	Well Child

Previous Balance	Today's Charges	Total Due	Amount Paid	New Balance		
	88.00	88.00	∅	88.00	PRN _____ Weeks _3_	Follow Up Months _____ Units _____
					Next Appointment Date:	Time:

I hereby authorize release of any information acquired in the course of
examination or treatment and allow a photocopy of my signature to be used.

_____

PORTFOLIO FIGURE IV-6

Sydney Carrington & Associates P.A.

34 Sycamore Street Suite 300
Madison, CA 95653

To the student:
This should be the next
number in your system
↓

Date: 2/17/—

Time: 1:00

Patient: Arash Bonaker

Guarantor: Bonaker

Voucher No.:

Patient No:

Doctor: 3 - S. Carrington, M.D.

☐	CPT	DESCRIPTION	FEE	☐	CPT	DESCRIPTION	FEE	☐	CPT	DESCRIPTION	FEE
☐	99211	Office Visit Minimal	____	☐	72110	X-Ray Lumbrosacral Complete	____	☐	99070	Supplies and Materials	____
☐	99212	Office Visit Focused	____	☐	73030	X-Ray Shoulder, Complete (3)	____	☐	99070.1	Sling	____
☒	99213	Office Visit Expanded	40.00	☐	73070	X-Ray Elbow Ap & Lat Views	____	☐	99070.2	Catheterization Supplier	____
☐	99214	Office Visit Detailed	____	☐	73560	X-Ray Knee Ap & Lat	____	☐	68900	Cast Application - Lower Leg	____
☐	99215	Exam Comprehensive Hist/Phys	____	☐	76088	Mammary Ductogram Complete	____	☐	68902	Cast Application - Upper Leg	____
☐	90086	Exam Complex Hist Phys	____	☐	76140	X-Ray Interpret & Consult	____	☐	29075	Cast Application - Lower Arm	____
☐	90606	Exam & Evaluate Intermediate	____	☐	76300	Thermography	____	☐	68906	Cast Application - Up Arm/Shld	____
☐	90610	Exam & Evaluate Extended	____	☐	76499	X-Ray Entire Spine, (4) Views	____	☐	68915	Cast Application - Wrist-Ankle	____
☐	90620	Exam Compre. W/Hist & Phys	____	☐	81000	Urinalysis	____	☐	68920	Body Cast	____
☐	90642	Exam Follow-up Intermediate	____	☐	82951	Glucose Tolerance Test	____	☐	69050	Cast Charge	____
☐	90643	Exam Follow-up Extended	____	☐	84550	Uric Acid: Blood Chemistry	____	☐	29700	Cast Removal W/Exam	____
☐	92002	Exam Intermediate (New Pat)	____	☒	85014	Hematocrit *done for the anemia	18.00	☐	30930	Fract Nasal Turbinate Therap	____
☐	95860	Electromyography 1 Extremity	____	☐	85022	CBC	____	☐	35001	Repair of Aneurysm	____
☐	95869	Electromyography: Ltd. Spec M	____	☐	85031	Hemogram, Comp Blood Work	____	☐	42826	Tonsillectomy - Age 12 or Over	____
☐	99032	Counseling - 50 Minutes	____	☐	86287	Hepatitis B Surface Antigen	____	☐	66830	Removal of 2nd Mem Cataract	____
☐	99033	Counseling - 25 Minutes	____	☐	86289	Hepatitis B Antibody Core	____	☐	97010	Treatment - Hot	____
☐	90110	Home Care Service (New Pat)	____	☐	86291	Hepatitis B Antibody	____	☐	97110	Exercise Therapeutic	____
☐	90150	Home Care Service (Estab Pat)	____	☐	86296	Hepatitis A Antibody	____	☐	97124	Massage	____
☐	90215	Admiss Hist/Phys Intermediate	____	☐	87070	Culture	____	☐	97128	Ultrasound	____
☐	99223	Admiss Hist/Phys Comprehen	____	☐	87210	Wet Mount	____	☐	97720	Extremity testing for strength	____
☐	99232	Hospital Visit Expanded	____	☐	88150	Pap Smear	____	☐	97752	Muscle Testing, Torque Curves	____
☐	90260	Hospital Visit Intermediate	____	☐	93000	Electrocardiogram	____	☐	53670	Catheterization Incl Supplies	____
☐	90270	Hospital Visit Extended	____	☐	99000	Lab Special Handling	____	☐	77263	Treatment Planning - Complex	____
☐	99238	Hospital Visit Discharge Exam	____	☐	-583	Hepatitis Profile # 1	____	☐	77290	Simulation - Complex	____
☐	90510	Emergency Room Care Limited	____	☐	femlab	Female Lab Series	____	☐	77300	Central Axis Dose	____
☐	90515	Emerg Room Care Intermediate	____	☐	-gtt-3	Glucose Tolerance Test - 3 hour	____	☐	77305	Simple Isodose Plan	____
☐	90941	Homodialysis	____	☐	-gtt-5	Glucose Tolerance Test - 5 hour	____	☐	77333	Shielding Block - Regular	____
☐	71020	X-Ray Chest Pa B Lat	____	☐	pre-op	Pre-operative Routine Labs	____	☐	77336	Continuing Physics/Week	____
☐	71010	Radiological Exam Entire Spine	____	☐	90701	Immunization	____	☐	77415	Port Film Verification	____
				☐	90749	Injection	____	☐	77420	3-B MEV, Daily, Complex	____

	ICDA CODE DIAGNOSIS			ICDA CODE DIAGNOSIS			ICDA CODE DIAGNOSIS	
☐	783.1	Abnormal Weight Gain	☐	921.1	Contusions of Eyelids/Periocular	☐	575.2	Obstruction of Gallbladder
☐	783.2	Abnormal Weight Loss	☐	780.3	Convulsions	☐	742.2	Pain: Lower back
☐	461.9	Acute Sinusitis	☐	352.9	Cranial Neuralgia	☐	481.0	Pneumococcal Pneumonia
☐	346.2	Allergic Headache	☐	300.4	Depression	☐	V22.2	Pregnancy
☐	006.3	Amebic Liver Abscess	☐	311	Depression	☐	722.0	Prolapse/Protrusion Cervical IVD
☒	285.9	Anemia	☐	830.6	Dislocated Hip	☐	593.9	Renal Insufficiency
☐	783.	Anorexia	☐	830.5	Dislocated Shoulder	☐	727.6	Rupture Achilles Tendon
☐	440.0	Atherosclerosis	☐	487.0	Flu	☐	727.8	Rupture Flexor Tendon Hand/Wrist
☐	353.0	Brachial Plexus Irritation	☐	802.0	Fracture - Nasal Closed	☐	355.0	Sciatic Nerve Root Lesion
☐	174.9	Breast Cancer	☐	892.0	Fractured Fibula	☐	564.1	Spastic Colon
☐	185.0	Cancer of the Prostate	☐	891.2	Fractured Tibia	☐	842.5	Sprained Ankle
☐	442.81	Carotid Artery	☐	780.1	Hallucinations	☐	841.2	Sprained Wrist
☐	354.0	Carpal Tunnel Syndrome	☐	477.9	Hay Fever	☐	538.8	Stomach Pain
☐	366.9	Cataract	☐	573.3	Hepatitis	☐	918.1	Superficial Injury to Eye (Cornea)
☐	353.9	Cervical Dorsal Outlet Syndrome	☐	553.3	Hiatal Hernia	☐	524.6	Temporo-Mand Joint Syndrome
☐	721.0	Cervical Osteo/Spondyloarthritis	☐	009.0	Ill-defined Intestinal Infections	☐	353.3	Thoratic Nerve Root Compression
☐	571.4	Chronic Hepatitis	☐	919.5	Insect Bite, Nonvenom, Infected	☐	721.2	Thoratic Spondylo/Osteoarthritis
☐	473.9	Chronic Sinusitis	☐	721.3	Lumbar Osteo/Spondyloarthritis	☐	474.0	Tonsillitis
☒	571.5	Cirrhosis of the Liver	☐	353.1	Lumbosacral Plexus Lesion	☐	386.0	Vertigo
☐	892.5	Combo Fibula/Tibia Fracture	☐	346.9	Migraine Headache	☐	480.0	Viral Pneumonia
☐	460.0	Common Cold	☐	721.1	Neuro-Vascular Compression	☐	V20.2	Well Child

Previous Balance	Today's Charges	Total Due	Amount Paid	New Balance	PRN _____ Weeks	Follow Up
____	58.00	____	____	____	Next Appointment Date: 2/17/—	Months _____ Units _____ Time: 10 a.m.

I hereby authorize release of any information acquired in the course of
examination or treatment and allow a photocopy of my signature to be used.

PORTFOLIO FIGURE IV-7

Sydney Carrington & Associates P.A.
34 Sycamore Street Suite 300
Madison, CA 95653

To the student:
This should be the next
number in your system
↓

Date: 2/17/—

Time: 11:00

Patient: Sandra Hight

Guarantor: Hight

Voucher No.:

Patient No:

Doctor: 3 - S. Carrington, M.D.

☐	CPT	DESCRIPTION	FEE	☐	CPT	DESCRIPTION	FEE	☐	CPT	DESCRIPTION	FEE
☐	99211	Office Visit Minimal	___	☐	72110	X-Ray Lumbosacral Complete	___	☐	99070	Supplies and Materials	___
☐	99212	Office Visit Focused	___	☐	73030	X-Ray Shoulder, Complete (3)	___	☐	99070.1	Sling	___
☒	99213	Office Visit Expanded	40.00	☐	73070	X-Ray Elbow Ap & Lat Views	___	☐	99070.2	Catheterization Supplier	___
☐	99214	Office Visit Detailed	___	☐	73560	X-Ray Knee Ap & Lat	___	☐	68900	Cast Application - Lower Leg	___
☐	99215	Exam Comprehensive Hist/Phys	___	☐	76088	Mammary Ductogram Complete	___	☐	68902	Cast Application - Upper Leg	___
☐	90086	Exam Complex Hist Phys	___	☐	76140	X-Ray Interpret & Consult	___	☐	29075	Cast Application - Lower Arm	___
☐	90606	Exam & Evaluate Intermediate	___	☐	76300	Thermography	___	☐	68906	Cast Application - Up Arm/Shld	___
☐	90610	Exam & Evaluate Extended	___	☐	76499	X-Ray Entire Spine, (4) Views	___	☐	68915	Cast Application - Wrist-Ankle	___
☐	90620	Exam Compre. W/Hist & Phys	___	☐	81000	Urinalysis	___	☐	68920	Body Cast	___
☐	90642	Exam Follow-up Intermediate	___	☐	82951	Glucose Tolerance Test	___	☐	69050	Cast Charge	___
☐	90643	Exam Follow-up Extended	___	☐	84550	Uric Acid: Blood Chemistry	___	☐	29700	Cast Removal W/Exam	___
☐	92002	Exam Intermediate (New Pat)	___	☐	85014	Hematocrit	___	☐	30930	Fract Nasal Turbinate Therap	___
☐	95860	Electromyography 1 Extremity	___	☐	85022	CBC	___	☐	35001	Repair of Aneurysm	___
☐	95869	Electromyography: Ltd. Spec M	___	☐	85031	Hemogram, Comp Blood Work	___	☐	42826	Tonsillectomy - Age 12 or Over	___
☐	99032	Counseling - 50 Minutes	___	☐	86287	Hepatitis B Surface Antigen	___	☐	66830	Removal of 2nd Mem Cataract	___
☐	99033	Counseling - 25 Minutes	___	☐	86289	Hepatitis B Antibody Core	___	☐	97010	Treatment - Hot	___
☐	90110	Home Care Service (New Pat)	___	☐	86291	Hepatitis B Antibody	___	☐	97110	Exercise Therapeutic	___
☐	90150	Home Care Service (Estab Pat)	___	☐	86296	Hepatitis A Antibody	___	☐	97124	Massage	___
☐	90215	Admiss Hist/Phys Intermediate	___	☐	87070	Culture	___	☐	97128	Ultrasound	___
☐	99223	Admiss Hist/Phys Comprehen	___	☐	87210	Wet Mount	___	☐	97720	Extremity testing for strength	___
☐	99232	Hospital Visit Expanded	___	☐	88150	Pap Smear	___	☐	97752	Muscle Testing, Torque Curves	___
☐	90260	Hospital Visit Intermediate	___	☐	93000	Electrocardiogram	___	☐	53670	Catheterization Incl Supplies	___
☐	90270	Hospital Visit Extended	___	☐	99000	Lab Special Handling	___	☐	77263	Treatment Planning - Complex	___
☐	99238	Hospital Visit Discharge Exam	___	☐	-583	Hepatitis Profile # 1	___	☐	77290	Simulation - Complex	___
☐	90510	Emergency Room Care Limited	___	☐	femlab	Female Lab Series	___	☐	77300	Central Axis Dose	___
☐	90515	Emerg Room Care Intermediate	___	☐	-gtt-3	Glucose Tolerance Test - 3 hour	___	☐	77305	Simple Isodose Plan	___
☐	90941	Homodialysis	___	☐	-gtt-5	Glucose Tolerance Test - 5 hour	___	☐	77333	Shielding Block - Regular	___
☐	71020	X-Ray Chest Pa B Lat	___	☐	pre-op	Pre-operative Routine Labs	___	☐	77336	Continuing Physics/Week	___
☐	71010	Radiological Exam Entire Spine	___	☐	90701	Immunization	___	☐	77415	Port Film Verification	___
				☐	90749	Injection	___	☐	77420	3-B MEV, Daily, Complex	___

	ICDA CODE DIAGNOSIS			ICDA CODE DIAGNOSIS			ICDA CODE DIAGNOSIS	
☐	783.1	Abnormal Weight Gain	☐	921.1	Contusions of Eyelids/Periocular	☐	575.2	Obstruction of Gallbladder
☐	783.2	Abnormal Weight Loss	☐	780.3	Convulsions	☐	742.2	Pain: Lower back
☒	461.9	Acute Sinusitis	☐	352.9	Cranial Neuralgia	☐	481.0	Pneumococcal Pneumonia
☐	346.2	Allergic Headache	☐	300.4	Depression	☐	V22.2	Pregnancy
☐	006.3	Amebic Liver Abscess	☐	311	Depression	☐	722.0	Prolapse/Protrusion Cervical IVD
☐	285.9	Anemia	☐	830.6	Dislocated Hip	☐	593.9	Renal Insufficiency
☐	783.0	Anorexia	☐	830.9	Dislocated Shoulder	☐	727.6	Rupture Achilles Tendon
☐	440.0	Atherosclerosis	☐	487.0	Flu	☐	727.8	Rupture Flexor Tendon Hand/Wrist
☐	353.0	Brachial Plexus Irritation	☐	802.0	Fracture - Nasal Closed	☐	355.0	Sciatic Nerve Root Lesion
☐	174.9	Breast Cancer	☐	892.0	Fractured Fibula	☐	564.1	Spastic Colon
☐	185.0	Cancer of the Prostate	☐	891.2	Fractured Tibia	☐	842.5	Sprained Ankle
☐	442.81	Carotid Artery	☐	780.1	Hallucinations	☐	841.2	Sprained Wrist
☐	354.0	Carpal Tunnel Syndrome	☐	477.9	Hay Fever	☐	538.8	Stomach Pain
☐	366.9	Cataract	☐	573.3	Hepatitis	☐	918.1	Superficial Injury to Eye (Cornea)
☐	353.9	Cervical Dorsal Outlet Syndrome	☐	553.3	Hiatal Hernia	☐	524.6	Temporo-Mand Joint Syndrome
☐	721.0	Cervical Osteo/Spondyloarthritis	☐	009.0	Ill-defined Intestinal Infections	☐	353.3	Thoratic Nerve Root Compression
☐	571.4	Chronic Hepatitis	☐	919.5	Insect Bite, Nonvenom, Infected	☐	721.2	Thoratic Spondylo/Osteoarthritis
☐	473.9	Chronic Sinusitis	☐	721.3	Lumbar Osteo/Spondyloarthritis	☐	474.0	Tonsillitis
☐	571.5	Cirrhosis of the Liver	☐	353.1	Lumbosacral Plexus Lesion	☐	386.0	Vertigo
☐	892.5	Combo Fibula/Tibia Fracture	☐	346.9	Migraine Headache	☐	480.0	Viral Pneumonia
☐	460.0	Common Cold	☐	721.1	Neuro-Vascular Compression	☐	V20.2	Well Child

Previous Balance	Today's Charges	Total Due	Amount Paid	New Balance		
___	40.00	___	___	___	PRN ___ Weeks ___	Follow Up Months ___ Units ___
					Next Appointment Date:	Time:

I hereby authorize release of any information acquired in the course of examination or treatment and allow a photocopy of my signature to be used.

_____

PORTFOLIO FIGURE IV-8

Sydney Carrington & Associates P.A.

34 Sycamore Street Suite 300
Madison, CA 95653

To the student:
This should be the next number in your system
↓

Date: 2/17/—
Time: 10:00
Patient: Cynthia Rambo
Guarantor: James H. Rambo

Voucher No.:

Patient No:
Doctor: 3 - S. Carrington, M.D.

	CPT	DESCRIPTION	FEE		CPT	DESCRIPTION	FEE		CPT	DESCRIPTION	FEE
☒	99211	Office Visit Minimal	30.00	☐	72110	X-Ray Lumbrosacral Complete	___	☐	99070	Supplies and Materials	___
☐	99212	Office Visit Focused	___	☐	73030	X-Ray Shoulder, Complete (3)	___	☐	99070.1	Sling	___
☐	99213	Office Visit Expanded	___	☐	73070	X-Ray Elbow Ap & Lat Views	___	☐	99070.2	Catheterization Supplier	___
☐	99214	Office Visit Detailed	___	☐	73560	X-Ray Knee Ap & Lat	___	☐	68900	Cast Application - Lower Leg	___
☐	99215	Exam Comprehensive Hist/Phys	___	☐	76088	Mammary Ductogram Complete	___	☐	68902	Cast Application - Upper Leg	___
☐	90086	Exam Complex Hist Phys	___	☐	76140	X-Ray Interpret & Consult	___	☐	29075	Cast Application - Lower Arm	___
☐	90606	Exam & Evaluate Intermediate	___	☐	76300	Thermography	___	☐	68906	Cast Application - Up Arm/Shld	___
☐	90610	Exam & Evaluate Extended	___	☐	76499	X-Ray Entire Spine, (4) Views	___	☐	68915	Cast Application - Wrist-Ankle	___
☐	90620	Exam Compre. W/Hist & Phys	___	☐	81000	Urinalysis	___	☐	68920	Body Cast	___
☐	90642	Exam Follow-up Intermediate	___	☐	82951	Glucose Tolerance Test	___	☐	69050	Cast Charge	___
☐	90643	Exam Follow-up Extended	___	☐	84550	Uric Acid: Blood Chemistry	___	☐	29700	Cast Removal W/Exam	___
☐	92002	Exam Intermediate (New Pat)	___	☐	85014	Hematocrit	___	☐	30930	Fract Nasal Turbinate Therap	___
☐	95860	Electromyography 1 Extremity	___	☐	85022	CBC	___	☐	35001	Repair of Aneurysm	___
☐	95869	Electromyography: Ltd. Spec M	___	☐	85031	Hemogram, Comp Blood Work	___	☐	42826	Tonsillectomy - Age 12 or Over	___
☐	99032	Counseling - 50 Minutes	___	☐	86287	Hepatitis B Surface Antigen	___	☐	66830	Removal of 2nd Mem Cataract	___
☐	99033	Counseling - 25 Minutes	___	☐	86289	Hepatitis B Antibody Core	___	☐	97010	Treatment - Hot	___
☐	90110	Home Care Service (New Pat)	___	☐	86291	Hepatitis B Antibody	___	☐	97110	Exercise Therapeutic	___
☐	90150	Home Care Service (Estab Pat)	___	☐	86296	Hepatitis A Antibody	___	☐	97124	Massage	___
☐	90215	Admiss Hist/Phys Intermediate	___	☐	87070	Culture	___	☐	97128	Ultrasound	___
☐	99223	Admiss Hist/Phys Comprehen	___	☐	87210	Wet Mount	___	☐	97720	Extremity testing for strength	___
☐	99232	Hospital Visit Expanded	___	☐	88150	Pap Smear	___	☐	97752	Muscle Testing, Torque Curves	___
☐	90260	Hospital Visit Intermediate	___	☐	93000	Electrocardiogram	___	☐	53670	Catheterization Incl Supplies	___
☐	90270	Hospital Visit Extended	___	☐	99000	Lab Special Handling	___	☐	77263	Treatment Planning - Complex	___
☐	99238	Hospital Visit Discharge Exam	___	☐	-583	Hepatitis Profile # 1	___	☐	77290	Simulation - Complex	___
☐	90510	Emergency Room Care Limited	___	☐	femlab	Female Lab Series	___	☐	77300	Central Axis Dose	___
☐	90515	Emerg Room Care Intermediate	___	☐	-gtt-3	Glucose Tolerance Test - 3 hour	___	☐	77305	Simple Isodose Plan	___
☐	90941	Homodialysis	___	☐	-gtt-5	Glucose Tolerance Test - 5 hour	___	☐	77333	Shielding Block - Regular	___
☐	71020	X-Ray Chest Pa B Lat	___	☐	pre-op	Pre-operative Routine Labs	___	☐	77336	Continuing Physics/Week	___
☐	71010	Radiological Exam Entire Spine	___	☐	90701	Immunization	___	☐	77415	Port Film Verification	___
				☐	90749	Injection	___	☐	77420	3-B MEV, Daily, Complex	___

	ICDA CODE DIAGNOSIS			ICDA CODE DIAGNOSIS			ICDA CODE DIAGNOSIS	
☐	783.1	Abnormal Weight Gain	☐	921.1	Contusions of Eyelids/Periocular	☐	575.2	Obstruction of Gallbladder
☐	783.2	Abnormal Weight Loss	☐	780.3	Convulsions	☐	742.2	Pain: Lower back
☐	461.9	Acute Sinusitis	☐	352.9	Cranial Neuralgia	☐	481.0	Pneumococcal Pneumonia
☐	346.2	Allergic Headache	☐	300.4	Depression	☐	V22.2	Pregnancy
☐	006.3	Amebic Liver Abscess	☐	311	Depression	☐	722.0	Prolapse/Protrusion Cervical IVD
☐	285.9	Anemia	☐	830.6	Dislocated Hip	☐	593.9	Renal Insufficiency
☐	783.0	Anorexia	☐	830.9	Dislocated Shoulder	☐	727.6	Rupture Achilles Tendon
☐	440.0	Atherosclerosis	☐	487.0	Flu	☐	727.8	Rupture Flexor Tendon Hand/Wrist
☐	353.0	Brachial Plexus Irritation	☐	802.0	Fracture - Nasal Closed	☐	355.0	Sciatic Nerve Root Lesion
☐	174.9	Breast Cancer	☐	892.0	Fractured Fibula	☐	564.1	Spastic Colon
☐	185.0	Cancer of the Prostate	☐	891.2	Fractured Tibia	☐	842.5	Sprained Ankle
☐	442.81	Carotid Artery	☐	780.1	Hallucinations	☐	841.2	Sprained Wrist
☐	354.0	Carpal Tunnel Syndrome	☐	477.9	Hay Fever	☐	538.8	Stomach Pain
☐	366.9	Cataract	☐	573.3	Hepatitis	☐	918.1	Superficial Injury to Eye (Cornea)
☐	353.9	Cervical Dorsal Outlet Syndrome	☐	553.3	Hiatal Hernia	☐	524.6	Temporo-Mand Joint Syndrome
☐	721.0	Cervical Osteo/Spondyloarthritis	☐	009.0	Ill-defined Intestinal Infections	☐	353.3	Thoratic Nerve Root Compression
☐	571.4	Chronic Hepatitis	☐	919.5	Insect Bite, Nonvenom, Infected	☐	721.2	Thoratic Spondylo/Osteoarthritis
☐	473.9	Chronic Sinusitis	☐	721.3	Lumbar Osteo/Spondyloarthritis	☐	474.0	Tonsillitis
☐	571.5	Cirrhosis of the Liver	☐	353.1	Lumbosacral Plexus Lesion	☐	386.0	Vertigo
☐	892.5	Combo Fibula/Tibia Fracture	☐	346.9	Migraine Headache	☐	480.0	Viral Pneumonia
☐	460.0	Common Cold	☐	721.1	Neuro-Vascular Compression	☒	V20.2	Well Child

Previous Balance	Today's Charges	Total Due	Amount Paid	New Balance		PRN _____ Weeks _____	Follow Up Months _____ Units _____
___	30.00	___	___	___		Next Appointment Date:	Time:

I hereby authorize release of any information acquired in the course of examination or treatment and allow a photocopy of my signature to be used.

PORTFOLIO FIGURE IV-9

Sydney Carrington & Associates P.A.
34 Sycamore Street Suite 300
Madison, CA 95653

To the student:
This should be the next
number in your system
↓

Date: 2/17/—

Time: 11:00

Patient: Margaret Stryker

Guarantor: Margaret Stryker

Voucher No.:

Patient No:

Doctor: 3 - S. Carrington, M.D.

☐	CPT	DESCRIPTION	FEE	☐	CPT	DESCRIPTION	FEE	☐	CPT	DESCRIPTION	FEE
☐	99211	Office Visit Minimal	___	☐	72110	X-Ray Lumbrosacral Complete	___	☐	99070	Supplies and Materials	___
☐	99212	Office Visit Focused	___	☐	73030	X-Ray Shoulder, Complete (3)	___	☐	99070.1	Sling	___
☐	99213	Office Visit Expanded	___	☐	73070	X-Ray Elbow Ap & Lat Views	___	☐	99070.2	Catheterization Supplier	___
☐	99214	Office Visit Detailed	___	☐	73560	X-Ray Knee Ap & Lat	___	☐	68900	Cast Application - Lower Leg	___
☒	99215	Exam Comprehensive Hist/Phys	85.00	☐	76088	Mammary Ductogram Complete	___	☐	68902	Cast Application - Upper Leg	___
☐	90086	Exam Complex Hist Phys	___	☐	76140	X-Ray Interpret & Consult	___	☐	29075	Cast Application - Lower Arm	___
☐	90606	Exam & Evaluate Intermediate	___	☐	76300	Thermography	___	☐	68906	Cast Application - Up Arm/Shld	___
☐	90610	Exam & Evaluate Extended	___	☒	76499	X-Ray Entire Spine, (4) Views	150.00	☐	68915	Cast Application - Wrist-Ankle	___
☐	90620	Exam Compre. W/Hist & Phys	___	☒	81000	Urinalysis	8.00	☐	68920	Body Cast	___
☐	90642	Exam Follow-up Intermediate	___	☐	82951	Glucose Tolerance Test	___	☐	69050	Cast Charge	___
☐	90643	Exam Follow-up Extended	___	☐	84550	Uric Acid: Blood Chemistry	___	☐	29700	Cast Removal W/Exam	___
☐	92002	Exam Intermediate (New Pat)	___	☒	85014	Hematocrit	18.00	☐	30930	Fract Nasal Turbinate Therap	___
☐	95860	Electromyography 1 Extremity	___	☐	85022	CBC	___	☐	35001	Repair of Aneurysm	___
☐	95869	Electromyography: Ltd. Spec M	___	☐	85031	Hemogram, Comp Blood Work	___	☐	42826	Tonsillectomy - Age 12 or Over	___
☐	99032	Counseling - 50 Minutes	___	☐	86287	Hepatitis B Surface Antigen	___	☐	66830	Removal of 2nd Mem Cataract	___
☐	99033	Counseling - 25 Minutes	___	☐	86289	Hepatitis B Antibody Core	___	☐	97010	Treatment - Hot	___
☐	90110	Home Care Service (New Pat)	___	☐	86291	Hepatitis B Antibody	___	☐	97110	Exercise Therapeutic	___
☐	90150	Home Care Service (Estab Pat)	___	☐	86296	Hepatitis A Antibody	___	☐	97124	Massage	___
☐	90215	Admiss Hist/Phys Intermediate	___	☐	87070	Culture	___	☐	97128	Ultrasound	___
☐	99223	Admiss Hist/Phys Comprehen	___	☐	87210	Wet Mount	___	☐	97720	Extremity testing for strength	___
☐	99232	Hospital Visit Expanded	___	☐	88150	Pap Smear	___	☐	97752	Muscle Testing, Torque Curves	___
☐	90260	Hospital Visit Intermediate	___	☒	93000	Electrocardiogram	57.00	☐	53670	Catheterization Incl Supplies	___
☐	90270	Hospital Visit Extended	___	☐	99000	Lab Special Handling	___	☐	77263	Treatment Planning - Complex	___
☐	99238	Hospital Visit Discharge Exam	___	☐	-583	Hepatitis Profile # 1	___	☐	77290	Simulation - Complex	___
☐	90510	Emergency Room Care Limited	___	☐	femlab	Female Lab Series	___	☐	77300	Central Axis Dose	___
☐	90515	Emerg Room Care Intermediate	___	☐	-gtt-3	Glucose Tolerance Test - 3 hour	___	☐	77305	Simple Isodose Plan	___
☐	90941	Homodialysis	___	☐	-gtt-5	Glucose Tolerance Test - 5 hour	___	☐	77333	Shielding Block - Regular	___
☐	71020	X-Ray Chest Pa B Lat	___	☐	pre-op	Pre-operative Routine Labs	___	☐	77336	Continuing Physics/Week	___
☐	71010	Radiological Exam Entire Spine	___	☐	90701	Immunization	___	☐	77415	Port Film Verification	___
				☐	90749	Injection	___	☐	77420	3-B MEV, Daily, Complex	___

☐	ICDA CODE DIAGNOSIS		☐	ICDA CODE DIAGNOSIS		☐	ICDA CODE DIAGNOSIS	
☐	783.1	Abnormal Weight Gain	☐	921.1	Contusions of Eyelids/Periocular	☐	575.2	Obstruction of Gallbladder
☐	783.2	Abnormal Weight Loss	☐	780.3	Convulsions	☐	742.2	Pain: Lower back
☐	461.9	Acute Sinusitis	☐	352.9	Cranial Neuralgia	☐	481.0	Pneumococcal Pneumonia
☐	346.2	Allergic Headache	☐	300.4	Depression	☐	V22.2	Pregnancy
☐	006.3	Amebic Liver Abscess	☐	311	Depression	☐	722.0	Prolapse/Protrusion Cervical IVD
☐	285.9	Anemia	☐	830.6	Dislocated Hip	☐	593.9	Renal Insufficiency
☐	783.0	Anorexia	☐	830.9	Dislocated Shoulder	☐	727.6	Rupture Achilles Tendon
☐	440.0	Atherosclerosis	☐	487.0	Flu	☐	727.8	Rupture Flexor Tendon Hand/Wrist
☐	353.0	Brachial Plexus Irritation	☐	802.0	Fracture - Nasal Closed	☐	355.5	Sciatic Nerve Root Lesion
☐	174.9	Breast Cancer	☐	892.1	Fractured Fibula	☐	564.1	Spastic Colon
☐	185.0	Cancer of the Prostate	☐	891.2	Fractured Tibia	☐	842.5	Sprained Ankle
☐	442.81	Carotid Artery	☐	780.1	Hallucinations	☐	841.2	Sprained Wrist
☐	354.0	Carpal Tunnel Syndrome	☐	477.9	Hay Fever	☐	538.8	Stomach Pain
☐	366.9	Cataract	☐	573.3	Hepatitis	☐	918.1	Superficial Injury to Eye (Cornea)
☐	353.9	Cervical Dorsal Outlet Syndrome	☐	553.3	Hiatal Hernia	☐	524.6	Temporo-Mand Joint Syndrome
☐	721.0	Cervical Osteo/Spondyloarthritis	☐	009.0	Ill-defined Intestinal Infections	☐	353.3	Thoratic Nerve Root Compression
☐	571.4	Chronic Hepatitis	☐	919.5	Insect Bite, Nonvenom, Infected	☐	721.2	Thoratic Spondylo/Osteoarthritis
☐	473.9	Chronic Sinusitis	☐	721.3	Lumbar Osteo/Spondyloarthritis	☐	474.0	Tonsillitis
☐	571.5	Cirrhosis of the Liver	☐	353.1	Lumbosacral Plexus Lesion	☐	386.0	Vertigo
☒	892.5	Combo Fibula/Tibia Fracture	☒	346.9	Migraine Headache	☐	480.0	Viral Pneumonia
☐	460.0	Common Cold	☐	721.1	Neuro-Vascular Compression	☐	V20.2	Well Child

Previous Balance	Today's Charges	Total Due	Amount Paid	New Balance		
___	318.00	___	___	___	PRN ___ Weeks ___	Follow Up
					Next Appointment Date:	Months ___ Units ___
						Time:

I hereby authorize release of any information acquired in the course of
examination or treatment and allow a photocopy of my signature to be used.

_____

DAILY LOG *for 2/17*

S. Carrington, M.D.

DATE	PATIENT	PROFESSIONAL SERVICES	TODAY'S CHARGE		PAYMENT		CURRENT BALANCE		PREVIOUS BALANCE		NAME
2/17	Jake	99213, 68906	80	00							Marley
2/17	Bijan	99215, 93000	57	00							Dimek
2/17	Ashley	99211, 88150	60	00							Wagner
2/17	Mike	99213, 81000	50	00							Herndon
TOTALS											

PORTFOLIO FIGURE IV-11

APPROVED OMB-0938-0008

CARRIER

PICA ☐☐

HEALTH INSURANCE CLAIM FORM

PICA ☐☐

1. MEDICARE	MEDICAID	CHAMPUS	CHAMPVA	GROUP HEALTH PLAN (SSN or ID)	FECA BLK LUNG (SSN)	OTHER	1a. INSURED'S I.D. NUMBER	(FOR PROGRAM IN ITEM 1)
☐ (Medicare #)	☐ (Medicaid #)	☐ (Sponsor's SSN)	☐ (VA File #)	☐	☐	☐ (ID)		

2. PATIENT'S NAME (Last Name, First Name, Middle Initial)

3. PATIENT'S BIRTH DATE
MM ꞉ DD ꞉ YY   SEX
M ☐   F ☐

4. INSURED'S NAME (Last Name, First Name, Middle Initial)

5. PATIENT'S ADDRESS (No., Street)

6. PATIENT RELATIONSHIP TO INSURED
Self ☐ Spouse ☐ Child ☐ Other ☐

7. INSURED'S ADDRESS (No., Street)

CITY   STATE

8. PATIENT STATUS
Single ☐   Married ☐   Other ☐

Employed ☐   Full-Time Student ☐   Part-Time Student ☐

CITY   STATE

ZIP CODE   TELEPHONE (Include Area Code)
(   )

ZIP CODE   TELEPHONE (INCLUDE AREA CODE)
(   )

9. OTHER INSURED'S NAME (Last Name, First Name, Middle Initial)

10. IS PATIENT'S CONDITION RELATED TO:

11. INSURED'S POLICY GROUP OR FECA NUMBER

a. OTHER INSURED'S POLICY OR GROUP NUMBER

a. EMPLOYMENT? (CURRENT OR PREVIOUS)
☐ YES   ☐ NO

a. INSURED'S DATE OF BIRTH
MM ꞉ DD ꞉ YY   SEX
M ☐   F ☐

b. OTHER INSURED'S DATE OF BIRTH
MM ꞉ DD ꞉ YY   SEX
M ☐   F ☐

b. AUTO ACCIDENT?   PLACE (State)
☐ YES   ☐ NO

b. EMPLOYER'S NAME OR SCHOOL NAME

c. EMPLOYER'S NAME OR SCHOOL NAME

c. OTHER ACCIDENT?
☐ YES   ☐ NO

c. INSURANCE PLAN NAME OR PROGRAM NAME

d. INSURANCE PLAN NAME OR PROGRAM NAME

10d. RESERVED FOR LOCAL USE

d. IS THERE ANOTHER HEALTH BENEFIT PLAN?
☐ YES   ☐ NO   If yes, return to and complete item 9 a-d.

READ BACK OF FORM BEFORE COMPLETING & SIGNING THIS FORM.
12. PATIENT'S OR AUTHORIZED PERSON'S SIGNATURE I authorize the release of any medical or other information necessary to process this claim. I also request payment of government benefits either to myself or to the party who accepts assignment below.

SIGNED _____ DATE _____

13. INSURED'S OR AUTHORIZED PERSON'S SIGNATURE I authorize payment of medical benefits to the undersigned physician or supplier for services described below.

SIGNED _____

PATIENT AND INSURED INFORMATION

14. DATE OF CURRENT: ILLNESS (First symptom) OR
MM ꞉ DD ꞉ YY   INJURY (Accident) OR
PREGNANCY(LMP)

15. IF PATIENT HAS HAD SAME OR SIMILAR ILLNESS.
GIVE FIRST DATE   MM ꞉ DD ꞉ YY

16. DATES PATIENT UNABLE TO WORK IN CURRENT OCCUPATION
MM ꞉ DD ꞉ YY   MM ꞉ DD ꞉ YY
FROM   TO

17. NAME OF REFERRING PHYSICIAN OR OTHER SOURCE

17a. I.D. NUMBER OF REFERRING PHYSICIAN

18. HOSPITALIZATION DATES RELATED TO CURRENT SERVICES
MM ꞉ DD ꞉ YY   MM ꞉ DD ꞉ YY
FROM   TO

19. RESERVED FOR LOCAL USE

20. OUTSIDE LAB? $ CHARGES
☐ YES   ☐ NO

21. DIAGNOSIS OR NATURE OF ILLNESS OR INJURY. (RELATE ITEMS 1,2,3 OR 4 TO ITEM 24E BY LINE)

1. L___ . __   3. L___ . __

2. L___ . __   4. L___ . __

22. MEDICAID RESUBMISSION
CODE   ORIGINAL REF. NO.

23. PRIOR AUTHORIZATION NUMBER

24. A							B	C	D		E	F	G	H	I	J	K
		DATE(S) OF SERVICE					Place of Service	Type of Service	PROCEDURES, SERVICES, OR SUPPLIES (Explain Unusual Circumstances)		DIAGNOSIS CODE	$ CHARGES	DAYS OR UNITS	EPSDT Family Plan	EMG	COB	RESERVED FOR LOCAL USE
	From			To					CPT/HCPCS	MODIFIER							
	MM	DD	YY	MM	DD	YY											
1																	
2																	
3																	
4																	
5																	
6																	

PHYSICIAN OR SUPPLIER INFORMATION

25. FEDERAL TAX I.D. NUMBER   SSN ☐ EIN ☐

26. PATIENT'S ACCOUNT NO.

27. ACCEPT ASSIGNMENT?
(For govt. claims, see back)
☐ YES   ☐ NO

28. TOTAL CHARGE
$

29. AMOUNT PAID
$

30. BALANCE DUE
$

31. SIGNATURE OF PHYSICIAN OR SUPPLIER INCLUDING DEGREES OR CREDENTIALS
(I certify that the statements on the reverse apply to this bill and are made a part thereof.)

SIGNED _____ DATE _____

32. NAME AND ADDRESS OF FACILITY WHERE SERVICES WERE RENDERED (If other than home or office)

33. PHYSICIAN'S, SUPPLIER'S BILLING NAME, ADDRESS, ZIP CODE & PHONE #

PIN#   GRP#

(APPROVED BY AMA COUNCIL ON MEDICAL SERVICE 8/88)

PLEASE PRINT OR TYPE

FORM HCFA-1500 (U2) (12-90)
FORM OWCP-1500   FORM RRB-1500

PORTFOLIO FIGURE IV-12

Becoming a Career Medical Assistant

Health care reform will have a dramatic impact on the field of medical assisting. If, as expected, family physicians and internists become the primary point of entry into the health care system, the employment market will expand for medical assistants who have general knowledge of how to run a medical office and basic knowledge of terminology, body systems, and clinical procedures.

A medical assistant must possess far more than medical assisting skills, however, in order to be successful in today's job market. Employability, communication, and technology skills are named at the top of the list of required attributes by people who hire entry-level staff. This means you must be at work every day, give a full day's work for a full day's pay, perform as a team member, possess outstanding ability to get along with people, and operate computers and related high technology equipment.

First, though, you must get a job. This means preparing a well-written, attractive resume, making a professional impression during an interview, and negotiating a salary that meets your needs and matches your experience and education. Seeking employment is an intensive, invigorating, demanding, and sometimes frustrating activity. Ultimately, however, the reward of a challenging medical assisting job is worth all the energy you put into the search.

Once you are employed, you must continue your education in order to grow professionally and increase your income. You should consider credentialing, returning to school for additional courses, and becoming a member of a professional medical assisting association.

Chapters 16 and 17 start you on your way to becoming employed as a medical assistant. Good luck!

Chapter 16

Workplace Readiness

OKLAHOMA CITY, OKLAHOMA

My biggest on-the-job challenge isn't insurance forms or bookkeeping. It's human relations and staying up to date on all the changes in procedures and technology. I can scarcely believe how much has changed in the short time since I completed my training, and many more changes are in sight. The professional journals are filled with new and developing telecommunications and computer applications. Every day, the news is full of new societal developments, both in our country and abroad, that affect health care management, procedures, and documentation. *What* I learned in school is not nearly as important as that I learned *how* to learn.

I am also continually challenged to be attentive and patient with supervisors, calm and supportive with patients, and friendly to co-workers. Every day, my co-workers and I encounter patients who are upset, irritable, depressed, and anxious. We even feel that way ourselves, sometimes.

I've learned many things they don't teach in school—to take notes when someone gives me instructions, not to be defensive when my work is criticized, and never to express my bad moods to patients or staff. It's quite a challenge, and I can always improve!

Sasha Fredericks
Medical Assistant

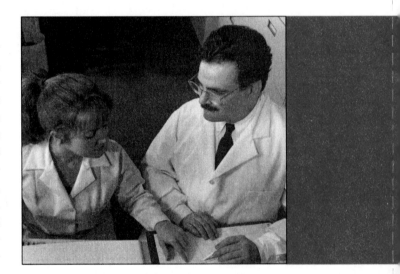

PERFORMANCE BASED COMPETENCIES

At the end of this chapter, you should be able to:
1. Create a plan for enhancing your work readiness skills. (DACUM 1.0, Advanced Skill)
2. Deliver a short talk on the skills that are most important for job success today. (DACUM 2.0, Advanced Skill)
3. Discuss the major studies that identify what employers look for in employees. (DACUM 7.0)

Employers say that "being ready to work" is far more important than having training as a medical assistant. In fact, they say that a medical background is secondary when it comes to getting and keeping a job. You may find this surprising since most of your training focuses on the clinical or administrative aspects of being a medical assistant.

The three crucial workplace readiness skills named by physicians and others who hire are (1) employability, (2) communications ability, and (3) proficiency in using technology, especially computers. You might look at these as an umbrella for success. If you have good work-place readiness skills and also possess a strong medical assisting background, plus proficiency in the basic skills of language usage and math, you can almost certainly guarantee a successful career.

The workplace readiness skills are discussed in detail on the following pages. Figure 16-1 illustrates the umbrella of skills necessary for a successful career.

What Is Employability?

Doctors often refer to employability as "caring" about the work. Employability is the hardest of the workplace readiness components to describe because it has to do with attitude. It's the distinction between *being able* to do a job well and *wanting* to do the job well.

Employability means that you care about being on time and are at work every day; you care about the image of the practice, and you work hard to leave a good impression with patients. Your employability shows when you work cooperatively with other people, refrain from asking special favors for yourself, and look upon constructive criticism as an opportunity to improve. Dressing correctly for the situation, behaving professionally, taking pride in your work, perseverance, self-motivation and an interest in self-improvement are other aspects of employability.

According to one physician, "Employability is the difference between working for money and working because you want to make a contribution to the practice." In a talk to a class of medical assisting students, this doctor said, "You are not worth much to me if I can't depend on you. That means I want to be able to trust your judgment, your ethics, your sense of responsibility, your attention to detail, and your professionalism. If I can't count on you in these ways, then nothing else matters, not how smart you are, the good grades you made in school, or how terrific you are at billing and collection or clinical assistance."

Although physicians are not always able to give a good description of employability, they know when a medical assistant possesses it, and

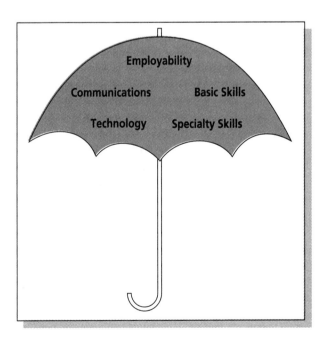

FIGURE 16-1 Umbrella of work readiness skills

Employability Skills
Exhibiting loyalty to the company
Being at work on time
Evidencing a desire to learn
Taking pride in details
Showing flexibility, adaptability
Seeing the big picture
Organizing work
Dressing appropriately
Adapting to diversity of tasks and people
Working cooperatively with others
Participating as a member of a team
Exhibiting a good attitude
Dealing with organizational change
Managing time
Exhibiting discipline in work habits
Thinking creatively
Solving problems
Making decisions
Understanding organizational dynamics
Learning new skills and duties
Persevering until job completion
Prioritizing work
Handling multiple priorities
Dealing with stress

FIGURE 16-2 Employability skills

they are usually willing to pay a premium salary to keep such a person. When the people who work with you like you, in addition to respecting your ability, then you surely possess good employability skills. Figure 16-2 lists employability skills that are frequently mentioned by physicians and other employers as most important to job success.

Communication Ability

Some people always seem to communicate well, orally, nonverbally, and in written form. These individuals have developed a priceless skill because the ability to communicate effectively is highly valued in our society. Good health care communicators often are leaders because they size up situations correctly, articulate their positions well, and are able to give instructions to others in a precise, friendly manner.

Good communicators get along well with others, say the right thing at the right time, and refrain from saying the wrong thing at the wrong time. Strong communicators are generous with praise and sparse with criticism. When they criticize, they do it in a constructive way that reduces offensiveness. Good health care communicators perceive patients' needs and are good at satisfying them. A medical assistant who is a good communicator might ask, for example, "Would you like a magazine while you wait?" or "Dr. Amos is running thirty minutes behind. I know you're on your lunch hour. Will that cause you a problem?"

Listening is an important component of interpersonal skills, yet most people never have a course or a unit in listening during all the time they are in school. Figures 16-3 and 16-4 show the role that listening plays in our daily communication. Although 40 percent of our day is spent listening, we spend at most only one and one-half years of our education in listening training.

Conducting meetings in a professional manner, coaching other staff, using appropriate grammar, asking questions, and matching non-

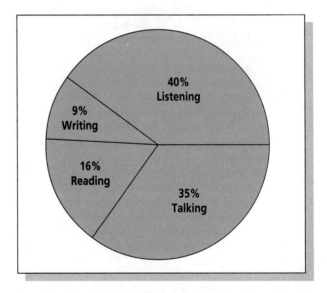

FIGURE 16-3 The majority of the time we spend communicating is spent listening.

Formal Training in Communication

Type of Communication	Formal Years Training
Writing	12 years
Reading	6–8 years
Speaking	1–2 years
Listening	0–½ years

FIGURE 16-4 Formal training in communication

verbal behaviors with oral comments are all communication skills. Interpersonal relations, or the way people interact with other people, is highly dependent on these.

Co-workers and others like to be around good communicators because they make them feel comfortable. Even when the message is negative or offers a contrary point of view, good communicators deliver it in such a way that listeners are not made to feel uncomfortable.

You may have heard that someone is a "born communicator." Don't be misled; communicators develop their strengths, they aren't born with them. Good communication is a series of skills that can be developed by anyone, and like any other skill, such as playing a musical instrument or water skiing, good communication must be practiced. Look at the list of communication skills given in Figure 16-5. Analyze whether you need to develop or practice any of these.

Technology Skills

After completing the chapters in this book, you can see how important computers are to a medical office. Beginning with the patient's first visit when personal information is used to create a file through all of the patient's succeeding visits, computer records identify the diagnoses, treatments, charges, and payments. Other documents related to patients, including letters, reports, and claim forms, plus practice reports, financial analyses, and employment records also are maintained by computer.

As a medical assistant, you will be expected to use a computer efficiently, troubleshoot simple software and hardware problems, and interact with peripheral equipment such as printers, FAX machines, telephone systems, e-mail, and voice mail. In addition, you will be expected to use the medical technology related to your specialty.

One of the best ways to become a key employee in your practice is to possess outstanding technology skills. Technology changes very quickly. Predictions indicate that 50 percent of the technology that will be used by today's eighth graders when they go to work has not been invented yet. This means the technology you use in the next thirty or forty years of your career will change many times.

You should build technology seminars and training into your continuing education plan. By maintaining up-to-date knowledge of computer usage, you can bring authority and leadership to the practice's computer operations. Figure 16-6 provides a list of technology skills important in medical practices.

Communication Skills

Writing general documents
Writing technical documents
Communicating orally
Using language effectively
Following instructions
Giving instructions
Reading and interpreting technical manuals
Listening
Analyzing customer needs
Serving customers
Conducting meetings
Handling telephone conversations
Accepting and giving criticism
Handling conflict
Supervising others
Leading others
Managing projects
Coaching other staff

FIGURE 16-5 Communication skills

Technology Skills

Ability to use computer for:

- Using word processing
- Using databases
- Creating databases
- Using spreadsheets
- Creating spreadsheets
- Using other software
- Accessing and using
  - E-mail
  - Company networks
  - Public networks, such as Prodigy, Source

Ability to use other communications technology:

- FAX
- Voice mail

FIGURE 16-6 Technology skills

IN YOUR OPINION

1. Prioritize the employability skills shown in Figure 16-2. Include additional skills you consider important.
2. Which of the communications skills shown in Figure 16-5 can be used to improve interpersonal relationships?
3. What changes have you seen in computer technology since you entered high school?

What the World Tells Us Is Needed for Career Success

The economy of the world is changing dramatically and quickly. This affects every occupation and employee. Evidence of the upheaval that this time of economic change is bringing can be seen in the powerful health care reform movement taking place today. Many of the rules, guidelines, financial payment systems, and paperwork procedures are changing dramatically. All of this will influence your work as a medical assistant.

In addition, careers are changing. People in mid-life in all types of careers outside health care who thought they had careers until retirement are losing their jobs. Many are forced to take new jobs at lower pay after many months without employment. In some cases, their new positions require retraining in a completely different field. Some specialties, such as internal medicine, are becoming more desirable, while others may become less desirable. You, in fact, can expect to have at least three major career changes during your employment life, even though you may continue as a medical assistant. An example is the person who, until a few years ago, worked for a sole practitioner but today works in a ten-physician group while still assigned to the same doctor.

Over the last ten years, a great deal of attention has been given by professional organizations, research firms, and government agencies to identifying what leads to job success and continuing employment. The work readiness skills summarized in Figures 16-2, 16-5, and 16-6 appear as very important in each of these studies. It is valuable for you to know about the studies and understand what the research organizations learned from them.

DACUM

The DACUM (Developing a CUrriculuM) chart of skills was presented first in Chapter 2, and all the Performance Based Competencies identified at the beginning of each chapter in this book are based on DACUM skills. The DACUM is a process that draws knowledgeable employers, teachers, and employees from a specific field together for one to two days to develop a road map of skills, knowledge, behaviors, and characteristics that lead to success in the field being studied. The medical assisting DACUM is presented in Figure 2-3 on pages 24 and 25 and in the Appendix on pages 384 and 385. Compare it to the work readiness skills and to your own administrative and clinical background to determine if you need to pay special attention to any areas of career preparation.

REGISTERED MEDICAL ASSISTANT GUIDELINES

The American Medical Technologists has created guidelines for career preparation as a medical records manager. These are reproduced in Figure 16-7. Review these guidelines to ensure that you are competent in all areas the RMA considers valuable.

I. General Medical Assisting Knowledge
A. Anatomy and Physiology
  1. Body systems
     a. Know the structure and function of the skeletal system
     b. Know the structure and function of the muscular system
     c. Know the structure and function of the endocrine system
     d. Know the structure and function of the urinary system
     e. Know the structure and function of the reproductive system
     f. Know the structure and function of the gastro-intestinal system
     g. Know the structure and function of the nervous system
     h. Know the structure and function of the respiratory system
     i. Know the structure and function of the cardio-vascular system
     j. Know the structure and function of the integumentary system
     k. Know the structure and function of the special senses system
  2. Disorders of the body
     a. Identify various diseases
     b. Identify various conditions
     c. Identify various syndromes
B. Medical Terminology
  1. Word parts
     a. Identify word parts: root, prefixes, and suffixes
  2. Definitions
     a. Define medical terms
  3. Common abbreviations and symbols
     a. Know medical abbreviations and symbols
  4. Spelling
     a. Spell medical terms correctly
C. Medical Law
  1. Medical law
     a. Identify the various types of consent, and how and when to obtain each
     b. Know disclosure laws (i.e., what information must be reported to proper agency), what constitutes confidential information, and what information may be disclosed under certain circumstances
     c. Recognize legal responsibilities of the medical assistant
     d. Know the various medically-related laws (i.e., Good Samaritan, Anatomical Gift Act, Drug storage and record maintenance, Drug Enforcement Agency regulations)
     e. Define legal terminology associated with medical law
  2. Licensure, certification, and registration
     a. Know credentialing requirements of medical professionals

D. Medical Ethics
  1. Principles of medical ethics
     a. Know the principles of medical ethics established by the American Medical Association
     b. Define terminology associated with medical ethics
  2. Ethical conduct
     a. Identify the ethical response for the various situations in a medical facility
     b. Recognize unethical practices
E. Human Relations
  1. Patient relations
     a. Identify emotional reactions of various age groups
     b. Respond appropriately to emotional needs of patients
  2. Other interpersonal relations
     a. Employ appropriate interpersonal skills in the workplace
F. Patient Education
  1. Patient instruction
     a. Employ various methods to instruct patients (i.e., echo method, verbal, and written instructions)
     b. Instruct patients, as directed, in areas of nutrition, diet, medications, body mechanics, and treatment procedures
     c. Document patient instructions properly
  2. Patient resource materials
     a. Maintain patient resource materials

II. Administrative Medical Assisting
A. Insurance
  1. Terminology
     a. Assist patients with insurance inquiries
     b. Know terminology associated with health and accident insurance in the medical office
  2. Plans
     a. Know the major types of medical insurance programs encountered in the medical office including government-sponsored, group, individual, and workers' compensation programs
  3. Claim forms
     a. Complete and file forms for insurance claims
     b. Evaluate claims rejection
     c. Complete "first" reports
  4. Coding
     a. Know coding systems used in insurance processing
     b. Code diagnoses and procedures
  5. Financial aspects of medical insurance
     a. Know billing requirements for insurance programs
     b. Process insurance payments
     c. Track unpaid claims
B. Financial Bookkeeping
  1. Terminology
     a. Know terminology associated with financial bookkeeping in the medical office
  2. Patient Billing
     a. Maintain and explain physician's fee schedules

FIGURE 16-7 Registered medical assistant career guidelines for administrative medical assistants (Adapted from American Medical Technologists, RMA Certification Exam Construction Parameters)

b. Collect and post payments; manage patient ledgers
c. Make financial arrangements with patients
d. Prepare and mail itemized statements
e. Know methods of billing
f. Cycle billing procedures
3. Collections
    a. Identify delinquent accounts; take appropriate steps for collection
    b. Perform skip tracing
    c. Perform telephone collection procedures
    d. Know collection as related to bankruptcy and small claims cases
4. Fundamental medical office accounting procedures
    a. Employ appropriate accounting procedures (e.g., pegboard)
    b. Employ daily balancing procedures
    c. Prepare monthly trial balance
    d. Know accounts payable/receivable procedures
5. Banking
    a. Manage petty cash
    b. Prepare and make bank deposits
    c. Reconcile bank statements
    d. Use and process checks appropriately (including NSF and endorsement requirements)
    e. Maintain checking account
    f. Process payables (office bills)
6. Employee payroll
    a. Prepare employee payroll
    b. Maintain payroll tax deduction records, prepare employee tax forms, and prepare payroll tax deduction reports
    c. Know terminology pertaining to payroll and taxes
7. Financial mathematics
    a. Perform calculations related to patient and practice accounts

C. **Medical Secretarial-Receptionist**
1. Terminology
    a. Know terminology associated with medical secretarial and receptionist duties
2. Reception
    a. Receive and greet patients and visitors under non-emergency conditions
    b. Screen visitors and sales persons requesting to see physician
    c. Obtain patient information
    d. Call/assist patients into examination rooms
3. Scheduling
    a. Employ appointment scheduling system (maintain appointment book, type daily schedule, review schedule with physician)
    b. Prepare information for referrals
    c. Arrange hospital admissions and surgery, and schedule patients for out-patient diagnostic tests
    d. Manage recall system and file
    e. Employ procedures for handling cancellations and missed appointments

4. Oral and written communications
    a. Answer and place telephone calls employing proper etiquette
    b. Manage telephone calls requiring special attention (including lab and x-ray reports, angry callers, and personal calls)
    c. Instruct patients by telephone regarding emergency treatment and medications
    d. Inform patients of laboratory results
    e. Employ effective intra-office oral communication skills (including employee supervision and patient handling)
    f. Compose correspondence according to acceptable business format
    g. Type bills, statements, medical records, and other written materials, and proofread written material
    h. Manage mail
    i. Employ effective written communication skills
5. Records management
    a. Manage complete patient medical records system
    b. File records according to appropriate system (master calendars, tickler files, correspondence, financial records, physician's records, non-patient files)
    c. Transfer files
    d. Protect, store, and retain medical records according to appropriate conventions
6. Charts
    a. Arrange contents of patient charts in appropriate order and perform audits for accuracy
    b. Record laboratory results and patient communication in charts
    c. Maintain confidentiality of medical records and test results (e.g., HIV, pregnancy tests)
    d. Observe special regulations regarding the confidentiality of HIV results
7. Transcription and dictation
    a. Transcribe notes from dictaphone or tape recorder
    b. Transcribe notes from direct dictation
8. Supplies and equipment management
    a. Maintain inventory of medical and office supplies and equipment (reordering, order new supplies)
    b. Arrange for equipment maintenance and repair, and maintain warranty/services files
9. Computers for medical office applications
    a. Use computer for data entry and retrieval
    b. Use computer for word processing
    c. Use computer for billing and financial transactions
    d. Employ procedures for ensuring the integrity and confidentiality of computer-stored information
10. Office safety
    a. Maintain office cleanliness and comfort
    b. Maintain office safety (maintain office safety manual and post emergency instructions)
    c. Maintain records of biohazardous waste and hazardous chemicals
    d. Know and comply with Occupational Safety and Health Act (OSHA) guidelines and regulations

FIGURE 16-7 continued

SECRETARY'S COMMISSION ON ACHIEVING NECESSARY SKILLS

The SCANS report is a compilation of data developed over a year-long period and published in 1991 by former Department of Labor Secretary Lynn Martin and a group of 1,500 employers, labor leaders, managers, educators, and employees. SCANS is an acronym for Secretary's Commission on Achieving Necessary Skills. Its purpose was to identify the factors that are common to job success in all job categories and at all levels of the career ladder. The SCANS three-part foundation skills needed in all jobs are shown in Figure 16-8.

AMERICAN SOCIETY OF TRAINING AND DEVELOPMENT

The American Society of Training and Development (ASTD) is a professional organization made up of training managers from business and industry. These training managers are hired by corporations to develop and administer training programs for employees. In a study completed by ASTD, seven skills are named as most important for career success. They are listed in Figure 16-9.

TEN BEST-SELLING BOOKS

Training managers and corporate training instructors order books and videos to supplement their teaching. A list of the best selling books of 1994 from Crisp Publications, a company that provides corporate training materials, indicates where companies see the greatest need for additional training. The books are listed in Figure 16-10. How do you measure up in these categories?

Basic Skills:

A. Reading—locates, understands, and interprets written information in prose and in documents such as manuals, graphs, and schedules.

B. Writing—communicates thoughts, ideas, information, and messages in writing; and creates documents such as letters, directions, manuals, reports, graphs, and flow charts.

C. Arithmetic and Mathematics—performs basic computations and approaches practical problems by choosing appropriately from a variety of mathematical techniques.

D. Listening—receives, attends to, interprets, and responds to verbal messages and other cues.

E. Speaking—organizes ideas and communicates orally.

Thinking Skills:

A. Creative Thinking—generates new ideas.

B. Decision Making—specifies goals and constraints, generates alternatives, considers risks, and evaluates and chooses best alternative.

C. Problem Solving—recognizes problems and devises and implements plan of action.

D. Seeing Things in the Mind's Eye—organizes, and processes symbols, pictures, graphs, objects, and other information.

E. Knowing How to Learn—uses efficient learning techniques to acquire and apply new knowledge and skills.

F. Reasoning—discovers a rule or principle underlying the relationship between two or more objects and applies it when solving a problem.

Personal Qualities:

A. Responsibility—exerts a high level of effort and perseveres toward a goal attainment.

B. Self-Esteem—believes in own self-worth and maintains a positive view of self.

C. Sociability—demonstrates understanding, friendliness, adaptability, empathy, and politeness in group settings.

D. Self-Management—assesses self accurately, sets personal goals, monitors progress, and exhibits self-control.

E. Integrity/Honesty—chooses ethical courses of action.

FIGURE 16-8 SCANS three-part foundation skills (Adapted from the Department of Labor, Secretary's Commission on Achieving Necessary Skills, June 1991)

FIGURE 16-9 ASTD's seven most important skills for career success (Adapted from the American Society for Training and Development, U.S. Department of Labor, Employment and Training Adminstration)

Putting It All Together

Two activities will allow you to focus on your workplace readiness and prepare a plan for continued growth. One of these is the portfolio, which you are developing as a part of your study of this text, and the other is preparation for a mock interview with your mentor.

PORTFOLIO

Your portfolio, described on page xii and created in segments by you at the end of each part of this book provides evidence of your training in administrative medical assisting. Make sure that the portfolio presents the image you want to give employers. This is a communication tool that you will use to draw a picture of who you are and what you have to offer an employing practice.

1. Mentoring
2. Working Together
3. Team Building
4. Empowerment
5. Men and Women
6. Business of Listening
7. Coaching and Counseling
8. Time Management
9. Managing Change
10. Telephone Courtesy

FIGURE 16-10 Top ten best-selling books of 1994

MOCK INTERVIEW

You will be asked in an exercise at the end of this unit to compile all the items needed for an interview with your mentor; then you will be asked to arrange an interview so that you may practice your skills. Your interview should cover the following points:

1. Your interest in the position
2. Evidence of your knowledge of the position's requirements
3. Background support that you meet the requirements of the position
   a. Resume
   b. Portfolio
   c. The way you conduct yourself (communications)
4. Closure of the interview

Begin your planning now by reviewing the contents of this chapter and matching your skills to those named as most important for career success.

IN YOUR OPINION

1. Why are so many associations or organizations researching workplace issues?
2. What is the importance of the makeup of the groups involved in DACUM and SCANS?
3. Why is a portfolio an important item to have at an interview?

REFERENCES

Burley-Allen, Madelyn. *Listening, The Forgotten Skill,* New York. John Wiley & Sons, Inc., 1982.

Carnevale, Anthony, Leila J. Gainer, and Ann S. Meetzer. *Workplace Basics: The Skills Employers Want.* San Francisco: Jossey-Bass, 1988.

"The DACUM Revisited: The 1990 Update on the Profession of Medical Assisting," *The Professional Medical Assistant.* May/June 1990.

Hamlin, Sonya, *How to Talk So People Will Listen,* New York. Harper & Row, 1988.

"Top Ten Best Selling Books of 1994", Los Altos, California: Crisp Publications, Inc., 1994.

"What Work Requires of Schools—A SCANS Report for America 2000," U.S. Department of Labor, 1991.

Chapter Activities

PERFORMANCE BASED ACTIVITIES

1. Create a plan for enhancing the work readiness skills you possess. Include in the plan any new skills you need to develop.

Work Readiness Plan

Skills to Enhance	Skills to Develop	Plan	Time Line
_____	_____	_____	_____
_____	_____	_____	_____
_____	_____	_____	_____
_____	_____	_____	_____
_____	_____	_____	_____
_____	_____	_____	_____

2. Compare the skills, behaviors, and knowledge that are common to all the career success surveys discussed in this chapter. When an item is named by multiple organizations or studies, list it under each organization across the page on the same line in the chart. Write a one-page summary describing what you learned from the comparison.

Comparison of Success Skills

Medical Assisting DACUM	RMA Guidelines	SCANS	ASTD	Mentoring Practice
_____	_____	_____	_____	_____
_____	_____	_____	_____	_____
_____	_____	_____	_____	_____
_____	_____	_____	_____	_____
_____	_____	_____	_____	_____
_____	_____	_____	_____	_____

(DACUM 1.8, 2.7, 2.11)

3. Discuss with your mentor the factors that are important in being hired as a medical assistant in the mentoring practice. Add a fifth column to the chart in No. 2 comparing the guidelines from the organizations to the actual hiring standards in the mentoring practice. Record a three-minute talk on audio tape and give it to your instructor.

(DACUM 2.3, 2.7)

EXPANDING YOUR THINKING

1. Ask a school counselor to administer the Myers-Briggs Type Inventory or a similar personality indicator for you. Analyze the results with your counselor to determine your communication style. From the results, make a chart of your communication strengths and weaknesses with recommendations for improvement.

Communication Type	Strengths of This Type	Recommendations for Improvement
_____	_____	_____
_____	_____	_____
_____	_____	_____
_____	_____	_____
_____	_____	_____
_____	_____	_____

2. Review with your mentor the communication strengths and weaknesses you identified in No. 2. Ask your mentor for an opinion. You may be surprised that your strengths are greater than you think. Ask your mentor to recommend ways you can improve your effectiveness as a medical assistant. Then create a plan of action for addressing the improvements your mentor suggests. Use this as an exercise in accepting constructive criticism.

Chapter 17

Seeking Employment

WILMINGTON, NORTH CAROLINA

Last year when I was interviewing for jobs, my friends got tired of hearing me complain about dressing for interviews. I felt frustrated every time I put on my blue suit and blouse to go to an interview. I felt as though all of my individuality was eliminated by this "uniform."

One day a friend and I were having lunch together and I complained that I was going to get rid of my suit as soon as I got a job. She listened to me for a while; then she said, "You looked really great on Friday in your dress when you accepted your medical assisting award." I stopped and thought. "I liked the way those clothes let me express my personality. Why do I think I have to look dull for an interview?"

On the day I interviewed for this job I wore a dress and jacket, with pearl jewelry and medium-heel pumps. I thought that I looked organized, efficient, and capable and that my "look" reflected the skills on my resume. Dr. Braun must have thought so, too, because she offered me the job on the spot!

Stasia Merrill
Medical Receptionist

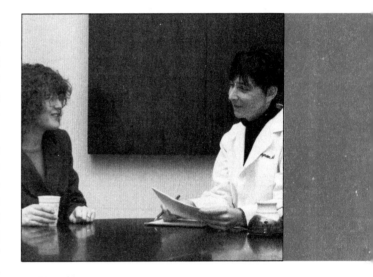

PERFORMANCE BASED COMPETENCIES

After completing this chapter, you should be able to:

1. Formulate a career objective. (DACUM 1.8, 1.9)
2. Prioritize the sources available to you for finding out about jobs that fulfill your career objective. (DACUM 2.6, 2.7)
3. Develop a resume, application letters, and follow-up letters that support your job search. (DACUM 2.11)
4. Use proper telephone technique to support your job search. (DACUM 2.8)
5. Manage the interview process. (DACUM 2.9)

HEALTHSPEAK

Fee-paid Employment agency practice that charges placement fees from employers rather than job seekers.
Networking Developing new contacts and keeping in touch with friends and acquaintances in the medical and related fields.
Resume Document that summarizes your background, education, and qualifications.

After spending many years in school preparing for a productive career, you are ready to go to work now. You know you want to be a medical assistant, and you have been told that many positions exist, but how do you locate a job?

Finding employment in a personally and financially rewarding position takes time, patience, perseverance, and confidence. In addition, locating the right job requires an understanding of (1) your skills and abilities, (2) the types of positions available in your area, and (3) your goals for the future.

Opportunities abound in many different types of medical offices, both large and small. You may choose to work for a private solo or group practice, a hospital, an outpatient clinic, an emergency center, a research center, a teaching center, or in some other medical setting. Whatever your ambitions, the decisions you make now will influence the rest of your life. Make your basic decisions only after thoughtful study of the job market and after considering the implications for your career. Talk over your questions and concerns with someone you trust, preferably someone who is knowledgeable about the medical assisting field and who has several years of experience. Since your future happiness may depend on selecting a good first job, do not take any position unless it feels right to you.

The following sections provide suggestions to help you in the job search process. Follow the step-by-step procedures, and your search will be much easier.

Researching Employment Opportunities

The time you spend now investigating the medical assisting job market will yield dividends later in saved time, reduced frustration and fatigue, and a good understanding of what positions are available. Begin your research while you are still in school and have access to both your instructors and library facilities. By beginning early, you will be able to discuss your questions and concerns with instructors who can provide insight and objectivity about prospective employers. Your best sources for job information are (1) your school placement office, (2) newspaper classified advertisements, (3) professional organizations, (4) acquaintances, (5) employment agencies, (6) instructors at your school, (7) medical societies, and (8) the yellow pages directory.

SCHOOL EMPLOYMENT OFFICES

Colleges, universities, trade schools, and other educational institutions keep a list of employers who are actively recruiting. In many cases, these listings include complete details about specific jobs. Be sure to visit the employment office of your school and review the job listings because good positions are sometimes overlooked when students fail to take advantage of this excellent source (Figure 17-1). The office may also list alumni who are willing to speak with job seekers.

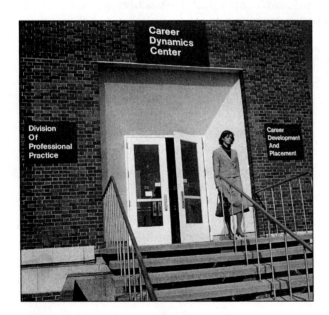

FIGURE 17-1 School employment offices are an excellent source for locating job opportunities.

NEWSPAPER CLASSIFIED ADVERTISEMENTS

Employers routinely advertise positions in the classified section of the newspaper because they recognize that this is the fastest way of reaching a large number of prospective employees. The Sunday edition's classified advertisements are an especially rich source of opportunities. While you are looking for a position, you should spend several hours reviewing each Sunday's ads.

Advertisements for medical assistants may be found under many headings, including (1) medical assistant, (2) phlebotomist (3) medical secretary, (4) secretary, (5) EKG technician, (6) receptionist, (7) nurse assistant, (8) bookkeeper, (9) billing clerk, (10) administrative assistant, (11) medical office manager, (12) insurance clerk, or (13) transcriptionist. Do not overlook an advertisement just because it does not have "medical" in the title. The "medical" reference may be buried in the body of the copy, or it may be identifiable only from the company or institution named. For example, an advertise-ment for an "administrative assistant in a psychiatric clinic" clearly would be worth investigating even though the word "medical" is not used. In large cities newspapers may print a special section called "Health Care Opportunities" or some similar label. Be sure also to review this section thoroughly (Figure 17-2).

As you read the ads, review the skills and abilities required and match your own to those listed. In addition, you may have special skills that will be helpful in some positions and that will give you an advantage over other applicants. For example, a knowledge of Spanish is helpful for medical assistants in Miami, the Southwest, and in many large cities where a large number of residents are Hispanic.

Furthermore, do not dismiss an ad just because the position does not sound exactly like the one you are seeking. After all, it is very difficult for a personnel manager to describe fully the features of a job in only a few lines. In your initial research, you cannot afford to overlook any potentially worthwhile prospects.

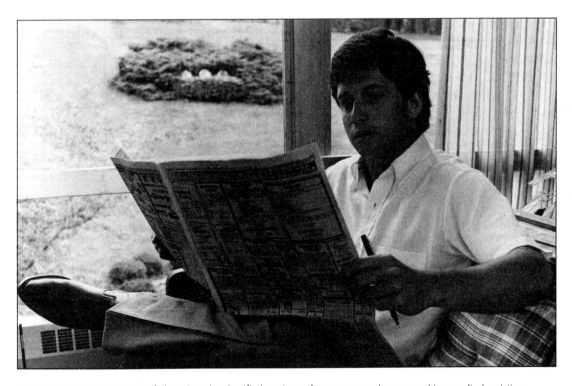

FIGURE 17-2 Be sure to carefully review the classified sections of newspapers when researching medical assisting employment opportunities. Not all job titles list the word "medical."

PROFESSIONAL ORGANIZATIONS

Members of the local chapters of professional medical assisting organizations such as the American Association of Medical Assistants (AAMA) and the American Association of Medical Transcriptionists are usually employees in medical institutions. Sometimes they also do hiring. By becoming acquainted with members of a local organization, you may hear of positions in your area. If you do not personally know any members, determine the name of the organization's president through the local AAMA chapter and give that person a call. Usually, these people are very willing to help new employees get started in the field.

ACQUAINTANCES

Friends and acquaintances can also offer information about potential openings before an announcement is made in the newspaper. Word-of-mouth is a valuable source of information, because the person who hears of a job by this means may also learn important details that would not be printed in an advertisement. Keeping in touch with friends and acquaintances in the field is called networking.

EMPLOYMENT AGENCIES

Employment agencies match employment opportunities and prospective employees. The prospective employee registers with an agency, which has many job listings from physicians, medical companies, and other related institutions. The agency tests applicants and provides pre-employment screening for the employer. When the agency is satisfied that an applicant meets the qualifications specified by an employer, it makes a referral. The prospective employer then interviews the applicant, who may be required to undergo a second series of tests.

Public organizations, such as state or city employment departments, provide their services at no charge. However, private employment agencies charge a fee, usually a percentage of the employee's beginning salary. The amount can become quite large when the beginning salary is large. Some companies pay the agency's fee, since they think the best-qualified applicants have many employment opportunities and will not take a job for which they must pay. Fortunately, in the last few years, more and more agencies are advertising "fee-paid" jobs. The fee is an important consideration that you should discuss with an employment agency before registering for its service (Figure 17-3).

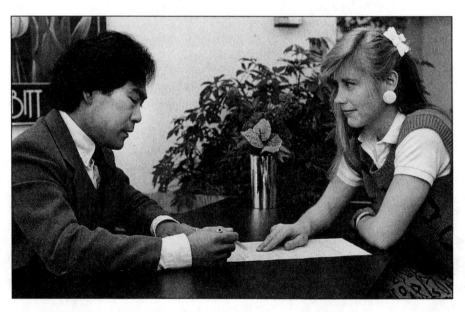

FIGURE 17-3 Before signing a contract with a private employment agency, read the document and study its terms carefully.

When using a private employment agency, you will probably be asked to sign a legally binding contract that holds you to certain requirements. Do not sign a contract unless you have read it carefully and are fully satisfied with its terms. A typical binding clause states that you cannot tell other people about the position. If you do and someone else takes the job, you may be held responsible for paying the agency fee. The contract may also state that you are not allowed to take the job at a later date to avoid paying the agency's fee.

YELLOW PAGES

Medical assistants have a distinct advantage over many other job-seekers because physicians, hospitals, and other medical facilities have specialized listings in the yellow pages. Although going through the yellow pages and dropping a resume in person to each physician or facility is not recommended as a first source of employment, this method could be used with selected physicians. This type of contact also has word-of-mouth potential, and you may learn of prospects in other medical offices when you make random calls. Most medical office managers are willing to talk with potential applicants.

IN YOUR OPINION

1. What sources will you use when you start your first job search?
2. How can you begin to form a network of acquaintances while you are still in school who can help with employment?
3. Considering your skills and abilities, which medical assistant-related job titles appeal to you?

The Job Application Process

The process of applying for a job requires several steps. The person who methodically and confidently works through each step will likely find worthwhile employment, while those who attempt to shortcut the process will undermine their own efforts and not do justice to their training and preparation.

THE RESUME

The most important document you will prepare for an interview is a resume, which is a thorough, yet concise, summary of your background, education, and abilities. A resume is an advertisement for the product you wish to sell, and the product is you. Just as companies spend a great deal of time and effort ensuring that their advertisements deliver the right message to the people they want to reach, you should take care that your resume promotes you honestly and advantageously. Before you distribute a resume, you should rewrite it, edit it, and proofread it, perhaps several times, before you send it out.

Preparing a Resume

Just as the packaging for a product should be attractive, neat, and visually appealing, so should your resume. Use good quality buff or off-white bond paper, a business-like typeface, and an attractive format. Write objective, brief sentences that clearly describe your background; then ask a friend or a relative to proofread the resume for you. Grammatical or typographical mistakes, carelessly done corrections, misspelled words, wrinkled or poor quality paper, ribbon smudges, and awkward placement leave the impression that you are incapable of submitting a quality document or that you do not care about quality. Word processing programs, especially those with graphics features, are very helpful in preparing attractive resumes. One page is sufficient for a beginner's resume.

Parts of a Resume

The parts of a resume are (1) personal information, including name, address, and telephone number; (2) career objective; (3) special skills; (4) work experience; (5) education; (6) awards and honors; (7) extracurricular activities; and (8) references. If you are a student, you may have very little work experience; therefore, the education portion of your resume should list a complete record of the coursework you have completed that prepares you for a medical assisting position.

Personal Information List your full name, address, and telephone number as the heading for a resume. Discrimination laws prohibit employers from requiring personal information, so it is unnecessary to provide age, height, weight, sex, and marital status.

Career Objective Make a concise statement about your career objective. Since you may use the resume for a variety of interviews, do not make the statement so specific that it will eliminate you from competition for a variety of positions.

Special Strengths Compile a list of what makes you special to an employer. Be honest and list only the items that you are sure you possess. Your list should include some of the employability skills listed in Chapter 16.

Work Experience Work experience is a yardstick against which prospective employers measure an applicant's abilities to perform in another job. As a standard that employers understand, work experience indicates how valuable you will be to an organization, how broad your background is, and whether your experience was in a related area. In considering you for a prospective job, a future employer will look at the type of work you did, the number of years you stayed at the company, and any promotions you received.

On your resume, you should list the dates of all employment, beginning with the most recent, and give a brief description of your responsibilities for each job. Include details about any previous jobs that have a connection with the prospective position or that show professional growth. If you received promotions, describe them and your new responsibilities. In short, use the best points of your background to sell your abilities to a prospective employer.

Many students are so busy attending school that they often do not have a broad employment background. Although experience in a related job is very helpful, all job experience is valuable and should be listed, including employment at fast food restaurants, babysitting, lifeguarding, volunteer work, or camp-related employment. List any employment that shows a work ethic, a sense of responsibility, or the development of skills and hobbies.

Education List your college, university, business school, or other postsecondary education. If you have attended more than one school, give the most recent first, even if you did not graduate, and list other institutions and dates of attendance in reverse chronological order. Include the dates of graduation and a list of any degrees, licenses, or applicable certification. Emphasize your clinical training and externship.

Honors and Awards If you have received honors and awards that demonstrate resourcefulness, hard work, or a good attitude, you should list them, especially if they relate to the job for which you are applying.

Extracurricular Activities Many students participate in valuable extracurricular activities because they represent commitment and a sense of responsibility. You should list these activities so that you demonstrate the value of the experience to future employment. You might include in this portion of a resume some of these extracurricular activities: president of a club, band or chorus member, stage crew member for a class play, member of a sports team, or editor of the school newspaper or yearbook.

References References are names of people who know your work habits and skills. Previous employers or supervisors are the best references, followed by teachers or club advisors. Never use a parent or other relative, a minister, or a friend as a reference. These personal references cannot evaluate your abilities objectively, and using them leaves an impression that you do not know about appropriate business practices.

Some applicants do not list names of references on their resume; instead, they use the phrase, "References Upon Request." Unless you have a specific reason not to name a reference, it is good practice to list the names directly on the resume and relieve the employer of the annoyance of having to call you for the names. If you wish to keep your employment search confidential, you will want to be selective in listing references. Figure 17-4 shows a sample form for collecting the information needed for a resume. Figure 17-5 shows an example of a completed resume.

1. Your name, address, and telephone number(s).

2. Employment objective—your career goal.

3. Special Skills—what makes you unique.

4. Work experience—list the name of the job, description of duties, and dates of employment.

   Employer   *Job Title*   *Job Duties*   *Dates of Employment*

5. Education—list the type of diploma, major, and schools attended with dates. You need go no further back than high school. List courses and projects related to the job you want, especially those that have to do with your clinical experience.

   School   *Major*   *Dates Attended*   *Special Projects*

6. Certificates and licenses related to the job.

7. Awards and honors.

8. References—list three references.

   Name   *Phone*   *How Known*

FIGURE 17-4 Resume data collection form

WRITING AN APPLICATION LETTER

The application letter accompanying your resume provides an opportunity to emphasize important parts of your background and offers one more way to sell yourself to a prospective employer. To be effective, it must be well written, visually attractive, error free, and relatively short. The letter should not review all the information provided in your resume, but it should explain why you are interested in the job and why your background has prepared you for the particular position. Mention both front office and back office skills that qualify you for the position.

Although you may copy a resume and use it to apply for several different positions, each application letter should be an original document written for the specific position. The letter should be easy to read and unique without being clever or cute. Above all, it should be interesting, since a dull application letter may discourage an employer from thoroughly reviewing a resume. Refer to Figure 17-6 for a sample cover letter. Use the following procedures for writing your application letter.

Karen Beyer
78 Justine Lane
Nashville, TN 19087
(615) 555-2836

CAREER OBJECTIVE: An office position in the medical field that allows an opportunity to use medical terminology and secretarial skills.

EDUCATION: Volunteer Community College, Nashville, TN.
Associate Degree in Medical Assisting, June 1994.

Major Courses:

Medical Terminology	Machine Transcription
Anatomy and Physiology	Medical Word Processing
Medical Law and Ethics	Computer Applications
Business English	Medical Office Procedures
Business Communication	Human Relations

Internship Program: Participated in a one-year, half-day internship program as a medical assistant trainee for Adele R. Matz, M.D.

WORK EXPERIENCE:

1993–94 Adele R. Matz, M.D., 804 Oakdale Drive, Lebanon, TN 37087 (615) 555-7432. Internship Employer. Transcribed case histories, answered telephone, substituted at reception desk during lunch hour and other special times.

1986-87 McDonald's, 1801 Main Street, Lebanon, TN 37087 (615) 555-2945. Part-time work during summer and after school. Waited on customers.

HONORS AND AWARDS:

Outstanding Office Administration Student, Volunteer Community College, 1994.

EXTRACURRICULAR ACTIVITIES

Representative, Radnor High School Student Council, 1990–92.

Member, Future Business Leaders of America, 1991–92.

REFERENCES:

Adele R. Matz, M.D., 804 Oakdale Drive, Lebanon, TN 37087 (615) 555-7432

Mr. Ralph Gallagher, Office Manager, Adele R. Matz, M.D., 804 Oakdale Drive, Lebanon, TN 37087

Ms. Rachel Sellers, Supervisor, McDonald's, 1801 Main Street, Lebanon, TN 37087 (615) 555-2945

FIGURE 17-5 Completed resume example

78 Justine Lane
Lebanon, TN 37087

June 16, 19—

Ms. Anna Capodici, CMA
Office Manager
Orthopedic Associates, P.C.
20-A Medical Arts Building
Nashville, TN 19087

Dear Ms. Capodici:

Your advertisement for a medical assistant in the June 15 <u>Nashville Tennessean</u>
seeks an employee with the skills and abilities I possess, and I would like to be
considered for the position. The enclosed resume describes thoroughly my education
and work background that prepare me for employment in your medical office.

At Volunteer Community College, I majored in Medical Assisting. The curriculum
focused on medical terminology, office technology, and human relations in the
medical office. As a high B student, I was able to participate in the college's
Internship Program, attending school half time each day and working in the medical
office of Dr. Adele Matz the other half.

Dr. Matz and her office manager, Ralph Gallagher, made certain that I received a
thorough orientation in medical office work. Initially, my job was to transcribe case
histories and other dictation; however, by the end of my internship year, I had
gained broad experience in all areas of medical office work. Frequently, I was asked
to fill in for other employees during their lunch hour or absence from work. Dr. Matz
and Mr. Gallagher both encouraged me to use their names as references.

May I come to your office for an interview, so we can further discuss how my background and your needs for a skilled employee are similar? You may call me at
555-2836; however, since I am sometimes difficult to reach, I will call your office
next Tuesday morning. I look forward to discussing your position further.

Sincerely,

Karen Beyer
Enclosure

FIGURE 17-6 Sample cover letter

Procedures for Writing an Application Letter

1. Send the letter to a specific person, using the person's title. If you do not know the name or title, call the office, and ask the person who answers the telephone for the information you need. ("Hello, this is Alison Rivers. I wish to write a letter to your office manager, but I don't have a name. Will you please tell me the name of the office manager?")
2. Use the "You" viewpoint. Do not overuse "I."
3. Begin with a brief first paragraph describing how you heard of the job and why you are interested. Explain the reasons that you would be good for the job, not the reasons that the job would be good for you. Refer to the resume for brief details about your background.
4. Summarize pertinent information about your education or background and employment history that have prepared you for the job. This is the "selling" section of your letter, so include important details that distinguish you from other applicants. Use two paragraphs if you have enough to say that is different, but do not repeat everything already stated in the resume.
5. Request a personal interview so that you can discuss how your background and the employer's needs match. Make the situation easy by offering to call the employer within a few days to set an appointment; then follow through on the call.
6. Make a copy of the letter for your file. See Figure 17-7.

COMPLETING AN APPLICATION FORM

As a matter of policy, some employers require all applicants to complete an application form in addition to submitting an application letter and resume. Transferring information from your resume to an application form is a relatively simple matter, but remembering all the dates of employment and years of education can be difficult if you do not have a resume handy. Therefore, it is a good idea to take a copy of your resume with you before leaving for an interview. Answer each question on the application form fully; do not skip any questions. If a question does not apply to you, write "N/A" for "not applicable." Write

your answers neatly. This is a sample of your penmanship for the manager to read.

PROVIDING DOCUMENTATION

Some employers may require you to submit an official school transcript as documentation of your education. Since obtaining a transcript may be a lengthy process at some schools, you should begin this step immediately after graduation. Ask for one official copy of your transcript as soon as you are allowed and then make several additional copies that you can give to employers. You will not want to postpone employment because of bureaucratic delays.

```
Your Address

Date


Name of Person
Title
Company Name
Street Address
City, State, Zip Code

Dear_____:

Opening Paragraph:
    Your purpose in writing the letter.

Middle Paragraph:
    Why this employer should consider
    you for this job.

Closing Paragraph:
    Thanks, and plan for your future
    contact with this employer.

Sincerely,



Your Name
```

FIGURE 17-7 Cover letter form

If you have been employed previously, you may have achieved special recognition or professional certification. You should have any important professional certifications or supporting documents available in case an employer asks for them. For example, the Certified Medical Assistant, Certified Professional Secretary, Registered Medical Assistant, and other similar certifications are valuable recognitions of your extensive background that an employer may wish to include in your file.

IN YOUR OPINION

1. As a student who does not yet have a broad work background, how can you convince an employer that you would make a good medical assistant?
2. How can you write a letter accompanying a resume and use the "You" viewpoint?
3. What initial steps can you take while still in school to prepare for interviewing?

Interviewing for a Position

A personal interview is an important part of the employment process because both the employer and prospective employee get a chance to evaluate one another. Personal "chemistry," or the way the interviewer and applicant relate to each other, plays a subtle, yet crucial, role in any interview. Although the employer is responsible for helping the applicant relax, the applicant must be at his or her best. The employer will dismiss an impressive resume and a wonderfully written application letter if the interview does not go well.

APPEARANCE

When a prospective employee walks through the door, an interviewer immediately evaluates the person's appearance. Any negative reactions will subconsciously affect the interviewer's opinion and the outcome of the interview. You should look rested, alert, comfortable, and businesslike. Dress conservatively and neatly. If you own a tailored suit, this is the time to wear it; if not, wear a jacket over tailored clothes. Wear a white or light-colored blouse or shirt, a tie if you are male, and clean, polished shoes. You should eliminate clothes that are too tight, too baggy, too faddish, or "too" anything from your business wardrobe.

Style your hair in a conservative, becoming manner. Long, flowing, or unkempt hair will project a casual, nonbusiness-like image. Use makeup and jewelry sparingly. Any makeup or jewelry should enhance your general appearance and not stand out as gaudy or heavy. Very trendy or provocative styles announce that you are unsophisticated in the ways of business. Dress in a way that reinforces the message that you would be a valuable addition to the employer's staff (Figure 17-8).

To add a measure of polish to your image, carry an 8½" by 11" portfolio. The folder holds extra copies of your resume, provides paper for taking notes, gives you something to do with your hands, and projects a businesslike feeling. Taking a briefcase to an interview, however, is not recommended because it may appear pretentious. For women, matching your purse, shoes, and portfolio color in black, navy, brown, or burgundy will give you an especially polished, pulled-together appearance.

CONDUCT

An interviewer will pay close attention to your behavior during an interview because it shows how you react under pressure. Conducting yourself in a confident, natural manner will help reduce any anxiety you feel. Be honest, and answer all questions thoroughly, but refrain from talking too much or speaking too loudly. Shake hands when you meet the interviewer and make confident eye contact without appearing bold. Your facial expression should be pleasant and attentive.

An applicant who appears nervous, aloof, inattentive, or arrogant during an interview will spoil any positive impressions that the resume generated. Although a certain amount of nervousness may provide the edge that makes for a strong interview, try to control your nervousness instead of letting it control you. Be mindful of nervous habits like running your fingers through your hair, biting your nails, fiddling with jewel-

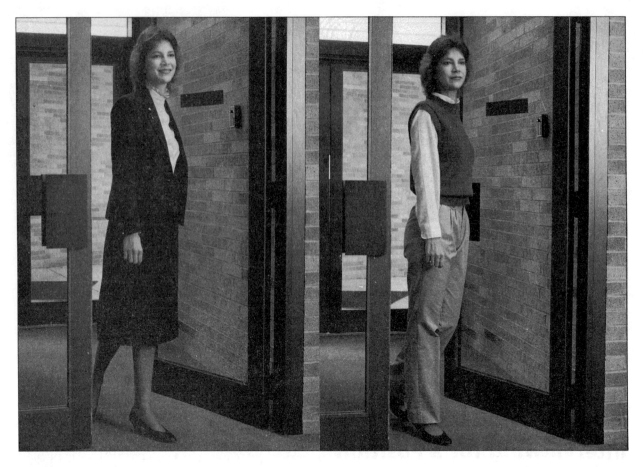

FIGURE 17-8 A neat, conservative, businesslike appearance (left) is preferable for an interview. Sport or casual clothes (right) are too informal.

ry, or swinging your foot. These nervous reactions are unconscious, and they may be annoying to the interviewer. They will certainly show that you are ill at ease and not in control.

You should sit so that you face the interviewer squarely, with your arms in a relaxed, "open" posture. Hands should rest in your lap or on the arms of the chair (Figure 17-9).

KNOWLEDGE OF THE EMPLOYER

Before going for an interview, obtain as much information as possible about the company or medical office and about the position for which you are being interviewed. A good place to seek information about a practice is from your medical assisting instructors. They may know the physicians or someone on the staff. If not, they may be able to direct you to another person who can share information about the practice.

You may also call the Physician Licensing Department in your state for routine information, such as the year the physician started the practice and number of years at the current address, and related information. Another source of information is your local chapter of the AAMA. Obtain the name of the president or another officer from a local hospital personnel office, or if necessary, contact the national office of the AAMA at 20 North Wacker Drive, Chicago, Illinois 60606, and ask for the name of the president of your local chapter.

You may want to obtain these names before you begin the actual search so that you can obtain the information more quickly. Use the officers as resource people to answer questions you may have about a particular practice or position. Most professionals are pleased to be able to help one another find employment, and medical assistants are no different. You will quickly

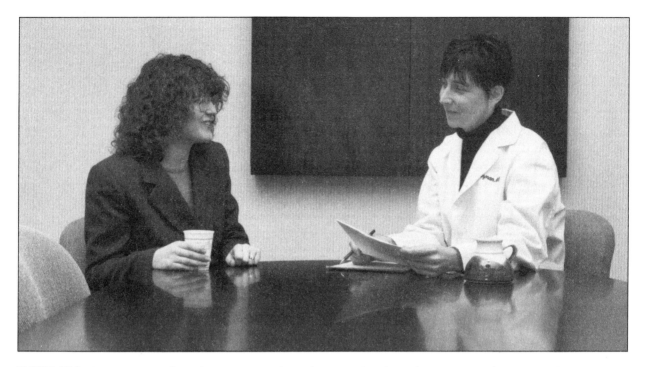

FIGURE 17-9 The interviewer will pay close attention to the applicant's conduct during their meeting. An honest, natural manner is most effective.

build a network of acquaintances through these valuable sources. Here are several questions that you should find answers for before attending an interview:

- What is the physician/practice's specialty?
- How large is the practice?
- How many staff members does the practice employ?
- What hospitals does the physician(s) serve as staff member (if applicable), or at which hospital(s) does the physician(s) have privileges?
- What medical product or service does the company make or sell (if appropriate)?
- How long has the company or practice been operating?
- What is the "style" of the office; family-like or professional? Hectic or relaxed?

ASKING THE RIGHT QUESTIONS

The purpose of an interview is to provide information that both you and the employer can use to make a sound decision about employment. The employer should cover basic facts, such as responsibilities of the position, office hours, benefits, and salary. You are expected to have additional questions and to ask them with confidence. However, you should be careful not to appear overly concerned about a high salary, the number of days off, coffee breaks, and other matters that are too "me-oriented."

If an employer asks you how much you want to be paid, it is best not to give an exact number. A good answer to this question is, "I expect to be compensated in line with your community standards for compensation, given my background and experience." In fact, this is the best compensation policy for all concerned; if you are paid unfairly more than others in the office, they will find out and resent it. If you are paid unfairly less, *you* will find out and resent it!

The interviewer will most likely address the list of questions given in the next section; if not, you may tactfully ask the questions that are appropriate to the size of the practice. Review the list and add questions of your own that you would like answered before agreeing to assume a new position.

- What are the responsibilities of the position?
- To whom will you report?
- What is the potential for career growth?
- Does the office promote from within?

- Is the practice growing?
- What does the employer envision for the practice in five years?
- What is the "style" or culture of the office?
- What is the salary range? Are increases automatic or based on merit?
- What are the benefits? Are continuing education units (CEUs) paid for, and is membership in AAMA included?
- Are health and/or dental insurance offered? Who pays?
- What is the sick leave policy?
- How much vacation time is allowed each year?
- How is vacation time accrued?
- Are there any education benefits? Will the company reimburse for college courses? Will the cost of textbooks be included?
- How many days of released time to attend professional conferences per year are given?
- Who pays for registration and travel expenses?

Illegal Questions

Prospective employers are prohibited by law from asking certain questions. As an interviewee, you should know (1) which questions are illegal, and (2) how to handle the situation gracefully if you are asked an illegal question.

Religion Employers cannot ask your religious faith. They can, however, ask if your faith will interfere with your ability to execute the duties of the job for which you are interviewing. If asked your religion, respond this way, "If you are asking me if my faith will prevent me from being able to do this job, let me assure you that it will not." If, in fact, your religion prohibits you from working on certain days or from carrying out any duties in the job description, you should discuss this with your employer. "My faith prohibits me from working on a Saturday. Would this present a problem?" The discussion should be about the job requirements, not about your personal beliefs.

Marital Status An employer cannot ask if you are married, if you have children, or if you plan to have children. The employer may ask a question similar to the one on religion; "Will your obligations prevent you from being able to execute the duties of this job?"

If asked if you have small children or plan to become pregnant soon, you could answer, "I have no family commitments that will interfere with this job as described." If you do have a responsibility that compels you to leave work promptly, for example, to pick up a child at daycare, do not give personal details. Say, "I will need to leave work at 5:00 p.m. unless we arrange an alternative schedule that allows me to meet family responsibilities."

Arrests Employers can ask if you have been *convicted* of a crime, but cannot ask if you have been *arrested*. This is unlikely to be asked on an interview, but a question about conviction will almost certainly be included on a written application.

Drug Testing An employer is allowed to, and often does, ask for drug testing as a part of a pre-employment physical exam.

In general, if a question seems too personal, or seems unrelated to the job for which you are interviewing, it is perfectly correct to ask, "Can I ask you how this would affect the job we are discussing?"

WRITING A FOLLOW-UP LETTER

If you are interested in a position after the interview, write a courteous follow-up letter to the interviewer. The letter should thank the person for the interview, express your interest in the position, and further sell your abilities. Since many people do not write follow-up letters, yours will remind the interviewer of you and perhaps give you an advantage over other applicants. Figure 17-10 shows a sample follow-up letter.

IN YOUR OPINION

1. If two applicants appear to be equally qualified for a job, what factors might influence the physician in favor of one or the other applicant?
2. How can a medical assistant ask the right questions about a position without appearing too aggressive?
3. How can a medical assistant ask the right questions about a position without appearing over-anxious?

June 25, 19—

Ms. Anna Capodici, CMA
Office Manager
Orthopedic Associates, P.C.
20-A Medical Arts Building
Nashville, TN 19087

Dear Ms. Capodici:

Thank you for discussing your
opening for a medical assistant with
me. As a result of our conversation,
I am convinced that my experience as
a medical transcriptionist and as an
internship student has prepared me
well for your position. I hope we have
the opportunity to work together and
look forward to hearing from you
soon.

Sincerely,

Karen Beyer

FIGURE 17-10 Sample follow-up letter

Continuing the Education Process

College was traditionally viewed as the end of formal education and the beginning of a career. Graduates happily received their diplomas and then went about their business of being employees. Those days are gone for the medical assistant and others in the allied health professions. Advances in technology, changes in the health care delivery system, and other trends discussed in the previous section create modifications, new procedures, and increased paper work almost daily. Today's medical assistant should understand this "challenge of change" before entering the career field and be prepared to continually upgrade skills and knowledge.

Several resources exist for continuing education; from formal college and university courses leading to a degree to informal courses, seminars, and workshops conducted by vendors, professional organizations, employers, and medical institutions. Courses may be taken for a variety of reasons including (1) intrinsic value and the satisfaction they offer to the student, (2) advancement potential and salary increase, (3) necessity to keep current with the field, (4) certification, and (5) revalidation. Figure 17-11 shows the educational background of medical assistants.

CERTIFICATION

Although licensing is not yet required nationally for medical assistants, some states have licensing guidelines. A person may gain credentials voluntarily through one of the professional organizations after successfully completing a certifying examination. The AAMA awards the Certified Medical Assistant (CMA) credential; the American Medical Technologists awards the Registered Medical Assistant (RMA) credential; and the Commission on Allied Health Personnel in Ophthalmology awards the Ophthalmic Medical Assistant (OMA) credential.

Certification is considered the mark of a professional, offering proof that the person has been evaluated and found qualified in the field. The Certifying Board of the AAMA notes that the CMA credential identifies and recognizes those who have the "knowledge and skills to perform competently the routine clinical and administra-

Occupational Training	Percentage
On-the-job training	46
Certificate/diploma in medical assisting	46
Associate degree in medical assisting	22
Training in related discipline	20
High school medical assisting program	4
Others	18

FIGURE 17-11 Educational background of medical assistants

tive duties in the office of a primary care physician." The entry-level competencies for a CMA, discussed in Chapter 2 as a part of the DACUM project, are measured by a certification examination sponsored by the AAMA. Certification by any of the professional organizations offers several advantages:

1. It affirms to employers that you are a skilled professional who has gained recognition through formal procedures conducted by a professional organization.
2. It offers prestige among your contemporaries in the field.
3. It often leads to a higher salary.
4. It provides personal satisfaction for achieving a professional standard.

Do not underestimate the importance of certification. If you were a potential employer choosing between a certified medical assistant and a noncertified medical assistant, which candidate would you select? As you begin your career as a medical assistant, check with the local chapter of your professional organization about dates and procedures for testing.

Revalidation

Revalidation of certification attests to a medical assistant's or other health practitioner's continued competency and commitment. Since the CMA certification examination of the AAMA is based on entry-level competency and is not a measure of continued competency, the Certifying Board of the AAMA developed a revalidation program based on continuing education. For this program, the certified medical assistant is required to obtain a given number of continuing education credits in specified subject areas

over a five-year period. Credits may be obtained through continuing education units (CEUs) attached to continuing education or through seminars, noncredit college courses, and conferences sponsored by professional associations.

Continuing education units are widely used at colleges and universities and among professional organizations to measure informal continuing education programs (as opposed to formal college or university credit courses). Professional organizations that accept CEUs usually approve a large number of chapter and society programs; home study courses; seminars and workshops sponsored by colleges and universities; special conferences sponsored by medical supply firms, manufacturers, and insurance companies; video courses; and many other programs. The CEU places a standard value on informal education. After accruing a specified number of CEUs in named subject areas over a given period of time, an allied health worker can have his or her credential revalidated by the sponsoring organization. Revalidation provides formal recognition of lifelong learning.

REFERENCES

The Medical Assistant: Your Partner in Professionalism. Chicago: American Association of Medical Assistants.

"Analysis of Employment Opportunities," *Philadelphia Inquirer,* April 29, 1993.

"What High Tech Can't Accomplish," *Newsweek,* October 10, 1993.

Zedlitz, Robert. *Getting a Job in Health Care.* Cincinnati, Ohio: South-Western Publishing Co., 1987.*

*Currently published by Delmar Publishers.

Chapter Activities

PERFORMANCE BASED ACTIVITIES

1. Following the example shown on page 368, prepare and key your resume. Include all sections that relate to your background. Make sure your document is perfect with no typographical mistakes, messy corrections, bad grammar, or misspelled words. Begin by completing the information sheet below, then transfer the information to the resume form and key and print the completed resume.

RESUME DATA COLLECTION FORM

(1) Your name, address, and telephone number(s).

(2) Employment objective—your career goal. Make it clear and short.

(3) Special Skills—characteristics and skills that make you special and that will be valuable to an employer.

(4) Work experience—any jobs you have done, including work at home and volunteer work or community projects. List the name of the job, description of duties, and dates of employment. List your clinical externship.

	Employer	*Job Title*	*Job Duties*	*Dates of Employment*
1.	_____	_____	_____	_____
2.	_____	_____	_____	_____
3.	_____	_____	_____	_____
4.	_____	_____	_____	_____

(5) Education—type of diploma, major, all schools attended with dates of attendance and graduation. List courses and projects related to the job you want, especially those that have to do with your clinical experience.

School	*Major*	*Dates Attended*	*Special Projects*

(6) Certificates and licenses related to the job

(7) Awards and honors

(8) References—include full names, phone numbers, and how you know the person. List at least three references.

	Name	*Phone*	*How Known*
1.	_____	_____	_____
2.	_____	_____	_____
3.	_____	_____	_____

(DACUM 1.9, 2.11)

2. Find a position that appeals to you in the classified advertisements of your local newspaper. Write a cover letter applying for the position. Use the format below to compose your letter, then key and print a final copy.

COVER LETTER FORM

Your Address
Date

Name of Person
Title
Company Name
Street Address
City, State, ZIP Code

Dear _____:

Opening Paragraph:
   (Your ad in the Sunday <u>Inquirer</u> for the position of medical assistant interests...)

Middle Paragraph:
   (Your practice is known for its good rapport with patients. I have experience in...)

Closing Paragraph:
   May I come for an interview? I will call your office...)

Sincerely,

Your Name

(DACUM 2.6, 2.11)

3. Using the classified advertisement from No. 2 above, develop a list of questions you think the interviewer might ask an applicant. Prepare answers to the questions based on your background. (DACUM 1.8, 2.9)

4. Select a classmate to serve as interviewer in a mock interview with you. Give your classmate the advertisement from No. 2 above and the list of questions you developed for No. 3. Ask the classmate to add other questions and keep them secret. Conduct a mock interview for the class. Dress appropriately for the interview. At the conclusion, ask for a critique of the interview from other class members.

INTERVIEW CRITIQUE FORM

(1) Did each person sit straight and face the other person?

(2) Did each speak clearly?

(3) Did the interviewee make good eye contact?

(4) Did the interviewer listen and pay attention?

(5) What kind of impression did the interviewee make?

(6) Did either person seem to be uncomfortable? Why?

(7) Did the interviewer ask good questions and were they appropriate to the job?

(8) Did the interviewee give good answers? What made them good?

(9) Did the interviewer ask any illegal questions? If so, how well did the interviewee handle them?

(10) What suggestions would you make to help each person improve?

(DACUM 2.9)

5. Analyze the Sunday advertisements in your local newspaper and compare the skills and abilities required for five medical office positions. Using the following chart as an example, develop a list of the requirements for each position. Tally the number of positions, naming each individual skill or ability. Make a priority list of skills needed based on your tally.

Skills and Abilities Required for Medical Office Employment

	Title of Position	*Skills and Abilities Needed*
Job No. 1	_____	_____
Job No. 2	_____	_____
Job No. 3	_____	_____

(DACUM 1.8, 1.9, 2.6, 2.7)

EXPANDING YOUR THINKING

1. Assume that you are ready to begin a job search. Compile your "network" of friends and acquaintances who might help you learn of available positions. Include family members, current and former employers, teachers, classmates, your friends' parents, and people you know through civic organizations, sports, church, scouts, or clubs.

Networking Data Collection Form

Name of Person	How Known	Questions to Ask, or Information to Seek	Follow-Up or Referral
1.			
2.			
3.			
4.			
5.			
6.			
7.			
8.			
9.			
10.			
11.			
12.			
13.			
14.			
15.			
16.			
17.			
18.			
19.			
20.			
21.			
22.			
23.			
24.			
25.			

2. Identify several habits you have seen among people you know and explain how they might be annoying to an interviewer. Classify by type in the following chart.

Distracting Behaviors

Related to Speech

1. _____
2. _____
3. _____
4. _____
5. _____

Related to Eye Contact

1. _____
2. _____
3. _____
4. _____
5. _____

Related to Posture and Movement

1. _____
2. _____
3. _____
4. _____
5. _____

Other

1. _____
2. _____
3. _____
4. _____
5. _____

3. Create a list of information you should have about employers before attending an interview. Add other information you might want to learn about a prospective employer.

Information About Job Duties

1. _____
2. _____
3. _____
4. _____
5. _____

Information About Working Conditions, Hours, and Overtime

1. _____
2. _____
3. _____
4. _____
5. _____

Information About Computers and Software

1. _____
2. _____
3. _____
4. _____
5. _____

Information About Career Planning and Continuing Education

1. _____
2. _____
3. _____

Information About Practice Type and Specialty

1. _____
2. _____

4. Investigate continuing education opportunities advertised in your Sunday newspaper. Compile a list giving the following information for all continuing education offerings:

a. Topic

b. Time

c. Location

d. Fee

e. Instructor

f. Result of training

Portfolio Assessment

(DACUM 2.3, 2.4, 2.7)

1. Ask your mentor to interview you for a fictitious position as a medical assistant in the mentoring practice. Arrange a time for the interview, dress appropriately, take your resume, and interview for the position.

(DACUM 2.3, 2.4, 2.7)

2. Ask your mentor to critique your performance in the interview and critique your own performance. Prepare a summary of what you would do differently in the future.

APPENDIX

1990 DACUM Analysis of the Medical Assisting Profession

1.0	1.1	1.2	1.3	1.4	1.5	1.6	1.7
Display Professionalism	Project a positive attitude	Perform within ethical boundaries	Practice within the scope of education, training, and personal capabilities	Maintain confidentiality	Work as a team member	Conduct oneself in a courteous and diplomatic manner	Adapt to change

2.0	2.1	2.2	2.3	2.4	2.5	2.6	2.7
Communicate	Listen and observe	Treat all patients with empathy and impartiality	Adapt communication to individuals' abilities to understand	Recognize and respond to verbal and non-verbal communication	Serve as liaison between physician and others	Evaluate understanding of communication	Receive, organize, prioritize, and transmit information

3.0	3.1	3.2	3.3	3.4	3.5	3.6	3.7
Perform Administrative Duties	Perform basic secretarial skills	Schedule and monitor appointments	Prepare and maintain medical records	Apply computer concepts for office procedures	Perform medical transcription	Locate resources and information for patients and employers	Manage physician's professional schedule and travel

4.0	4.1	4.2	4.3	4.4	4.5	4.6	4.7
Perform Clinical Duties	Apply principals of aseptic technique and infection control	Take vital signs	Recognize emergencies	Perform first aid and CPR	Prepare and maintain examination and treatment area	Interview and take patient history	Prepare patients for procedures

5.0	5.1	5.2	5.3	5.4	5.5	5.6	5.7
Apply Legal Concepts to Practice	Document accurately	Determine needs for documentation and reporting	Use appropriate guidelines when releasing records or information	Follow established policy in initiating or terminating medical treatment	Dispose of controlled substances in compliance with government regulations	Maintain licenses and accreditation	Monitor legislation related to current healthcare issues and practices

6.0	6.1	6.2	6.3	6.4	6.5	6.6	
Manage the Office	Maintain the physical plant	Operate and maintain facilities and equipment safely	Inventory equipment and supplies	Evaluate and recommend equipment and supplies for a practice	Maintain liability coverage	Exercise efficient time management	*Supervise personnel

7.0	7.1	7.2	7.3	7.4			
Provide Instruction	Orient patients to office policies and procedures	Instruct patients with special needs	Teach patients methods of health promotion and disease prevention	Orient and train personnel	*Provide health information for public use	*Supervise student practicums	*Conduct continuing education activities

8.0	8.1	8.2	8.3	8.4	8.5	8.6	8.7
Manage Practice Finances	Use manual bookkeeping systems	Implement current procedural terminology and ICD-9 coding	Analyze and use current third-party guidelines for reimbursement	Manage accounts receivable	Manage accounts payable	Maintain records for accounting and banking purposes	Process employee payroll

1.8	1.9						
Show initiative and responsibility	Promote the profession	*Enhance skills through continuing education					

2.8	2.9	2.10	2.11				
Use proper telephone technique	Interview effectively	Use medical terminology appropriately	Compose written communication using correct grammar, spelling, and format	*Develop and conduct public relations activities to market professional services			

4.8	4.9	4.10	4.11	4.12	4.13	4.14	
Assist physician with examinations and treatments	Use quality control	Collect and process specimens	Perform selected tests that assist with diagnosis and treatment	Screen and follow-up patient test results	Prepare and administer medications as directed by physician	Maintain medication records	*Respond to medical emergencies
*Develop and maintain policy and procedure manuals	*Establish risk management protocol for the practice						

*Develop job descriptions	*Interview and recommend new personnel	*Negotiate leases and prices for equipment and supply contracts
*Develop educational materials		
*Manage personnel benefits and records		

*Denotes advanced-level skills.
The medical assistant should be able to perform all other skills after completing a CAIIEA-accredited program and starting a first job.

Developed by:
The American Association of Medical Assistants, Inc.,
20 North Wacker Drive, Suite 1575,
Chicago, IL 60606.
312-899-1500;
toll-free 800-228-2262.
Consultants: Mary Lee Seibert, EdD, CMA, and Patricia A. Amos, MS

Glossary

account aging Method for reporting how long an account has been due

active listening Conscious attention to the speaker, asking open-ended questions that elicit additional information, and using verbal and nonverbal skills to provide feedback

advance directives Patient's wishes regarding future treatment if the patient is incapacitated

allocation Deciding how to divide available resources, such as time, among conflicting demands

ambulatory care centers Twenty-four-hour medical centers that treat patients with minor illnesses or injuries

answering service Twenty-four-hour service that answers phones for a fee

association Organization that advocates special interests through information or lobbying

basic insurance Insurance benefits that cover physicians' fees, hospital expenses, and surgical fees as determined by the plan contract, usually after payment of a deductible

bibliography List of books or articles about a subject, including the author, title, publisher, date, and page of the information

bioethics Branch of medical ethics concerned with moral issues resulting from high technology and sophisticated medical research. Social issues such as abortion, fetal research, artificial insemination, and euthanasia are important bioethical questions

block Letter format in which all lines begin at the left margin

blood tests Analysis of blood to determine whether infection is present, excessive urea is evident, or glucose or other substances are present in too high or too low a concentration

Blue Cross and Blue Shield Nonprofit insurers organized under the laws of individual states; generally, Blue Shield pays for physicians' services and Blue Cross covers hospital costs

business class Flight class that offers more amenities than coach, but fewer than first

case history Analysis of the patient's complaint, examination results, lab results, diagnosis, prescribed treatment, and family and personal history

cellular phone Portable telephone that operates by means of batteries, independent of any fixed location

Centers for Disease Control and Prevention Federal medical research center located in Atlanta, Georgia

central processing unit (CPU) Electronic circuitry that performs computer instructions

civil law Rights and obligations that people have toward one another, usually concerned with a wrong or injury one person inflicts upon another

closed files Medical records of patients who are no longer under the physician's care because they have moved, changed doctors, or died

CMA Certified Medical Assistant, a credential earned through the American Association of Medical Assistants

collection Process for expediting overdue accounts

commercial insurance For-profit companies offering individual or group health insurance

communication skills Ability to speak, listen, and write in a manner that gets one's point across and leaves a favorable impression

comprehensive insurance Combination of basic and major medical insurance

computer scheduling Scheduling patient appointments with computer software

copayment Percent of medical expenses beyond the deductible for which the patient is responsible

CPT Current Procedural Terminology

credentialing Examination that certifies the medical assistant in administrative and clinical procedures

criminal law Rights and obligations people have toward society

Current Procedural Terminology (CPT) Industry coding standard recognized by most insurance companies and widely used in medical offices to identify procedures and services performed

cycle billing Method for spreading billing over the whole month instead of sending all bills at the same time

DACUM Acronym for Developing A CUrriculuM

daily list of appointments List showing names of all patients who will be seen in one day

daily log The day's summary of patient transactions

data Numbers and letters keyed into a computer

database Software application for sorting and summarizing large amounts of data

data processing Organization of data into understandable information that can be used in decision making

DDD Direct Distance Dialing; placing long-distance calls directly, without intervention of an operator

deductible Amount paid by a patient prior to initiation of insurance benefits

direct flight Flight that connects two cities without a plane change

diagnosis-related group (DRG) Method of classifying patients into categories based on the primary diagnosis

disk drive Internal or external storage device for computer documents and programs

DNR Do Not Resuscitate order permits the patient to die without cardiopulmonary resuscitation. This order is commonly used in treating terminally ill or elderly patients

doctor's notes, or progress notes Doctor's comments that are added to the medical record each time the patient is treated

drug schedules Categories of drugs divided according to their potential for abuse

durable power of attorney Document that provides broad powers of medical authority to an individual, often either a family member or an attorney, who is given legal power to decide what extraordinary measures should be taken with a patient when the patient is too sick to decide. A durable power of attorney usually accompanies a DNR in the patient's hospital record

effective Achieving the mission of the practice in serving patients, whether or not resources are used efficiently

efficient Making good use of available resources

electrocardiogram Graphic illustration of the heart's activity

e-mail Electronic mail; computer network allowing persons at different computer terminals to leave messages for others on the network

empathy Mentally putting oneself in another's situation

employability A measurement of the combined attitudes, behaviors, personal characteristics, motivation, appearance, and work ethic that one brings to a job

FAX Facsimile transmission of documents by telephone line from one location to another

feedback Responses that provide direction

fee-for-service Payment system in which the full bill is paid each time a patient visits the physician

fee-paid Employment agency practice that charges placement fees from employers rather than job seekers

formatting Placement of the parts of a letter or medical document

function keys Extra keys that expand the computer's capacity

gender bias Subtle form of verbal sex discrimination

gender neutral Language that is not biased toward either sex

genetic counseling Counseling related to gene disorders. Prospective parents often receive genetic counseling regarding the likelihood of bearing a child with genetic disorders

genetic engineering Advanced, complex, and often controversial means of isolating and replacing part or all of a "mutant" gene to reduce or eliminate the chances that a person will develop a particular disease

genetics Study of genes and their role in illness and disease. Gene therapy is an exciting, emerging field of medical study because it promises cures for some illnesses now considered terminal

Good Samaritan laws Laws that protect physicians and other health care professionals who assist people in unusual emergency situations

graphics Pictures or charts designed on a computer

group insurance Coverage of a group of people based on a common characteristic, such as employment at a company

hardware Machines in a computer system

hold Telephone function that allows a call to be kept waiting on the line

ICD codes Diagnosis codes from the *International Classification of Diseases,* Ninth Edition, used to identify the patient's medical problem

inactive files Medical records of patients who have not visited the physician for an extended period

informed consent Law that states a patient must be given medical information about risk before undergoing a procedure

interpersonal From one person to another

inventory Store of supplies

inventory issue Taking an item out of inventory to use it

inventory receipt Taking an item into inventory

invoice Statement of services

itinerary Schedule of travel, including departure and arrival times, flight numbers, lodging, and telephone numbers

keyboard Input device that allows the operator to key data into the computer

laboratory request Test to be administered and the name of the attending physician

lead time The delay between placing a purchase order and receiving the item

ledger card Chronological listing of one family's financial activity with the practice

literature search Review of published sources at the library or by computer to find articles on specified topic

lliving will Legal document, signed by an individual, that provides precise instructions about the amount of extraordinary care to be delivered in the event of a life-threatening medical situation

major medical insurance Insurance designed to offset potentially catastrophic expenses from a lengthy illness or accident

managed competition Medical care in which physicians and hospitals compete for patients

Medicaid Government health insurance program that protects the poor

medical ethics Term applied to the principles governing medical conduct. Medical ethics deals with the relationship of the physician to the patient, the patient's family, fellow physicians, and society

medical law Standards set by elected officials in the state and nation. An illegal act is always unethical, according to the American Medical Association's Principles of Medical Ethics, but an unethical act may not be illegal

medical specialties Branches of medicine that concentrate on specific body systems

Medicare Government health insurance program that protects the elderly

micrographics Photographic process that miniaturizes documents and stores them on magnetic film or cards

modem Hardware that connects a computer, via phone lines, to other computers; this device that converts a sender's computer signals into telephone signals

modified block Format in which the date and closing lines begin at the center

monitor Television-like screen on which words, charts, letters, and other data appear

multi-functional medical assistant Medical assistant who is trained in both administrative and clinical duties

networking Developing new contacts and keeping in touch with friends and acquaintances in the medical and related fields

non-stop Flight that connects two cities without making intermediate stops

nonverbal communication The signals humans send out without speaking, including facial expressions, gestures, posture, and appearance

obsolete supplies Inventory items that are no longer used

objective The intent of the process

OMA Ophthalmic Medical Assistant, a credential earned through the Joint Commission on Allied Health Personnel in Ophthalmology

optical character recognition Process by which handwritten or printed characters are converted into electronic impulses that a computer or word processor can understand

optimal Making the best use of a resource

orient To provide an informational overview

overbooking Scheduling more patients than the physician can see in the time available

pathology and cytopathology Field of laboratory testing that shows the results of studies of body tissue and body cells

patient information form Form completed by a patient immediately upon arriving at the medical office for the initial visit

patient health questionnaire Questions about the patient's previous health and surgical history and family history

Patient's Bill of Rights Established by the American Hospital Association in 1972, the Patient's Bill of Rights provides basic guidelines for the care of hospitalized patients

Patient Self-Determination Act Federal law requiring all hospitals and nursing homes to explain in detail the extraordinary care their state permits. These facilities must alert patients of their right to execute living wills or appoint health care proxies through a durable power of attorney

payables Amount of money owed by the practice to those from whom it purchases goods and services

PC Personal computer

pegboard accounting Traditional method of maintaining accounts, named for the flat writing board on which accounting papers are prepared

physician extenders Paramedical staff trained to support the physician by performing some tasks previously performed only by the physician

practice analysis Overview of procedures and treatments provided and income derived during a specified period

problem-oriented medical record Patient's complaints identified in list form

process Activity that includes input, modification or change to the input, and output; input can include people, materials, or information

progress appointments Follow-up appointments that monitor the progress of treatment

proof of posting Verification of the calculation of columns in the daily log

proofread To examine a document for errors

prospective payment Term describing a method of flat fee pricing

receivables Amount of money owed to a practice by those who purchase its services

redundancy Unnecessary repetition of words

referral Determination by a physician that a patient should see a specialist or subspecialist for a consultation

reprographics Process of making copies

residency Three years of specialty training that occurs after a physician finishes medical school

resume Document that summarizes an individual's background, education, and qualifications

reversed charges Collect call

root medical word Basic medical word used in combination with other words or prefixes and suffixes

screening Evaluation of a call for proper referral

secondary research Study of sources already published

shingling Method of filing small reports

SOAP Method of reporting patient's diagnosis and treatment plan: subjective examination (S), objective test results (O), doctor's assessment (A), and treatment plan (P)

software Programs or instructions that operate computers

source-oriented medical record Information grouped according to its source

spreadsheet Software application for rows and columns of numbers and their calculation

stored letter parts Standard paragraphs that are stored in the computer's memory

superbill Patient charge slip or receipt listing the typical examinations, procedures, treatments, and services a patient might have during one visit

supply disposal Getting rid of out-of-date or obsolete items

tact Diplomacy in handling difficult situations

TAD Telephone answering device, or answering machine

technology skills Ability to use existing computers and medical equipment plus transferable skills that can be applied as technology is updated

thesaurus Reference book or word processing feature containing synonyms and antonyms

time zone Geographic area identified by its time of day in relation to time in other parts of the country or world

tone Sound of letters; what is said and how the writer chooses to say it

transcription To write from one source to another

urinalysis Routine laboratory test of urine often requested by physicians

vendor Supplier of products or services

wave scheduling Clustering appointments by time block; flow is maintained by rotating patients among needed procedures

word processing Processing of words to form narrative documents, using a computer and software package instead of a typewriter

workers' compensation insurance Employer-paid insurance that provides health care and income to employees and their dependents when employees suffer work-related injuries or illness

workplace readiness Specialty training and employability skills that prepare a person for employment

x-rays, CAT scans, and ultrasound Diagnostic tests to determine whether any unusual medical condition, such as a tissue mass, is present in the body

Index

Genetic engineering
  the law and, 54
  medical ethics and, 2, 35–36, 44–45
GENONE, 162
Geographic filing, 254
Good Samaritan laws, 71, 73
Government insurance programs, 289–290
Graphics, 181
Greeting patients, 95
Group practices, 5–6
Gynecologic oncology, as subspecialty, 13f
Gynecology, as specialty, 13f

H

Hard disk, computer, 152f, 153
Hardware, computer, 151–154
  central processing unit, 152–153
  disk drive, 152f, 153
  keyboard, 152
  modem, 153–154
  monitor, 152
  printer, 153
Health care
  costs, 1–2, 284–285
  types of coverage, 285, 287f
  types of delivery systems, 2
  See also Health insurance
Health Care Financing Administration (HCFA), 291
HCFA-1500 claim forms, 296f, 297f, 299–302
Health care professionals, licensure of, 54
Health care system, fraud/abuse in, 47
Health insurance, 283–305
  diagnosis-related groups (DRGs), 291, 293
  financing plans
    Blue Cross/Blue Shield, 286
    exclusive provider organization (EPO), 288
    government programs, 289–290
    health maintenance organizations (HMOs), 286–287
    Medicare/Medicaid, 288–289
    preferred provider organizations (PPOs), 287–288
    workers' compensation, 290–291, 292f
  prospective payment system, 291–292
Health insurance claims, 293–305
  completing HCFA-1500 claim forms, 296f, 297f, 299–302
  dental claim form, 298f
  establishing an audit trail
    claims register, 302–303
    computerizing the process, 304, 305f
    follow-up procedure, 303–304
    tickler file, 303, 304f
  filing a claim
    assignment of payment, 294
    coding systems
      CPT-4 codes, 294–295
      ICD-9-CM codes, 295, 299
    following the route of a claim, 293–294
    superbill as documentation, 299

place/type of service codes, 301f
Health maintenance organizations (HMOs), 286–287
Health resources, allocation of, medical ethics and, 41–42
Heart disease, genetic engineering and, 44
Hematology, as subspecialty, 12f
"Hemlock Society", 2
HIV testing, medical ethics and, 45–46
Hold function, 105–106, 107f
Honesty, medical assistant and, 27
Hospitals, 8–9
  computers in, 14–15
  scheduling patients for, 132–133
Huntington's disease, genetic engineering and, 44

I

ICD-9-CM codes, 26, 295, 299
Identidex™, 161
Illegal acts, by a physician, 63
Immunopathology, as subspecialty, 13f
Impatient behavior, medical assistant and, 89f
Inactive files, 244–245
Independent provider organizations (IPOs), 2
Infectious diseases, as subspecialty, 12f
Information cycle, 149, 150f
Information form, computerized, 274f
Information processing components, 154–159
  computer graphics, 156, 157f, 158f
  data processing, 154
  dictation, 156–157
  electronic communication, 158
  electronic mail (e-mail), 157–158
  micrographics, 155–156
  optical character recognition (OCR), 155
  reprographics, 156
  telephone technology, 157
  voice mail, 158
  word processing, 154–155
  See also Computer system
Informed consent, 59–60, 61f
Institutions
  hospitals, 8–9
  laboratories, 7–8
  nursing homes, 8
  research centers, 6–7
  specialized care centers, 8
Instruction, patient, 226–227
Insulin, 44
Insurance, professional liability, 57
  See also Health insurance
Insurance companies
  patient confidentiality and, 67, 68f
  payments by, 96
Insured mail, 164
Integumentary system, 10
Interferon, 44
Internal medicine, as specialty, 12f
International travel, 230
Internet, 162

by type of practice, 20f
ethics and, 49
multi-functional role of, 21
professional activities, 225–226
responsibilities of, 21–22
for patient confidentiality, 67, 69
for reporting crimes, 63
revalidation, 376
role in record keeping, 254–255
as witnesses, 71
working with the medical professionals
hospital staff, 30
other outside professionals, 30
physician and health care team, 26–27
See also Employment skills
Medical centers, 6
Medical ethics
computers and, 47–49
AMA position on computer security, 48–49, 50f
confidentiality, 48
the law and, 35–36
medical assistant's role and, 49
medical association statements
AMA Principles of Medical Ethics, 36–37
American Association of Medical Assistants, 38, 40f
American Hospital Association, 37–38
Code of Hammurabi, 36
social policy issues, 38–47
Medical Manager, The, 150
appointment scheduling, 125, 126, 127
daily transaction report, 183f
main menu screen, 151f
Medical microbiology, as subspecialty, 13f
Medical nuclear physics, as subspecialty, 13f
Medical oncology, as subspecialty, 12f
Medical Practice Acts
licensure, 54–55
renewal of license, 55
revocation/suspension of license, 55–56
Medical professionals
roles of, 22–23, 26
working with, 26–30
Medical records, malpractice and, 62
Medical records administrators, role of, 23, 26
Medical records management, 235–255
color coding the folder, 238–239
contents of the record
laboratory reports
blood test, 240–241, 247f
electrocardiogram, 240, 247f
pathology/cytopathology, 242, 249f
radiology, 241, 248f
urinalysis, 240, 246f
patient-completed forms, 239, 240f
patient health questionnaire, 239, 241f
physician-completed forms
case history, 239, 242f
doctor's notes, 239, 243f
laboratory request, 239, 244f

database management
computerized databases, 246, 251f
paper databases, 244–246
discussion, 235–237
medical assistant's role in record keeping, 254–255
medical record defined, 236
problem-oriented medical record (POMR), 243–244, 250f
SOAP formula, 244, 249f
source-oriented medical record (SOMR), 244
TAB Alpha Code system, 238f
trends and issues, 237
See also Filing
Medical records technicians, role of, 26
Medical reports, 209–210
Medical services telecommunications, 160
Medical specialties/subspecialties, 11–14
Medical technologist/technician, role of, 23
Medicare/Medicaid, 1, 96, 288–289
MedLine, 162
Memorandums, 209
Message taking
callback messages, 109, 110f, 111f
computer message screen, 112f
emergency calls, 111
procedures for prescription refill requests, 110
procedures for taking messages regarding an illness, 110–111
Metered mail, 164, 166, 166f
Microbiology, as subspecialty, 13f
Microcomputer, choosing and using, 177
Microfilm/microfiche, 155, 156f
Micrographics, 155–156
Micromedics, 162
Micromex, Inc., 161
Modem, computer, 153–154
Monitor, computer, 152
Muscular dystrophy, genetic engineering and, 44
Muscular system, 10

N

Narcotic drug records, 73
Negligence, concept of, 58
Nephrology, as subspecialty, 12f
Nervous system, 11
Networking, job search process and, 364
Neurofibromatosis, genetic engineering and, 44
Neurological surgery, as specialty, 13f
Neurology, 9
as specialty, 13f
Neuropathology, as subspecialty, 13f
Newspaper classified advertisements, job search process and, 363
Nexus, 162
Nonmedical databases, 162
Nonverbal communication, 90–91
Nuclear medicine, as specialty, 13f
Nuclear radiology, as subspecialty, 13f

Word processing, 154–155, 180, 197–217
  composing at the computer, 197, 198f
  input
    dictation and transcription, 201
    medical terminology, 202
    proofreader's marks, 199
    rough draft, 199–201
    sources of, 199
  output, 203–217
    business report formatting
      bibliography, 216
      footnotes, 216
      job instructions, 213, 215f
      margin guide, 213
      table of contents, 216
      title page, 216
    correspondence formatting, 203–212
      block/modified block formats, 204–207
      merged paragraphs, 208–209

      second-page headings, 208
      stored letter parts, 208
    medical report formatting, 209–210
    memorandums, 209, 210f
    proofreading, 216–217
    spell checkers, 216–217
  software, 202–203
    create/edit text, 203, 204f
Workers' compensation, 290–291, 292f

X

X-rays, 241
  packaging and mailing, 166

Y

Yellow pages, job search process and, 365
"You" viewpoint, 192–193

License Agreement for Delmar Publishers
An International Thomson Publishing Company

Educational Software/Data

You the customer, and Delmar incur certain benefits, rights, and obligations to each other when you open this package and use the software/data it contains. BE SURE YOU READ THE LICENSE AGREEMENT CAREFULLY, SINCE BY USING THE SOFTWARE/DATA YOU INDICATE YOU HAVE READ, UNDERSTOOD, AND ACCEPTED THE TERMS OF THIS AGREEMENT.

Your rights:

1. You enjoy a non-exclusive license to use the enclosed software/data on a single microcomputer that is not part of a network or multi-machine system in consideration for payment of the required license fee, (which may be included in the purchase price of an accompanying print component), or receipt of this software/data, and your acceptance of the terms and conditions of this agreement.

2. You own the media on which the software/data is recorded, but you acknowledge that you do not own the software/data recorded on them. You also acknowledge that the software/data is furnished "as is," and contains copyrighted and/or proprietary and confidential information of Delmar Publishers or its licensors.

3. If you do not accept the terms of this license agreement you may return the media within 30 days. However, you may not use the software during this period.

There are limitations on your rights:

1. You may not copy or print the software/data for any reason whatsoever, except to install it on a hard drive on a single microcomputer and to make one archival copy, unless copying or printing is expressly permitted in writing or statements recorded on the diskette(s).

2. You may not revise, translate, convert, disassemble or otherwise reverse engineer the software data except that you may add to or rearrange any data recorded on the media as part of the normal use of the software/data.

3. You may not sell, license, lease, rent, loan, or otherwise distribute or network the software/data except that you may give the software/data to a student or and instructor for use at school or, temporarily at home.

Should you fail to abide by the Copyright Law of the United States as it applies to this software/data your license to use it will become invalid. You agree to erase or otherwise destroy the software/data immediately after receiving note of Delmar Publisher's termination of this agreement for violation of its provisions.

Delmar gives you a LIMITED WARRANTY covering the enclosed software/data. The LIMITED WARRANTY can be found in this package and/or the instructor's manual that accompanies it.

This license is the entire agreement between you and Delmar Publishers interpreted and enforced under New York law.

Limited Warranty

Delmar Publishers warrants to the original licensee/purchaser of this copy of microcomputer software/data and the media on which it is recorded that the media will be free from defects in material and workmanship for ninety (90) days from the date of original purchase. All implied warranties are limited in duration to this ninety (90) day period. THEREAFTER, ANY IMPLIED WARRANTIES, INCLUDING IMPLIED WARRANTIES OF MERCHANTABILITY AND FITNESS FOR A PARTICULAR PURPOSE ARE EXCLUDED. THIS WARRANTY IS IN LEIU OF ALL OTHER WARRANTIES, WHETHER ORAL OR WRITTEN, EXPRESSED OR IMPLIED.

If you believe the media is defective, please return it during the ninety day period to the address shown below. A defective diskette will be replaced without charge provided that it has not been subjected to misuse or damage.

This warranty does not extend to the software or information recorded on the media. The software and information are provided "AS IS." Any statements made about the utility of the software or information are not to be considered as express or implied warranties. Delmar will not be liable for incidental or consequential damages of any kind incurred by you, the consumer, or any other user.

Some states do not allow the exclusion or limitation of incidental or consequential damages, or limitations on the duration of implied warranties, so the above limitation or exclusion may not apply to you. This warranty gives you specific legal rights, and you may also have other rights which vary from state to state. Address all correspondence to:

Delmar Publishers
3 Columbia Circle
P. O. Box 15015
Albany, NY 12212-5015